T0137895

Innovations in HIV Prevention Research and Practice through Community Engagement

Scott D. Rhodes
Editor

Innovations in HIV Prevention Research and Practice through Community Engagement

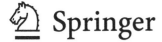 Springer

Editor
Scott D. Rhodes
Wake Forest University School of Medicine
Winston-Salem
North Carolina
USA

ISBN 978-1-4939-5336-3   ISBN 978-1-4939-0900-1 (eBook)
DOI 10.1007/978-1-4939-0900-1
Springer New York Heidelberg Dordrecht London

© Springer Science+Business Media New York 2014
Softcover reprint of the hardcover 1st edition 2014
This work is subject to copyright. All rights are reserved by the Publisher, whether the whole or part of the material is concerned, specifically the rights of translation, reprinting, reuse of illustrations, recitation, broadcasting, reproduction on microfilms or in any other physical way, and transmission or information storage and retrieval, electronic adaptation, computer software, or by similar or dissimilar methodology now known or hereafter developed. Exempted from this legal reservation are brief excerpts in connection with reviews or scholarly analysis or material supplied specifically for the purpose of being entered and executed on a computer system, for exclusive use by the purchaser of the work. Duplication of this publication or parts thereof is permitted only under the provisions of the Copyright Law of the Publisher's location, in its current version, and permission for use must always be obtained from Springer. Permissions for use may be obtained through RightsLink at the Copyright Clearance Center. Violations are liable to prosecution under the respective Copyright Law.
The use of general descriptive names, registered names, trademarks, service marks, etc. in this publication does not imply, even in the absence of a specific statement, that such names are exempt from the relevant protective laws and regulations and therefore free for general use.
While the advice and information in this book are believed to be true and accurate at the date of publication, neither the authors nor the editors nor the publisher can accept any legal responsibility for any errors or omissions that may be made. The publisher makes no warranty, express or implied, with respect to the material contained herein.

Printed on acid-free paper

Springer is part of Springer Science+Business Media (www.springer.com)

*To Dr. Curtis A. and Mrs. Suzanne H. Rhodes,
Who raised me to be who I am; And Glen
Troiano, Who loves me for who I am.*

Foreword

HIV continues to be a national and international challenge. Not all communities have benefited from the strides made in public health and medicine, and these differences have led to disparities across a variety of health concerns, including HIV. Although great progress has been made in both the prevention and treatment of HIV and its associated conditions, much more work is clearly needed. With more than 50,000 new HIV infections each year in the United States and the profound disproportionate burden borne by racial/ethnic and sexual minorities, including men who have sex with men (MSM), American Indians/Alaska Natives, African Americans/blacks, and Hispanics/Latinos, it is imperative that we further develop strategies that reach individuals, social networks, and communities, and change policies and promote social change to reduce risk.

Academic researchers and practitioners within local communities have developed and are implementing innovative approaches to reduce HIV exposure and transmission; the CDC's *Compendium of Evidence-based HIV Behavioral Interventions* (www.cdc.gov/hiv/topics/research/prs/compendium-evidence-based-interventions.htm), for example, provides a description of the currently available evidence-based interventions promoted and used across the country. The National Institutes of Health (NIH) also funds intervention research designed to move the science and practice of HIV prevention forward. The National Institute on Minority Health and Health Disparities (NIMHD) at NIH has several active studies designed to reduce risk among MSM, African Americans/blacks, and Hispanics/Latinos. Some of the progress highlighted within this important book, *Innovations in HIV Prevention Research and Practice through Community Engagement*, is a result of both CDC and NIH funding.

However, we must continue to develop even better approaches to reduce HIV exposure and transmission particularly for some of our most vulnerable and neglected communities. We cannot merely continue with what we have been doing; we know that what we have done is not enough. Rather, we must develop additional innovative approaches that are meaningful and authentic to communities; reach large numbers of community members at greatest risk; are sustainable; expand beyond HIV-related health disparities and build capacities that have potential to affect other health disparities.

An emerging approach that has gained traction within public health and medicine is community engagement. Community engagement is the process by which organizations, agencies, other types of institutions, and community members affiliated by geographic proximity, special interest, or similar situations build ongoing and permanent relationships to work collaboratively to reach a collective vision. Generally this vision includes addressing prioritized issues affecting the health and well-being of community members. Within the context of public health and medical research, community engagement can be powerful in bringing about changes that improve the health and well-being of communities and community members. At its core, community engagement involves partnerships and coalitions to mobilize resources and influence systems, change relationships among partners, and serve as catalysts for change. Community-based participatory research (CBPR) is based on the concept that community members' perspectives, experiences, and insights should be blended with sound science to produce the most promising interventions and programs to promote health and well-being and prevent disease.

This book comprises a compilation of innovative interventions and programs from across the United States that apply community engagement principles and approaches throughout HIV prevention intervention and program development. This book outlines both the successes and challenges faced when scientists and lay-experts from academic, government, and nongovernment institutions, including community-based organizations and businesses, and the community at large, partner and engage. It includes the perspectives, experiences, and insights gleaned from real-world examples of community engagement. It serves as a benchmark of the current state of the science and practice of community engagement for those from communities, community-based organizations, agencies (including health departments), businesses, and research institutions who want to better understand what community engagement is, what has been accomplished, and what the next steps might be in terms of community engagement as an approach to HIV-related disparities reduction and elimination. Chapters have been authored by outstanding leaders in HIV prevention and community engagement research and practice. The writing of the chapters and their compilation within this book represent unique partnerships of representatives from diverse communities, community-based organizations, agencies, businesses, and research institutions.

On a personal note, this book has been edited by a long-term mentee and colleague. I have known Dr. Scott D. Rhodes since 1990, when he was a graduate student and community activist in South Carolina. He and members of the CBPR partnership that he is part of in North Carolina have been on the forefront of authentic approaches to community engagement and partnership, and CBPR. Building on the firm foundation established by others in the field of CBPR, including Drs. Eugenia Eng, Barbara Israel, Meredith Minkler, and Nina Wallerstein, the unique and sustained partnership has multiple projects that cross race/ethnicity, sexual orientation, gender identity, assets, and risks.

Within public health and medicine we frequently hear of the need for community engagement, particularly as a strategy to address community priorities, build community capacity, and lead to a reduction in and subsequent elimination of health disparities. This book presents solid guidance for community engagement and partnership and CBPR. I am thrilled that this book has been realized; it will serve as an important resource as we work to prevent HIV within vulnerable and neglected communities.

Francisco S. Sy, MD, DrPH

Editor

AIDS Education and Prevention—An Interdisciplinary Journal

Contents

Contributors

Claire Abraham Department of Social Sciences and Health Policy, Division of Public Health Sciences, Wake Forest University School of Medicine, Winston-Salem, NC, USA

Aletha Akers Magee-Women's Hospital Department of Obstetrics, Gynecology and Reproductive Sciences, University of Pittsburgh School of Medicine, Pittsburg, PA, USA

Tashuna Albritton Center for Interdisciplinary Research on AIDS, Yale University, New Haven, CT, USA

Jorge Alonzo Department of Social Sciences and Health Policy, Division of Public Health Sciences, Wake Forest University School of Medicine, Winston-Salem, NC, USA

Robert E. Aronson Public Health Program, School of Natural and Applied Sciences, Taylor University, Upland, IN, USA

Adina Black North Carolina Translational and Clinical Sciences Institute, University of North Carolina at Chapel Hill, Chapel Hill, NC, USA

Fred R. Bloom Division of STD Prevention, National Center for HIV/AIDS, Viral Hepatitis, STD and TB Prevention, Centers for Disease Control and Prevention, Atlanta, GA, USA

Jaime M. Booth School of Social Work, University of Pittsburgh, Pittsburgh, PA, USA

Sheana Bull Department of Community and Behavioral Health, School of Public Health, University of Colorado, Aurora, CO, USA

Glenn Clark Behavioral Health Services, Whitman-Walker Health, Washington, DC, USA

Charles B. Collins Division of HIV/AIDS Prevention, National Center for HIV, Hepatitis, STD, and TB Prevention, Centers for Disease Control and Prevention, Atlanta, GA, USA

Giselle Corbie-Smith Department of Social Medicine, University of North Carolina at Chapel Hill School of Medicine, Chapel Hill, NC, USA

Jason Daniel-Ulloa Department of Community and Behavioral Health, University of Iowa College of Public Health, Iowa City, IA, USA

Mario Downs Department of Social Sciences and Health Policy, Division of Public Health Sciences, Wake Forest University School of Medicine, Winston-Salem, NC, USA

Danny Ellis Ellis Research & Consulting Service, LLC, Wilson, NC, USA

Arlinda Ellison North Carolina Translational and Clinical Sciences Institute, University of North Carolina at Chapel Hill, Chapel Hill, NC, USA

Eugenia Eng Department of Health Behavior, Gillings School of Global Public Health, University of North Carolina at Chapel Hill, Chapel Hill, NC, USA

John Gallagher Southwest Interdisciplinary Research Center, Arizona State University School of Social Work, Phoenix, AZ, USA

Steve Geishecker Behavioral Health Services, Whitman-Walker Health, Washington, DC, USA

Louis F. Graham Department of Public Health, University of Massachusetts Amherst, Amherst, MA, USA

Kenneth C. Hergenrather Department of Counseling and Human Development, Graduate School of Education and Human Development, The George Washington University, Washington, DC, USA

Stepheria Hodge-Sallah NC Department of Health and Human Services, Division of Public Health, Raleigh, NC, USA

Melvin Jackson Strengthening The Black Family, Inc., Raleigh, NC, USA

Deb Levine Youth Tech Health (YTH), Oakland, CA,USA

Alexandra Lightfoot Community Based Participatory Research Core Center for Health Promotion and Disease Prevention, University of North Carolina at Chapel Hill, Chapel Hill, NC, USA

Alice Ma Department of Public Health Education, University of North Carolina Greensboro, Greensboro, NC, USA

Lilli Mann Department of Social Sciences and Health Policy, Division of Public Health Sciences, Wake Forest University School of Medicine, Winston-Salem, NC, USA

Flavio F. Marsiglia Southwest Interdisciplinary Research Center, Arizona State University School of Social Work, Phoenix, AZ, USA

Cindy Miller   Public Health Sciences, Department of Social Sciences and Health Policy, Division of Public Health Sciences, Wake Forest University School of Medicine, Winston-Salem, NC, USA

Morgan M. Philbin   Department of Health, Behavior & Society, Johns Hopkins University School of Public Health, Baltimore, MD, USA

HIV Center for Clinical & Behavioral Studies, Columbia University and New York State Psychiatric Institute, New York, NY, USA

Regina McCoy Pulliam   Department of Public Health Education, University of North Carolina Greensboro, Greensboro, NC, USA

Barry Ramsey   Center for Health Promotion and Disease Prevention, University of North Carolina at Chapel Hill, Chapel Hill, NC, USA

Beth A. Reboussin   Department of Biostatistical Sciences, Division of Public Health Sciences, Wake Forest University School of Medicine, Winston-Salem, NC, USA

Dominica Rehbein   Department of Health Management and Policy, University of Iowa College of Public Health, Iowa City, IA, USA

Scott D. Rhodes   Department of Social Sciences and Health Policy, Division of Public Health Sciences, Wake Forest University School of Medicine, Winston-Salem, NC, USA

Linda Riggins   Focus on Youth Project, Strengthening the Black Family, Inc., Raleigh, NC, USA

Deborah Secakuku Baker   Southwest Interdisciplinary Research Center, Arizona State University School of Social Work, Phoenix, AZ, USA

Florence M. Simán   El Pueblo, Inc., Raleigh, NC, USA

Eunyoung Song   Department of Social Sciences and Health Policy, Division of Public Health Sciences, Wake Forest University School of Medicine, Winston-Salem, NC, USA

Jason Stowers   Triad Health Project, Greensboro, NC, USA

Amanda E. Tanner   Department of Public Health Education, University of North Carolina Greensboro, Greensboro, NC, USA

Hank L. Tomlinson   Division of HIV/AIDS Prevention, National Center for HIV, Hepatitis, STD, and TB Prevention, Centers for Disease Control and Prevention, Atlanta, GA, USA

Aaron T. Vissman   Department of Behavioral Sciences and Health, Rollins School of Public Health, Emory University, Atlanta, GA, USA

Tarik Walker   Department of Family Medicine and Colorado Area Health Education Center, University of Colorado, Aurora, CO, USA

David K. Whittier Division of HIV Prevention, National Center for HIV/AIDS, Viral Hepatitis, STD and TB Prevention, Centers for Disease Control and Prevention, Atlanta, GA, USA

Briana Woods-Jaeger Department of Community and Behavioral Health, University of Iowa College of Public Health, Iowa City, IA, USA

Mysha Wynn Project Momentum, Inc., Rocky Mount, NC, USA

Chapter 1
Authentic Community Engagement and Community-Based Participatory Research for Public Health and Medicine

Scott D. Rhodes

Complex problems in public health and medicine, including disparities in HIV, have been noted to be ill-suited for traditional outside-expert approaches to research and practice that often result in insufficient understanding of the factors key to health promotion and disease prevention and ineffective interventions and programs. Research aimed at understanding and eliminating health disparities and promoting community health has begun to focus attention on meaningful community engagement and authentic community partnership as integral processes throughout the entire research process. Blending the lived experiences of community members, the experiences of representatives from service- and practice-based organizations, and sound science has the potential to develop deeper and more informed understandings of health-related phenomena and produce more relevant and more likely successful and sustainable interventions to promote community health and reduce health disparities [1–8]. Community engagement and partnership and community-based participatory research (CBPR) recognize that a so-called outsider (e.g., academic researchers and practitioners) can work best with community members who themselves are experts. This book is a compilation of the state of the science of innovative behavioral HIV prevention interventions that use community engagement and partnership and CBPR.

Community Engagement and CBPR

As noted in the foreword of this book, community engagement is a process by which community members connected through geographic proximity, special interests, or similar situations; representatives from community-based organizations (e.g., churches, free clinics, and HIV-serving organizations); agencies (e.g., public health departments); businesses; and institutions (e.g., universities and

S. D. Rhodes (✉)
Department of Social Sciences and Health Policy, Division of Public Health Sciences,
Wake Forest University School of Medicine, Medical Center Blvd.,
Winston-Salem, NC 27157, USA
e-mail: srhodes@wakehealth.edu

S. D. Rhodes (ed.), *Innovations in HIV Prevention Research and Practice*
through Community Engagement, DOI 10.1007/978-1-4939-0900-1_1,
© Springer Science+Business Media New York 2014

other research institutions) establish, nurture, and sustain relationships to work in partnership to meet community priorities [9]. CBPR adds research to the mix. With community engagement and partnership in research through approaches such as CBPR, the notion is not to reduce knowledge gaps for the sake of reducing knowledge gaps; rather, the notion is to enhance understanding of health phenomena and translate this enhanced understanding into action to improve community health and well-being. Community-engaged approaches can be powerful in bringing about positive changes through multilevel action, including individual, group, community, policy, and social change, to improve the health and well-being of communities.

However, despite its advantages, community engagement is difficult. This book is designed to provide a survey in current innovative approaches to HIV prevention using community engagement in the USA. CBPR has emerged as an approach to community engagement, and within this book, examples of ways in which HIV prevention has harnessed engagement, partnership, and CBPR approaches are provided. Thus, within this book, we explore community engagement and partnership and CBPR as applied within highly innovative and significant intervention research. Chapter authors are experts in the field and have provided much detail in their current research.

Themes

Throughout this book, lay experts and scientists from academic, government, and nongovernment institutions, including community-based organizations and businesses, and the community at large share their perspectives, experiences, and insights in HIV intervention and program development, implementation, and evaluation within highly vulnerable and neglected communities. Several cross-cutting characteristics of community engagement and partnership and CBPR emerged across the chapters (Table 1.1).

Community engagement and partnership and CBPR are more expansive than merely community members serving on community advisory groups or community advisory boards. Within HIV, whether focusing on prevention or care, community advisory groups or boards are commonplace and expected; by themselves, they do not imply authentic engagement or partnership. In fact, they often are used to "rubberstamp" ideas that outsiders, including researchers and practitioners, have developed without much community input. Obtaining input and feedback after conceptualization of a study and/or receiving study funding does not reflect community engagement; rather, it tends to reflect "using" communities to meet predetermined research objectives and aims of outsiders. Such an approach is often perceived by community members as disrespectful and self-serving and maintains power imbalances that contribute to health disparities. Moreover, because of power imbalances, community members often do not have a structure to voice their concerns and make change within a research study. Even when researchers assume, believe, and assert that community members are onboard, they may not be, and indeed the study will not be, as

Table 1.1 Characteristics of community engagement and partnership and CBPR that emerged across chapters

Community engagement and partnership and CBPR are more expansive than merely community members serving on community advisory groups or community advisory boards
Community engagement and partnership and CBPR are processes that begin during conceptualization of the research question and continue throughout the entire research process
Community engagement and partnership and CBPR are democratic approaches to research
Community engagement and partnership and CBPR prevent researcher voyeurism and the pathologization of communities
Community engagement and partnership and CBPR increase community member skills and overall community capacity
Community engagement and partnership and CBPR promote social justice
Community engagement and partnership and CBPR promote translation and public health impact
Community engagement and partnership and CBPR require not only an established partnership but a sustained organizational capacity
Community engagement and partnership and CBPR bring diverse perspectives, experiences, and insights together
Community engagement and partnership and CBPR tend to harness existing community assets, including indigenous leadership
Community engagement and partnership and CBPR cannot be conducted by remaining within the walls of one's office
Language is key to engagement
Despite the potential of community engagement and partnership and CBPR in the prevention of HIV exposure and transmission, there may never be one answer to profound challenges such as HIV and other health disparities and inequities

successful as possible. We need all efforts to be as successful as possible. Not doing everything in our power to make our prevention research successful is analogous to providing less dosage than hypothesized as needed to test a new treatment.

Community engagement and partnership and CBPR are processes that begin during conceptualization of the research question and continue throughout the entire research process. It is through ongoing dialogue, interaction, and negotiation—engagement—that research questions are the most meaningful; methods are the most appropriate; interpretation of findings is the most accurate; and dissemination is the most comprehensive [1, 8, 10–12].

Community engagement and partnership and CBPR are democratic approaches to research. Engagement, partnership, and CBPR are strategies to re-distribute power and increase social justice [13]. Community members, organization representatives, and academic researchers are interactively linked in new ways through engagement and partnership that do not give the academic researcher exclusive power and ownership of the methods and products of research; all partners share in the methods of knowledge generation and the knowledge discovered, its application, and its dissemination [5].

Although sometimes power is shared and balanced without hierarchy and singular control, other times community partners may, in fact, hold more power. In the process of developing, implementing, and evaluating HIV prevention interventions through CBPR with soccer leagues in North Carolina [14], there were times when members of the partnership (including representatives from the soccer league) finalized decisions as a group, and those decisions were subsequently changed based on what other league members decided. In this case, partners had to be comfortable with both holding much less power and using an alternate decision-making process, because those most affected by the health problem and the research held more power.

Community engagement and partnership and CBPR prevent researcher voyeurism and the pathologization of communities. Voyeurism may occur or can be perceived to occur when outsiders "research" others, particularly when those others happen to be vulnerable or engaging in hidden behaviors, such as sexual and reproductive behaviors. Furthermore, just as behavioral science has moved from referring to research participants as "subjects," engagement and partnership ensure that community members, organization representatives, and academic researchers work shoulder-to-shoulder on behalf of community health and well-being; there is no room for a "them-versus-us" mentality or for seeing individuals, networks, and/or communities as problems. Voyeurism and pathologization are not respectful and have no role in community health and well-being.

Community engagement and partnership and CBPR increase community member skills and overall community capacity. Health disparities and health inequalities are related to underlying factors, including income, housing, education, skills, and employment. Engagement and partnership are designed to positively affect the underlying causes of health disparities and inequities through increasing understanding of available resources and how to access them, developing problem-solving and critical-thinking skills, and appreciating how systems function and policies are formed and learning how to influence them. The idea is to intervene upstream on the factors that underlie a variety of health issues rather than focusing downstream on each health issue individually (e.g., HIV, obesity, asthma, tobacco, and diabetes).

Community engagement and partnership and CBPR promote social justice. Social justice implies the fair distribution of resources (e.g., health care services, food, housing, education, employment, and income) and responsibilities among members of a population with a focus on the relative position of one social group in relation to others in society, the root causes of health disparities and inequities, and what can be done to eliminate them [15]. Social justice is based on the concepts of mutuality and interconnectedness, solidarity, fairness, and human dignity. Engagement, partnership, and CBPR are seen as approaches to promote social justice through the promotion of equity. Equity, which is often confused with equality, focuses on fairness and ensures the same opportunities for all, while equality focuses on sameness. Having the same thing (equality) only works if everyone starts at the same place. However, structural and historical discrimination based on race/ethnicity, sexual orientation, gender identity, poverty, and inadequate education, as examples, are not easily overcome and prevent everyone from starting at the same place. Thus, much work needs to be done to promote social justice.

Community engagement and partnership and CBPR promote translation and public health impact. It has been well acknowledged that through the inclusion of community members and organization representatives, the ecologic validity of interventions and programs and the potential for successful translation increase [1, 11, 16–20]. It may not matter much if an intervention and program is successful in the carefully controlled context of a laboratory; what is crucial is that it works within the community to promote health and prevent disease.

Community engagement and partnership and CBPR require not only an established partnership but a sustained organizational capacity. Changes in leadership or staff and/or organizational priorities can profoundly affect the ability of partners to work together authentically and productively. For example, a long-term and highly successful CBPR partnership faced a crisis when a new Executive Director took the helm at a small AIDS service organization. The Executive Director lacked the communication, leadership, supervision, and research skills that were required at the particular point of the partnership's CBPR. Despite efforts to get him "up to speed", it was decided through iterative discussion within the partnership and with the organization's Board of Directors that the organization needed to focus on practice and relinquish its research agenda; other partners stepped up to continue the CBPR.

Community engagement and partnership and CBPR bring diverse perspectives, experiences, and insights together. However, creating a space for engagement and partnership can be challenging. Identifiable differences among those involved in engagement and partnership include age, sexual orientation, gender identity, race/ethnicity, country of origin, educational attainment, time and place in life course, faith/spirituality, and socioeconomic status, among other differences. The challenge becomes how to work together in a meaningful way. Lessons from engagement and partnership suggest four key strategies to overcome the challenges and harness the strengths of how partners are different: engaging in open communication among all involved, being nonjudgmental about differing viewpoints, assuming best intentions, and prioritizing cultural humility.

Cultural humility is a concept that has re-emerged as individuals in public health, and medicine recognize the weaknesses of cultural competency [21]. Simply, cultural competency tends to suggest that there is a body of knowledge about "those who are different" that can be learned and then applied. The idea is that someone has learned to successfully work with gay men, Latinos lower-income populations, or adolescents, as examples. However, cultural humility suggests that there is no discrete endpoint for understanding, and in fact, when someone thinks he or she understands a group of people (e.g., gay men, Latinos, adolescents, or lower-income populations), he or she may make incorrect assumptions based on narrowly defined categories, and these assumptions often lead to stereotyping as opposed to understanding and productive interactions [21]. Cultural humility suggests that one should never assume; should continually self-reflect about one's own assumptions and perspectives to increase one's self-awareness; should apply learnings and increased awareness to change one's attitudes and behaviors; and should become a lifelong learner through ongoing interaction. Cultural humility is based on the idea that each of us is an expert in the intersections of who we are (our various identities and values) and our dynamic life experiences, and we must not assume to understand others, who are also experts of who they are. It is important to be humble and approach engagement, partnership, and CBPR as a learner. This can be particularly difficult for academic researchers and practitioners who have been trained to be experts and have been often told by others just like them that they are the experts.

Community engagement and partnership and CBPR tend to harness existing community assets, including indigenous leadership. The use of natural helpers, including lay health advisors and peer leaders, to reach other community members, for example, has been a common approach to health promotion and disease prevention, but only now are the health outcome data being collected to support these common sense approaches to community and population health [22–25].

Community engagement and partnership and CBPR cannot be conducted by remaining within the walls of one's office. Community engagement and partnership and CBPR require academic researchers and practitioners to be active participants in the communities in which they are working. Engagement is not a one-way street, and academic researchers and practitioners must be engaged within the community.

Language is key to engagement. In nonengaged approaches to research, the researcher, investigator, scientist, or practitioner is removed from community; the person represents the outside expert. However, engagement, partnership, and CBPR imply that representatives from the community, organizations, and businesses, as examples, also work as researchers, investigators, and scientists. Thus, the nomenclature can be confusing. In many CBPR partnerships, university-based partners are referred to as "academic researchers" because to simply refer to them as researchers can imply that community members are not researchers, and yet they are.

Despite the potential of community engagement and partnership and CBPR in the prevention of HIV exposure and transmission, there may never be one answer to profound challenges such as HIV and other health disparities and inequities. These types of challenges to health and well-being, in fact, require multi-pronged approaches. For example, within the USA, some, but not all, communities have access to preexposure prophylaxis; while some communities work to increase access and increase efficacy [26, 27], others strive to discover other approaches. We must recognize the limits of what we have done to prevent HIV, including the limits of clinical prevention.

Discussion

Although the early successes related to HIV prevention and care were very much linked to the community, overtime, academic researchers and practitioners within public health and medicine became less connected to communities; a gulf grew between outside experts and communities, and health disparities grew. We have created a chasm between knowledge generation and its translation and application for improved community health and well-being. However, there has been a pendulum swing in the direction of community engagement and partnership and CBPR. Community engagement and partnership, including CBPR, in public health and medicine are promoted as an approaches to better understand health phenomena. When such research is conducted well, this better understanding can yield more effective interventions and programs to reduce health disparities. HIV prevention research and practice have been at the forefront of community engagement and partnership and CBPR. Early on in the HIV epidemic, gay men and their close allies mobilized to promote action and lead the way in sound approaches to community engagement in the design, implementation, evaluation, translation, and dissemination of prevention interventions. In fact, we now have a critical mass of current and recent HIV prevention intervention studies that have applied innovative approaches to engagement, partnership, and CBPR; this book is designed to be a "go-to" state-of-the-art resource to which researchers, practitioners, students, and community and organization representatives can refer in order to bring the science and practice of community engagement to its next level.

Leaders in the field who are working at various points along the community-engagement continuum, with diverse populations, and different types of HIV prevention interventions (e.g., individual, community, and structural) have contributed important chapters that outline both innovative interventions designed to reduce HIV risk among some of the most affected communities and authentic and meaningful approaches to engagement, partnership, and CBPR. Chapter authors include community members who may come from communities greatly affected by HIV in the USA; organization representatives who are providing services to members of these communities; business representatives; federal scientists and practitioners; and academic researchers who must negotiate the challenges of their institutions (e.g., tenure and funding) and federal and foundation funders fully.

Contributions

Besides appreciating the commitment of the chapter authors and the risk they were willing to take to write candidly about their processes and expose both the successes and challenges faced, I thank past and current members of our local CBPR partnership and other colleagues for their patience and feedback during my own learning process over the past 13 years, including Jose Alegría-Ortega, Alex Boeving Allen, Jorge Alonzo, Mario Andrade, Ramiro A. Arceo, Tom Arcury, Jorge Elias Arellano, Robert E. Aronson, Laura H. Bachmann, Holly Baddour, Barbara Baquero, Precilla Belin, Fred R. Bloom, Rebecca Cashman, Suzanne Cashman, Jason Daniel-Ulloa, Ralph J. DiClemente, Mario Downs, Ilana Dubester, Ricky Duck, Stacy Duck, Jesse Duncan, Doug Easterling, Eugenia Eng, Kristie Long Foley, Arin Freeman, Raúl Gámez, Manuel Garcia, Paul A. Gilbert, Mark Hall, Anthony Hannah, Ellen Hendrix, Kenneth C. Hergenrather, Sheryl Hulme, Barbara Israel, Christine Jolly, Karen Klein, Emma Lawlor, Jami S. Leichliter, Laura C. Leviton, Kristin Lindstrom, Lilli Mann, Omar Martinez, Thomas McCoy, Cindy Miller, Meredith Minkler, Jaime Montaño, Addison Ore, Thomas Painter, Regina Pulliam, Sara Quandt, Barry Ramsey, Michael Reece, Beth A. Reboussin, Ivan Remnitz, Rodrigo Rodriguez-Celedon,

Michael Ross, Florence Simán, Eunyoung Song, Jason Stowers, Ron Strauss, Karen Strazza, Christina Sun, Erin Sutfin, Francisco Sy, Amanda Tanner, Scott Trent Aaron T. Vissman, Kim Wagoner, Debbie Warren, Aimee M. Wilkin, and Leland J. Yee.

I also thank the following individuals who reviewed and edited various chapters and provided much moral support during this process: Claire Abraham; Lori Alexander, MTPW; Robert E. Aronson, DrPH; Eugenia Eng, DrPH; Lilli Mann, MPH; and Aimee M. Wilkin, MD, MPH.

Conclusion

Since the HIV epidemic began, community involvement has been crucial to identifying priorities and meeting the needs of the most affected communities. This community involvement occurred before community engagement and partnership and CBPR were used to describe such efforts. In the early 1980s, community members came together not only to meet the immediate needs of those affected by HIV but to propel action. For example, community members organized and played a pivotal role in revising the process that the US Food and Drug Administration (FDA) used to test and approve medications for HIV and ensuring that women were included in HIV drug trials. They advocated for the inclusion of persons living with HIV/AIDS and those affected (e.g., partners and lovers, biologic families and families of choice, friends, and congregations) in decision-making, priority setting, research design and implementation, and evaluation. They sought out and partnered with health behavior experts, providers, and public health and medical researchers to initiate a process to explore developing effective approaches to understand and intervene on the psychosocial aspects of the epidemic. Thus, HIV has a long history of engagement and of fostering partnerships among community members, organization representatives, and academic researchers to promote health and prevention to reduce the burden of the epidemic.

The vision of the National HIV/AIDS Strategy is as follows:

> The United States will become a place where new HIV infections are rare and when they do occur, every person, regardless of age, gender, race/ethnicity, sexual orientation, gender identity or socio-economic circumstance, will have unfettered access to high quality, life-extending care, free from stigma and discrimination.

However, to reach this vision, community engagement and partnership and CBPR may be effective strategies to identify new meaningful and effective ways to reduce behavioral risk, seropositive infectivity, and/or biologic vulnerability to infection within communities at increased risk. This book provides examples of innovative behavioral HIV prevention interventions that use novel approaches to community engagement and partnership and CBPR.

References

1. Green LW. From research to "best practices" in other settings and populations. Am J Health Behav. 2001;25(3):165–78.
2. Institute of Medicine. Promoting health: intervention strategies from social and behavioral research. Washington, DC: National Academy Press; 2000.
3. Israel BA, Schulz AJ, Parker EA, Becker AB. Review of community-based research: assessing partnership approaches to improve public health. Annu Rev Public Health. 1998;19:173–202.
4. Minkler M, Wallerstein N. Introduction to community based participatory research. In: Minkler M, Wallerstein N, editors. Community-Based based participatory research for health. San Francisco: Jossey-Bass; 2003. p. 3–26.
5. Viswanathan M, Eng E, Ammerman A, Gartlehner G, Lohr KN, Griffith D, et al. Community-based participatory research: assessing the evidence. Evidence report/technology assessment. Rockville, MD: Agency for Healthcare Research and Quality, 2004 July. Report No.: 99.
6. Rhodes SD SD. Demonstrated effectiveness and potential of CBPR for preventing HIV in Latino populations. In: Organista KC, Editor. HIV prevention with Latinos: theory, research, and practice. New York: Oxford University Press; 2012. p. 83–102.
7. Rhodes SD, Duck S, Alonzo J, Daniel J, Aronson RE. Using community-based participatory research to prevent HIV disparities: assumptions and opportunities identified by the Latino partnership. J Acquir Immune Defic Syndr. 2013;63(Suppl 1):S32–5.
8. Rhodes SD, Duck S, Alonzo J, Downs M, Aronson RE. Intervention trials in community-based participatory research. In: Blumenthal D, DiClemente RJ, Braithwaite RL, Smith S, editors. Community-based participatory research: issues, methods, and translation to practice. New York: Springer; 2013. p. 157–80.
9. Fawcett SB, Paine-Andrews A, Francisco VT, Schultz JA, Richter KP, Lewis RK, et al. Using empowerment theory in collaborative partnerships for community health and development. Am J Community Psychol. 1995;23(5):677–97.
10. Bowie J, Eng E, Lichtenstein RR. A decade of postdoctoral training in CBPR and dedication to Thomas A. Bruce. Prog Community Health Partnersh. 2009;3(4):267–70.
11. Cashman SB, Adeky S, Allen AJ, Corburn J, Israel BA, Montaño J, et al. The power and the promise: working with communities to analyze data, interpret findings, and get to outcomes. Am J Public Health. 2008;98(8):1407–17.
12. Minkler M. Linking science and policy through community-based participatory research to study and address health disparities. Am J Public Health. 2010;100 (Suppl 1):S81–7.
13. Myser C. Community-based participaroty reserach in United States bioethics: steps toward more democratic theory and policy. Am J Bioethics. 2004;4(2):67–8.
14. Rhodes SD, Hergenrather KC, Bloom FR, Leichliter JS, Montano J. Outcomes from a community-based, participatory lay health adviser HIV/STD prevention intervention for recently arrived immigrant Latino men in rural North Carolina. AIDS Educ Prev. 2009;21(5 Suppl):103–8.
15. Commission on Social Determinants of Health. Closing the gap in a generation: Health health equity through action on the social determinants of health. Final report of the Comission on Social Determinants of Health. Geneva: World Health Organization; 2008.
16. Rhodes SD, Hergenrather KC, Vissman AT, Stowers J, Davis AB, Hannah A, et al. Boys must be men, and men must have sex with women: a qualitative CBPR study to explore sexual risk among African American, Latino, and white gay men and MSM. Am J Mens Health. 2011;5(2):140–51.
17. Rhodes SD, Malow RM, Jolly C. Community-based participatory research: a new and not-so-new approach to HIV/AIDS prevention, care, and treatment. AIDS Educ Prev. 2010;22(3):173–83.
18. Bogart LM, Uyeda K. Community-based participatory research: partnering with communities for effective and sustainable behavioral health interventions. Health Psychol. 2009;28(4):391–3.

19. Christens B, Perkins DD. Transdisciplinary, multilevel action research to enhance ecological and psychopolitical validity. J Community Psychol. 2008;36(2):214–31.
20. Green LW, Glasgow RE. Evaluating the relevance, generalization, and applicability of research: issues in external validation and translation methodology. Eval Health Prof. 2006;29(1):126–53.
21. Tervalon M, Murray-Garcia J. Cultural humility versus cultural competence: a critical distinction in defining physician training outcomes in multicultural education. J Health Care Poor Underserved. 1998;9(2):117–25.
22. Ayala GX, Vaz L, Earp JA, Elder JP, Cherrington A. Outcome effectiveness of the lay health advisor model among Latinos in the United States: an examination by role. Health Educ Res. 2010;25(5):815–40.
23. Eng E, Rhodes SD, Parker EA. Natural helper models to enhance a community's health and competence. In: Di Clemente RJ, Crosby RA, Kegler MC, editors. Emerging theories in health promotion practice and research. San Francisco: Jossey-Bass; 2009. p. 303–30.
24. Rhodes SD, Foley KL, Zometa CS, Bloom FR. Lay health advisor interventions among Hispanics/Latinos: a qualitative systematic review. Am J Prev Med. 2007;33(5):418–27.
25. Rhodes SD, Hergenrather KC, Bloom FR, Leichliter JS, Montaño J. Outcomes from a community-based, participatory lay health advisor HIV/STD prevention intervention for recently arrived immigrant Latino men in rural North Carolina, USA. AIDS Educ Prev. 2009;21(Suppl 1):104–9.
26. Baeten JM, Donnell D, Ndase P, Mugo NR, Campbell JD, Wangisi J, et al. Antiretroviral prophylaxis for HIV prevention in heterosexual men and women. N Engl J Med. 2012;367(5):399–410.
27. Baeten JM, Celum C. Antiretroviral preexposure prophylaxis for HIV prevention. N Engl J Med. 2013;368(1):83–4.

Chapter 2
HIV Prevention in a Rural Community: Project GRACE—A Multigenerational Approach to Community Engagement

Arlinda Ellison, Aletha Akers, Adina Black, Tashuna Albritton, Stepheria Hodge-Sallah, Mysha Wynn, Danny Ellis and Giselle Corbie-Smith

Advances in HIV prevention have great potential to reduce the incidence of HIV in USA, but to date, have had a limited impact on the epidemic in the communities most affected by the disease. Effectively preventing HIV within rural, racial/ethnic minority, and other underserved communities requires looking beyond strategies

A. Ellison (✉)
North Carolina Translational and Clinical Sciences Institute, University of North Carolina at Chapel Hill, 160 N. Medical Drive, Campus Box 7064, Chapel Hill, NC 27599, USA
e-mail: arlinda_ellison@med.unc.edu

A. Akers
Magee-Women's Hospital Department of Obstetrics, Gynecology and Reproductive Sciences, University of Pittsburgh School of Medicine, 300 Halket Street, Pittsburg, PA 15213, USA
e-mail: aakers@mail.magee.edu

A. Black
North Carolina Translational and Clinical Sciences Institute, University of North Carolina at Chapel Hill, 160 N. Medical Drive, Campus Box 7064, Chapel Hill, NC 27599, USA
e-mail: asblack@email.unc.edu

T. Albritton
Center for Interdisciplinary Research on AIDS, Yale University, 135 College Street, Suite 200, New Haven, CT 06510-2483, USA
e-mail: tashuna.albritton@yale.edu

S. Hodge-Sallah
NC Department of Health and Human Services, Division of Public Health, 225 N. McDowell Street, 1902 MSC Raleigh, NC 27601, USA
e-mail: stepheriasallah@gmail.com

M. Wynn
Project Momentum, Inc., P. O. Box 4053, Rocky Mount, NC 27803, USA
e-mail: projectmomentum@embarqmail.com

D. Ellis
Ellis Research & Consulting Service, LLC, 3514 Whetstone Place, Wilson, NC 27896, USA
e-mail: ruone@myglnc.com

G. Corbie-Smith
Department of Social Medicine, University of North Carolina at Chapel Hill School of Medicine, 333 S. Columbia Street, Chapel Hill, NC 27599, USA
e-mail: gcorbie@med.unc.edu

S. D. Rhodes (ed.), *Innovations in HIV Prevention Research and Practice through Community Engagement,* DOI 10.1007/978-1-4939-0900-1_2,
© Springer Science+Business Media New York 2014

that target individual-level risk determinants and considering strategies that target high-risk populations, address structural determinants of HIV risk, and harness social and sexual networks and interpersonal relationships [1, 2]. When considering what works best for a particular community, group, network, or other social unit, it is also important to examine key demographics and other characteristics of group members, as well as the contexts in which they live and work. These considerations represent potential areas for developing and tailoring interventions [3].

In this chapter, we explore the use of a community-based participatory research (CBPR) approach to develop, implement, and evaluate an intervention to prevent HIV in a rural community, highlighting the efforts of the Project GRACE (Growing, Reaching, Advocating for Change and Empowerment) Consortium, a community–academic partnership based in eastern North Carolina. The Project GRACE Consortium draws on the strengths of community, academic, and public partners with the goal of developing a multilevel, multigenerational, culturally specific, feasible, and sustainable prevention intervention to address the disproportionately high rates of HIV among African-American/black communities in two eastern North Carolina counties. This multigenerational approach to HIV prevention acknowledges that many social behaviors are learned by observing others [4] and builds on the strengths of multigenerational relationships and the existing interconnectedness among generations [5].

We begin this chapter by exploring the impact of HIV on the southeastern states and rural communities in North Carolina, particularly in African-American/black communities. We then highlight the unique process used to engage community members in the formation of the Project GRACE Consortium, the subsequent multigenerational intervention known as Teach One Reach One (TORO) that was born out of this Consortium, the lessons learned throughout the process, and recommendations for future research. Lastly, we describe research needs and priorities in terms of prevention and community engagement among African-American/black populations in the southeastern USA, particularly in rural communities.

The Impact of HIV on the Southeastern USA and Rural Communities

The disparate spread of HIV and other sexually transmitted infections (STIs) within African-American/black communities is a crucial problem in the USA. The US Centers for Disease Control and Prevention (CDC) estimates that 1.2 million persons are currently with HIV in the USA. The most severe burden of HIV continues to be in the African-American/black community, compared with all other races and ethnicities. African-Americans/black represented approximately 12–14 % of the US population in 2010, but in the same year accounted for an estimated 44 % of all new cases of HIV infection. In 2010, the estimated rate of new HIV infections among African-American/black men was six and a half times higher than that for white men, and more than two and a half times higher as that for Hispanic/Latino men and African-American/black women. In the same year, the estimated rate of new HIV infections among African-American/black women was 15 times that for white women and more than three times that for Hispanic/Latina women [6, 7].

Although often not well recognized outside the region, the HIV epidemic is especially profound in the southeastern USA. The South has the highest rate of new AIDS cases and the highest number of adults and youth living with and dying from AIDS. Although the South accounts for only 37 % of the US population, it accounts for more than half of the persons with HIV and 50 % of all new HIV infections in the USA. During the past several years, the number of persons with HIV in the South has exceeded those in all other regions of the country. In 2010, eight of the ten states in the country with the highest rates of HIV infection were in the South: Florida, Georgia, Louisiana, Mississippi, North Carolina, South Carolina, Tennessee, and Texas. Moreover, African-Americans/blacks in the South are disproportionately affected. Whereas African-Americans/blacks make up 20 % of the overall population in the South [8], more than half (56 %) of persons with HIV in the South are African-American/black [7, 9].

A large proportion of the southern population lives in rural areas, and most HIV/AIDS cases in the South are concentrated in these areas, with 65 % of all AIDS cases in the South being among rural populations [10]. Although some factors associated with HIV transmission, such as inconsistent condom use [11], limited partner selection options [12], poverty [12, 13], and poor access to care [13], can be similar in both rural and urban settings; other factors may be more common in rural settings, such as having an untested sex partner [11], believing that the untested partner is HIV negative [11], lack of HIV-prevention outreach [13], and higher rates of HIV stigma [13]. Additionally, limited recreational opportunities have been shown to be a contributor to HIV transmission in rural settings [14].

In 2009, African-American/black adults and adolescents represented 50 % of HIV diagnoses and 49 % of reported AIDS diagnoses in rural areas [6, 7]. Researchers and practitioners have identified contextual factors within rural communities that play significant roles in the disparate infection rates among minorities. These community-level challenges include economic hardship, racial/ethnic discrimination, and gender imbalance. However, other factors also contribute to racial disparities in HIV infection and are unique to rural communities, including limited access to health care, lack of perceived and real patient confidentiality in local health care settings, inadequate HIV-prevention outreach, HIV stigma, and community resistance to prevention efforts.

To date, HIV-prevention efforts designed for rural communities have largely targeted persons with HIV. These interventions have primarily focused on linking persons with HIV to care. Some interventions and programs focus on connecting people with HIV with skilled providers [15–18]. Other interventions and programs include medical care providers who provide brief, tailored HIV- and STI-prevention messages during the patient's regular care, educate patients about safer sex practices, screen patients for HIV- and STI-transmission risk behaviors, facilitate reductions in high-risk behaviors, and offer additional prevention services. Few interventions have been implemented in rural communities that focus specifically on the

Table 2.1 Demographic characteristics of counties of interest with high prevalence of HIV in 2006

County	Total population	African-Americans/black		Whites		Persons with HIV	
		Total percentage	Percentage living in poverty	Total percentage	Percentage living in poverty	Percentage African-Americans/blacks	Percentage white
Edgecombe[a]	55,606	58	27	40	9	86	11
Nash[a]	87,420	34	23	62	7	82	11
Halifax	57,370	53	34	43	11	85	14
Northampton	22,086	59	29	39	9	89	8
Wilson	73,814	39	30	40	9	90	8

[a] Partnership communities

prevention of HIV- and STI-transmission risk behaviors among those not infected with HIV. To our knowledge, the Hope Project [19], targeting rural men who have sex with men (MSM), the Students Together Against Negative Decisions (STAND) intervention [20], targeting rural youth, and the HoMBReS intervention [18], for immigrant Latino men who are members of rural recreational soccer teams, are the only three behavioral interventions that have been developed specifically within and for rural communities.

HIV in North Carolina

In North Carolina, the highest numbers of reported HIV/AIDS cases are found in urban/metropolitan counties; however, the counties with the highest incidence of HIV are rural [21]. Furthermore, some of the highest rates of HIV in the state and the most significant HIV and STI disparities are found in the community in which our partnership works, including both Nash and Edgecombe counties. These two counties are located in northeastern North Carolina and are bounded by Halifax, Northampton, and Wilson counties. In Edgecombe and Nash counties, HIV and poverty rates are all disproportionately higher among the African-American/black population than among other racial/ethnic populations (Table 2.1).

In Nash county, 82 % of people with HIV/AIDS in 2006 were African-American/black, although only 34 % of the county's population was African-American/black; the corresponding percentages for Edgecombe county were 86 and 58 % [15, 21]. Furthermore, 23 and 27 % of African-Americans/blacks live in poverty in Nash and Edgecombe counties, respectively, compared with 7 and 9 % of whites. The bordering counties of Halifax, Northampton, and Wilson are similar to Edgecombe and Nash counties in terms of demographic features and high rates of poverty and HIV [21, 22].

Nationally, the greatest HIV burden among all racial/ethnic groups is found among African-American/black youth, accounting for 55 % of reported HIV infections among those ages 13–24-years old. Between 2002 and 2006, 23 % of new HIV/AIDS cases in Edgecombe county and 21 % in Nash county were reported to occur in African-Americans/blacks 20–29-years old, whereas the rate of new cases was minimal among whites in the same age-group. Given the latency period from HIV infection to the development of AIDS, most persons with AIDS who are in their 20s likely acquired the infection in their teenage years [15, 23–25].

Project GRACE—Growing, Reaching and Advocating for Change and Empowerment

The CDC defines community engagement as "the process of working collaboratively with and through groups of people affiliated by geographic proximity, special interest, or similar situations to address issues affecting the well-being of those people" [26]. The Project GRACE Consortium was formed in 2005 in response to the concerns of community members about the profound impact of HIV in two neighboring counties: Edgecombe and Nash. Preexisting ties between the community stakeholders in these counties and the academic partners facilitated the development of this partnership. In prior formative work, HIV disparities had been identified as one of the top three major health concerns by both lay community members and representatives of community-based organizations. During the months leading up to the official formation of the Project GRACE Consortium, several stakeholders and community leaders from Nash and Edgecombe counties expressed a desire to begin addressing the HIV epidemic in their counties. In recognition of this health crisis, the decision was made to create a community–academic partnership with the explicit mission of addressing HIV disparities in these two counties [16].

There are many approaches to community engagement. To establish the Project GRACE Consortium, we used the 4-stage approach to partnership development articulated by Florin [15, 27, 28]. These four stages are (1) initial mobilization, (2) establishment of the organizational structure, (3) building capacity for action, and (4) developing an action plan. These initial stages lay the groundwork for action by engaging community partners, broadening the base of community support, identifying the strengths and capacity of community representatives, delineating roles for all partners, ensuring shared decision-making, developing organizational infrastructure, building capacity to support subsequent action steps, and planning for subsequent action and intervention development, implementation, and evaluation [16].

Initial Mobilization

Communities can be variably defined. In line with the CDC definition of community engagement, we define "community" as a group of people with existing relationships who share a common interest, live in the same geographic area, or share a similar ethnic/cultural background [15]. For the Project GRACE Consortium, we defined our community as individuals residing in or invested in the health of the African-American/black population in Nash and Edgecombe counties. As we developed the Consortium, we identified and invited a broad range of key stakeholders to participate in an initial planning meeting to ensure that a range of community perspectives were represented. There were 15 attendees at the initial meeting, including individual community members and representatives of local community-based education, health, social service organizations, as well as faith-based organizations. These attendees were encouraged to "spread the word" in the community about the formation of this community–academic partnership and to solicit participation from other organizations, agencies, and community activists [15].

Over time, the partnership grew and members worked collaboratively to solicit federal funding for the effort. In our grant writing efforts, we applied the principles of CBPR to ensure full engagement and participation of all members of the partnership. We developed teams composed of community members and academic investigators, who each provided insight into study design, feasibility, and evaluation plans. These efforts resulted in funding through a grant from the National Center on Minority Health and Health Disparities to UNC-Chapel Hill. After obtaining funding, we used subcontracts to community-based organizations to ensure that financial resources were divided equitably between community and academic partners.

Broad and appropriate representation in the Project GRACE Consortium has been essential to ensuring the acceptability and relevance of the intervention in the community. For example, although some of the organizations in our partnership have a health focus, others have missions that are not explicitly health related. Establishing broad representation requires effort, but our initial partners also recognized that maintaining such broad representation would be more challenging because membership and leadership at organizations tend to change fairly often. To gain and maintain broad representation, a community outreach specialist was hired from the community to work with the university-based project coordinator and representatives of the various subcontracting organizations to develop a matrix of community service providers, local leaders, and influential persons within both counties. The community outreach specialist contacted additional potential Project GRACE Consortium members to describe the project and invite them to attend one of the quarterly Consortium meetings. We created an e-mail Listserv that is still in use and can be accessed by all Project GRACE Consortium members to share information about upcoming community events and professional development activities. We also provide updates about Project GRACE-related activities through a regular newsletter. Consortium members drew on their knowledge of the community and on their professional and social networks to extend invitations to stakeholders that represented a broad range of community perspectives, experiences, and insights [15].

Establishing Organizational Structure

Although the Project GRACE Consortium engages a broad set of community partners, we recognized that we needed a core set of individuals who would be responsible for rigorous planning, oversight, and coordination of the long-term vision of the project. We decided to use the governing structure of a highly active Steering Committee that meets monthly. The Steering Committee consists of representatives from all contracting and subcontracting partner organizations and community leaders in each county [15]. The Project GRACE Consortium and Steering Committee provide a system of "checks and balances" on one another's decisions and activities. In addition, six subcommittees were created to tackle logistical aspects of Project GRACE activities. These six subcommittees are (1) Communications and Publications, (2) Research and Design, (3) Nominating, (4) Bylaws, (5) Events Planning, and (6) Fiscal and Budget. Each subcommittee is chaired by a community stakeholder and may be co-chaired by an academic partner. Subcommittee members represent our broader membership and are expected to report back to the Steering Committee [16]. This organizational structure, while complex, ensures a high degree of community engagement and participation at every level. This structure also builds sustainability, trust, and transparency.

Building Capacity for Action

The activities that occurred during the initial mobilization and establishment of organizational structure were necessary to ensure the development of strong and trusting relationships among Project GRACE Consortium members (including the Steering Committee). Efforts to build trust and capacity were also facilitated by structured and ongoing trust-building activities.

For example, all Consortium members—both community and academic partners—participated in a 4-day workshop called "Changing Racism and Other 'Isms': A Personal Approach to Multiculturalism." This workshop was conducted by consultants from VISIONS, Inc., an African-American/black, locally owned company based in Rocky Mount, North Carolina, that provides training and support to community-development projects. The workshop highlights, confronts, and challenges oppression of all types at the institutional, cultural, interpersonal, and personal levels.

We chose the "Isms" workshop for two reasons. First, it would help build the capacity of partnership members to recognize and address the various forms of oppression external to our Project GRACE Consortium that could represent a potential influence on the spread of HIV within the community. Second, it would allow us to see how different forms of oppression might operate with and between partnership members, thereby threatening the success of our efforts. This 4-day workshop is required of new project staff and members of the Project GRACE Consortium, to ensure that all involved have a shared vision and similar orientation to our partnership and work.

In addition to the 4-day "Isms" workshop by VISIONS, Inc., Project GRACE Consortium members also participated in an annual retreat to evaluate the CBPR process within the Consortium. Prior to each retreat, consultants from VISIONS, Inc. met with Consortium members to evaluate the extent and ways in which CBPR principles have been adhered to through the use of semi-structured interviews. This periodic process evaluation focuses on (1) community partners' knowledge of the project; (2) identified facilitators, barriers, and recommendations; (3) "Isms" and cultural differences; and (4) empowerment. During the retreat, the results of the evaluation are presented and used as a basis for strategic planning. It is at this annual retreat that changes in Consortium activities, procedures, and policies are discussed.

Planning for Action

In preparing to identify HIV-prevention efforts relevant to those living in Nash and Edgecombe counties, members of the Project GRACE Consortium conducted a needs and assets assessment. This assessment was conducted to identify community needs, resources, goals, and objectives to guide the choice of strategies and plans for intervention implementation and evaluation. This process underscores our mission to be facilitators of social change and community empowerment; we do not use a deficits approach to community health promotion and disease prevention.

The assessment consisted of focus groups and key informant interviews. During the spring and summer of 2006, we conducted a total of 11 focus groups with three main populations: community youth 16–24-years old, adults 25–45-years old, and formerly incarcerated adults (any age). These populations were selected because they represent the groups for which the rates of HIV are highest (e.g., youth and formerly incarcerated individuals) and those living with and caring for these individuals. We also conducted 37 key informant interviews in the fall and winter of 2006. The methods have been fully described elsewhere [29, 30]. Briefly, for both the focus groups and the interviews, we recruited through local community-based organizations and the use of flyers, print and radio advertising, and snowball sampling. In keeping with our desire to involve community members throughout the research process, we hired and trained interviewers and note-takers from the local community. These staff were trained by a professional, African-American/black-owned, qualitative research firm to conduct the focus groups and interviews.

In keeping with our CBPR principles, the research design and data interpretation and analysis processes were conducted collaboratively by both community and academic partners who were members of the Research and Design Subcommittee. Subcommittee members developed the guides for the moderators of the focus groups and interviews. After the data were collected, members of the Research and Design Subcommittee were divided into teams to review the data and develop the qualitative data-coding strategy. Here again, teams were always composed of both community and academic representatives, to ensure validity of the findings. To corroborate the validity of the findings, the data were presented at a quarterly Project GRACE Consortium meeting to a broader audience of community members and stakeholders.

From the focus groups and interviews conducted during our needs and assets assessment, a clear and consistent message emerged; simply, HIV-prevention efforts within our local community needed to focus on youth. Participants reported that the individual and social factors at the heart of the local epidemic (e.g., norms regarding sexual initiation and condom use, gender-based power differentials in relationships, and HIV stigma and its impact on HIV testing and health service utilization) were often learned across generations and therefore preventable or were amenable to change during adolescence. Participants also identified the need to place change in the context of the family and community. In order to reduce the rates of HIV and STIs, members of the Project GRACE Consortium decided that a family-based multigenerational intervention involving youth and their parents or primary caregivers (hereafter referred to as "caregivers") was needed and should be our priority.

The comprehensive approach to partnership development used by members of the Project GRACE Consortium provided a "collective confidence" that the future interventions we developed would be based on a thorough understanding of the needs of the target population and would build on existing community capacity to ensure sustainability [16]. In the sections that follow, we detail the process by which we integrated our CBPR approach with intervention mapping to develop our intervention [16, 31].

The Teach One, Reach One Intervention: A Multigenerational Approach

After collecting the formative data, we conducted intervention mapping to develop the intervention structure and content. Intervention mapping is a structured process for developing an intervention that is carried out in a series of steps that move from review of relevant literature and data to, ultimately, evaluation of the resulting intervention program [16, 31]. Step 1 involves conducting a needs and assets assessment. The structure and results of our needs and assets assessment were described earlier. Step 2 involves developing intervention goals, and in Step 3, the intervention methods are specified. Lastly, in Step 4, the program components are developed.

Preparation for Intervention Mapping: Co-learning on Applying Health Behavior Theory

After the formative data were collected, we proceeded with the next steps of intervention mapping with the Steering Committee and lay members of the community. This process consisted of intensive all-day workshops, group conference calls, and in-person meetings involving all partners in each step of the process, during May 2007 through January 2008. Our emphasis on capacity building and co-learning process included ensuring that all partners understood intervention mapping methods and had a working knowledge of health behavior theory. Thus, we conducted a half-day primer for partners that introduced several health behavior theories that could inform our work in effective intervention development. We used written condensed summaries of multiple major theories [16, 32], supplemented with abbreviated didactic sessions and small-group discussion. This format offered an opportunity for collective discussion about the importance of theoretically driven interventions and the relevance of constructs from different theoretical theories and models. It also allowed opportunities to discuss, answer clarifying questions about, and refine our process [16].

Intervention Mapping Workshop

Following the primer session to explore health behavior theory, we held an intensive 2-day workshop that initiated Step 2 of the intervention mapping process. The workshop was facilitated by a project staff with previous training and real-world experience using intervention mapping methods and by Steering Committee members who reviewed the formative research findings and facilitated the small-group sessions. During the first half of the first day of the workshop, we reviewed intervention mapping methods and recapped the findings from the formative research. During the second half of the first day, we organized a working group session wherein small groups consisting of both community and academic partners compiled lists of intervention goals to address the high rates of HIV in the local community. On the second day, we developed and refined the initial set of desired behavioral outcomes as well as drafted associated performance objectives required to achieve those outcomes, using a group consensus process [16].

Post-workshop Intervention Mapping Activities

Small groups of community and academic partners worked on other remaining tasks from Step 2 over the next 4 months. The remaining tasks included (a) refining performance objectives, (b) identifying determinants contributing to health behaviors, and (c) creating intervention matrices. Community and academic partners worked to further refine the proximal behavioral and performance objectives as they defined the behavioral determinants through an iterative process. All intervention matrices were reviewed as they were developed and presented to the larger group of collaborators until consensus on completeness was reached. To uphold the CBPR principles of co-learning and dissemination, early products from our collaborative work were periodically presented to the larger community at Project GRACE Consortium meetings. These presentations provided community members and leaders an opportunity to remain up-to-date on activities and structure to provide feedback [16].

Select Theory-based Methods and Strategies

Step 3 in the intervention mapping process focuses on matching the intervention methods to the performance objectives identified during Step 2. This task is accomplished by answering the key question: "*How* can we influence people to meet the performance objectives necessary for the desired behavioral outcomes?" Behavioral and social science theories directly address the behavioral determinants to inform intervention methods in any given intervention [16, 31]. Methods are general, more theoretical techniques that influence change in behavioral determinants, whereas strategies are specific pragmatic techniques for reaching the target community. In our partnership, subgroups of community and academic partners worked together to ensure that intervention methods aligned with the performance objectives.

Produce Program Components and Materials

Step 4 entails structuring and organizing strategies into a deliverable intervention or program. This step results in the actual design and details of an intervention or program, including the creation of the intervention training manuals and necessary guides and workbooks. In this intervention mapping step, we explored and decided on the program structure (e.g., scope and sequence), themes, channels for delivery, and intervention materials [16]. Again, upholding the CBPR principles within our intervention mapping process, a working group consisting of community and academic partners developed the curriculum lessons and conducted a community-wide pretest event. These processes led to the development of the Teach One, Reach One (TORO) intervention.

Results

Findings from the Needs and Assets Assessment

Participants in the focus groups and interviews described what they perceived to be the factors contributing to the high HIV rates in their communities and suggested ideas about how the HIV-prevention intervention should look. Participants unanimously stated that there was a profound need to focus on youth behavior, and that the intervention should take place specifically in the context of the family and community. Participants also noted individual and social factors that influence the sexual risk behaviors among youth in our community. In line with the feedback received from the focus groups and interviews, we determined that developing a collaborative family-based intervention was essential to HIV and STI risk reduction among youth in our local community. Additionally, to ensure sustainability, we chose to use a lay health advisor model in which individuals across generations (i.e., youth and caregivers) are trained and work in dyads to communicate HIV-prevention messages within their community. The lay health advisor model was the appropriate intervention framework because it is adaptable, targets change at multiple levels, is effective in developing trust and the capacity of community members, and has the ability to build on the strong sociocultural strengths and networks in rural African-American/black communities [16, 33].

Intervention Goals and Objectives

For both youth and their caregivers, intervention goals and objectives were created to reflect specific priorities of their respective group. Goals or desired behavioral outcomes for youth included delaying sexual initiation and following responsible sexual health practices (e.g., consistent condom use) for those who were sexually active. Desired outcomes for caregivers included improving parenting and communication skills. Literature suggests that focusing on parenting behaviors influences positive reproductive health outcomes for youth [16, 34–36]. We also identified several behavioral performance objectives identified as imperative to fully progress toward specific goals. For youth, those objectives included abstinence from sex, condom use among sexually active youth, and healthy dating and relationships. For caregivers, objectives included parental monitoring of youth-dating activities and parental communication about sex and healthy-dating relationships.

Theoretically-based Methods and Strategies

In the curricula, several methods were used to address each objective. Social learning and cognitive behavioral methods were used. The overall design of this intervention was based on the social ecologic framework [37]to address the individual-, social-, and community-level factors that affect behavior. Vicarious learning, guided practice, and self-efficacy were used to develop skills and attain goals [16, 31]. The curricula also incorporated teachable moments, in which participants were presented with a variety of situations and then given the opportunity to reflect on and demonstrate how they would address each situation. The strategies used to incorporate these teachable moments varied and included games, small-group discussions, individual activities, and storytelling.

Program Components and Materials

Our review of interventions and programs indicated that most existing interventions for youth targeted youth exclusively and neglected the caregiver. In order to be effective in addressing the behavioral objectives for the caregivers, we adapted many activities for caregivers using well-recognized theory-based methods and strategies to guide our process. Because of the creative nature of our study design (i.e., training youth and adult dyads as lay health advisors to deliver the multigenerational HIV-prevention intervention), it was important to reference those programs that had been tested in African-American/black and/or rural populations and considered to be successful. We drew from several evidence-based HIV- and STI-prevention interventions and programs: Focus on Kids, Safer Choices, Becoming a Responsible Teen, Making Proud Choices, Draw the Line, and Real AIDS Prevention Program [16, 38–42]. By integrating community input throughout the development process and building on the strengths of our community (i.e., strong social networks and natural helping), the intervention was designed with particular attention to cultural appropriateness, long-term sustainability within the community, and potential for dissemination to other communities and organizations [16].

After the completion of formative data collection and analysis and review of existing interventions, our end product was a multigenerational intervention that addressed the multiple factors that contributed to HIV and STI risk among African-American/black youth. Finalizing the intervention curricula consisted of a 1-day community-wide testing event, in which four youth and four caregiver sessions were conducted. Special attention was paid to assessing attitudes about taboo or controversial topics and activities such as condom use and condom demonstrations. Fifty-two participants were recruited by the Steering Committee and project staff to participate. Trained Steering Committee members served as facilitators and note-takers for each session. Each session had two facilitators, who led intervention activities and also conducted a scripted focus group at the end of each session to gather feedback. Note-takers were taught to observe the sessions thoroughly and to record detailed information about the participants and what occurred during implementation. Data collected from the sessions and the focus group discussions were useful in testing process evaluation methods, addressing cultural congruence, and identifying any logistic challenges. Steering Committee members were able to use these data to revise the intervention [16].

Further Engagement and Implementation

After developing the TORO intervention curricula, piloting the intervention, and creating matrices to both assess effectiveness of the intervention and measure outcomes, the intervention was implemented. TORO encompassed three focal points designed to engage the community and to teach other youth and adults about HIV and STIs: a lay health advisor component, instruction on positive communication skills and strategies, and reproductive health information. From the process of blending data and other feedback received during the process, the TORO intervention included the selection and training of youth 10–14-years old and their adult caregivers (at least 21-years old) to work in dyads to serve as lay health advisors to other members of the local community. These lay health advisors are known as "ambassadors," and the community members whom they reach out to are called their "allies." Allies are similar pairs of youth and adults who make up an outreach group for each ambassador dyad. In order to participate in the intervention as ambassadors, the youth and adult pair must possess certain key characteristics, such as natural leadership qualities, trustworthiness, ability to discuss "hot-button" and sensitive topics (such as HIV and human reproduction), and ability to commit the necessary time to the program [33, 43]. The ambassadors met with their allies monthly as a requirement of the program. Both the ambassadors and allies received monetary incentives for participating in meetings and data collection [16].

Creatively Expanding the Scope of TORO

After the implementation of TORO in 2008, we found other areas in which the intervention could be expanded in order to make a greater impact in the community. Members of the Project GRACE Consortium thought that it was important to address the disparities associated with HIV in rural communities in varying capacities and in different ways. During 2008, we conducted a photovoice project in which photographs were used to express how HIV was affecting the community through the eyes of the participants. In 2010, a postdoctoral fellow affiliated with Project GRACE added an advocacy and photovoice component to the TORO intervention and initiated a supplemental pilot program titled Making Healthy Change Happen [44]. This pilot program was designed as a health promotion tool to increase the TORO ambassadors' self-efficacy to make additional positive changes within their own communities.

During the winter of 2010, the female youth ambassadors of the TORO intervention were invited to participate in a project, designed and facilitated by a Project GRACE undergraduate research assistant conducting independent study, called Project Uplift My Sister. This project used the arts as a method of empowerment in reducing HIV risk among female African-American/black youth. These expansions on the TORO intervention were not anticipated at the inception nor during the development of the intervention, however, they reflect the desire and priority of Project GRACE Consortium members to creatively advance and further develop our HIV-prevention efforts in ways that meet community priorities using approaches that community members prefer.

Lessons Learned

During the early formation of our community–academic partnership, much of the available CBPR literature described the application of CBPR conducted in urban centers [15, 24, 45–47]. We found little in the scholarly literature to guide our work in rural communities and the application of CBPR in HIV prevention [15, 24, 48–52]. The use of CBPR to address the spread of HIV in rural African-American/black communities posed some unique challenges as well as interesting opportunities.

In the Shadow of HIV

The driving force for initiating our community–academic partnership was the impact of HIV on our local community. Moreover, the profound impact of HIV morbidity and mortality on this community has certainly helped to maintain the momentum of our partnership. Because much attention at the outset of Project GRACE was paid to the process of engagement, we were able to engender deep and true engagement of all partners, and this engagement has been sustained throughout the history of

Project GRACE. For example, all data collection, analysis, and interpretation were conducted collaboratively, and the intervention materials and evaluation tools were developed with the full participation of both community and academic partners. In fact, partners worked side-by-side to determine which components of successful interventions in the literature might be best adapted for and applied within our local context. It is also important to note that all products for dissemination—including this book chapter—are generated collaboratively and reviewed by a team of Steering Committee members before any presentations or submissions. However, as is typical in rural communities, HIV-related stigma presented a major barrier to engagement in particular sectors of the community. Although we have partnered on individual outreach events, members of the faith community have not been as widely or consistently represented as we had initially hoped.

Close-knit and Geographically Isolated Communities

Although it is important to acknowledge that all partnerships face some universal challenges to applying CBPR approaches, the social and geographic context of rural settings also provides a unique set of issues. Because of the smaller populations and the overlap between social and professional networks, the small community setting helped us to achieve our goal of ensuring that a wide range of perspectives, experiences, and insights were represented among the members of our Project GRACE Consortium. The community in which Project GRACE is situated has a close-knit social structure. We found that these prior and existing social relationships could readily facilitate our work. Although local organizations may experience turnover in particular staff positions, unlike in more urban environments, individuals in rural communities seldom rotate in or out of social, professional, or geographic circles, generating a sense of connectedness and spheres of influence that are unique to rural communities.

However, the density and overlapping nature of these networks became problematic at times. For example, in our efforts to be inclusive and egalitarian in the Steering Committee's decision-making, professional and social hierarchies sometimes became inadvertently inverted among members of the Project GRACE Consortium, creating unanticipated problems. In one instance, an employee of a community-based organization chaired a Project GRACE Consortium subcommittee on which his supervisor served as a member. This inversion of a professional hierarchy, where an employee in one setting took on a leadership role within the partnership, was exacerbated by the relatively small number of organizations and agencies to draw from in a rural setting.

Similarly, we learned that personal lives often intersect in communities with such dense social networks, which can complicate the work of the project. In our community, spouses and significant others often work for the same or complementary organizations. In instances in which their personal relationships became difficult, their employers (our partnering organizations) and/or Project GRACE staff had to actively avoid being drawn into these disputes or navigate the situations carefully.

Thus, issues of trust and trustworthiness were also magnified because of these over-lapping relationships. In more metropolitan areas, individuals and/or representatives from organizations might be known solely on the basis of their professional reputations. This was not our reality. Our partners had extensive knowledge of one another's professional and personal histories (including personally knowing other family members), their relationships, personalities, religious affiliations, and many other deeply personal details that at times affected the creation or maintenance of trust between partners.

The challenge of context and overlapping professional and social networks required us to pay particular attention to how reporting structures and power dynamics in one setting could negatively influence the work in another. Consultants from VISIONS, Inc. provided support in negotiating these types of conflicts so that the work of partners could continue despite difficulties between individuals or within organizations. Our process evolved to have a consultant from VISIONS, Inc. present at each Steering Committee meeting to facilitate discussions around sensitive issues and to address tension and conflict. Having a consultant skilled at conflict resolution and who understands and is respected by members of the community has been crucial to our success.

Multiple Roles of Partners

As in other partnerships, community members often held multiple roles in our community. As we thought about the needs of our partnership, we explicitly drew on the skills available among our partners to ensure strong and consistent community leadership. In the initial formation of the working committees, rather than asking for volunteers, our Steering Committee chair recruited specific community members to chair subcommittees, taking into account the unique needs of the subcommittee and the existing skills of potential chairpersons. For example, the chair of the By-laws Committee is an executive director of a community-based organization with prior experience drafting bylaws for nonprofit organizations. She was able to draw on that expertise in her role as chair. This deliberate and early attention to community leadership in the subcommittees set a positive tone for the partnership in decision-making for Project GRACE and allowed our partnership to benefit from the already existing expertise of individuals and organizations within the community.

Furthermore, it is important to recognize that roles change over time as capacity develops. For example, the first author of this chapter served on the Project GRACE Consortium as a community representative from the local health department. Over the course of the implementation of Project GRACE, she furthered her research experiences that she now applies working within an academic institution.

Advocacy, Research, and Conflicts of Interest

In addition, as might be expected, Steering Committee members are advocates for social change in a variety of roles and settings. Many members are community leaders who hold formal positions as elected officials and/or informal roles as community activists. Many are advocates for HIV prevention and treatment. Although the shared values and vision for change were essential to effective partnership, we found that at times lines could be blurred when community organizing and advocacy work were involved. Steering Committee members found themselves faced with answering complicated questions such as the following:

- Where does advocacy for the goals of the project begin and end?
- Are there potential conflicts of interests between an individual's advocacy work and efforts to accomplish project goals and how can we resolve such conflicts?
- How important is it to make distinctions between an individual's personal ideals and the goals of the partnership?
- How do we account for the multiple roles of some community members who serve as both Steering Committee members and project staff?
- How do we position ourselves for effective advocacy while avoiding being unwittingly drawn into local political issues?

As previously noted, these types of issues become magnified in smaller communities where there may be considerable overlap between professional and social roles and networks. For example, several Steering Committee members have run for political office and used the data collected in Project GRACE to support their political platform. The need to address environmental factors in HIV and STI prevention became a prominent issue in the elections in Edgecombe and Nash counties. We see this type of social action as an expected outcome of CBPR and have chosen to make these data as easily available as possible to all members of the Project GRACE Consortium and broader community for their use in striving for social change.

Designing the Intervention

The process of coming together to design the TORO intervention included three main challenges. First, one challenge faced by anyone planning to do community-based work is recognizing and planning for the relatively high turnover of staff at local community-based organizations. In this instance, leadership and staff turnover presented key challenges because new staff will, inevitably, lack knowledge about the community–academic partnership and CBPR, and they will have missed participating in both the trust-building phase and workshops orienting them to research and program-planning methods. This lack of familiarity can result in conflicts that challenge both partnership and project success. We addressed incidences of turnover by having multiple opportunities for continued involvement for individuals who are no longer employed by one of the partner organizations through subcommittee membership, ex officio positions on the Steering Committee, and continued membership in the Project GRACE Consortium. We also have tried to incorporate into our partnership strategies to avoid this challenge in the first place. For example, we included leadership from organizations that tend to experience less turnover sit on our Steering Committee to ensure their investment in the process and ongoing continuity of the process.

The second challenge was that community and academic partners had different lexicons and different perspectives on the development of Project GRACE. The academic partners were more versed in health behavior theory, research, and intervention and program-planning methods and had to ensure that community partners felt comfortable with this vocabulary. A half-day workshop was developed to address this challenge. As described earlier in this chapter, the workshop introduced theoretical frameworks and behavioral theories, thus allowing the process of intervention development to commence with both community and academic partners at the same table with a similar knowledge foundation. This was a time-intensive, but necessary process, and we recommend this to anyone wanting to use intervention mapping in a participatory framework.

Lastly, community partners were far more knowledgeable than academic partners about what was feasible and meaningful within the community. Community partners had a personal understanding of the community's collective capacity, resources, and informal relationships; they also had firsthand knowledge of which strategies would be most successful to effect change. For the research and the intervention to be successful, it was essential that academic partners learn from community partners in order to work together effectively and to integrate the real-world experiences of community members with the study design and intervention methods. This was addressed throughout the entire intervention mapping process; community input and involvement were present at every step. Our CBPR approach to intervention mapping led to the design of an intervention that was acceptable to all of the partners and culturally sensitive to the communities served.

Next Steps: HIV Prevention and Community Engagement

Scientific advances continue to bring us closer to ending the HIV epidemic, or at least transforming it to a low-level endemic disease; however, there remain highly vulnerable communities that continue to be disproportionately affected. These communities tend to be in the southeastern USA, particularly in rural areas, and to be composed of racial/ethnic minorities. There is much work to be done.

We must recognize that there are no magic bullets—no single prevention or curative intervention that will end the epidemic. Moreover, we must recognize that the epidemic, by its very nature, is a heterogeneous entity with different drivers in different populations and geographic settings. As such, different and innovative strategies and combinations of educational, biomedical, behavioral, structural, and policy approaches are necessary to reduce risk and control the disease. Developing effective HIV-prevention interventions that have broader, sustainable effects that extend beyond individual behavioral change remains an ongoing challenge for the field [53, 54]. Accomplishing these efforts in rural communities where the number of service providers and the HIV-advocacy communities are often small, where populations tend to be spread out, and where the local context is shaped by more conservative values and HIV-related stigma can make engaging community members more challenging [55]. However, as we have outlined in this chapter, efforts that bring together diverse local partners to identify sustainable, coordinated efforts to reduce HIV risk are possible.

The current US *National HIV/AIDS Strategy* calls on government agencies and their public and private partners to work collaboratively to address the needs of these populations to achieve a more coordinated national response to the HIV epidemic in the USA [56]. The *National HIV/AIDS Strategy* sets clear priorities for HIV prevention and care in the country and includes five main goals to be achieved over the next 5 years:

- Reduce the annual number of new infections by 25%
- Increase the percentage of people with HIV who know their HIV testing status from 79–90%
- Reduce the HIV transmission rate by 30%
- Increase the percentage of people with newly diagnosed HIV who are linked to care within 3 months from 65 to 85%
- Increase the proportion of HIV-diagnosed gay and bisexual men, African-Americans/black, and Hispanics/Latinos with undetectable viral load by 20%.

The *National HIV/AIDS Strategy* notes that prevention and care efforts should be a priority for populations in which either the incidence rates are highest or the disparities are greatest. These populations include gay and bisexual men, communities of color (including the African-American/black population), women, injection-drug users, transgender persons, and youth.

The *National HIV/AIDS Strategy* also articulates specific intervention strategies that should be emphasized. Community-based efforts to prevent HIV and to identify and care for those affected are an inherent part of the *National HIV/AIDS Strategy*. Such approaches build on shared values and norms, belief systems, and social practices to inform the development of more effective, culturally tailored intervention approaches. The nature and scope of such interventions will vary by community depending on the local context. This variation makes it crucial to have community engagement throughout the entire process, including in the selection of target populations and intervention strategies and in the development, implementation, and evaluation of interventions. Among many advantages, engaged and participatory efforts may be most successful at (1) identifying populations most at risk; (2) developing, implementing, and evaluating innovative strategies (e.g., the multigenerational TORO intervention) to reach members of vulnerable communities; (3) reducing stigma and discrimination; (4) changing social norms related to gender inequality and gender-based violence; (5) overturning local policies that restrict access to health care; (6) initiating and expanding advocacy programs to alter risk behaviors; (7) promoting HIV testing; and (8) connecting persons with HIV to high-quality confidential care and retaining them in care over time.

We know that for community-based HIV-prevention efforts to be effective, they need to be developed in conjunction with community members as well as government and private stakeholders, including academic institutions. Involving all parties from the outset in planning, designing, implementing, monitoring, and evaluating HIV-prevention efforts will increase the success and sustainability of these efforts over time. Because resources are limited, it is particularly important for community members to be involved in community HIV-prevention planning efforts. Those involved in community prevention planning efforts also need to ensure that resources target priority populations who are identified using reliable population-based epidemiologic data. Because diverse efforts may be needed, it is also important for a comprehensive plan be developed at the outset to delineate the engagement and partnership activities that will be emphasized during each phase of the HIV-prevention effort and the ways success will be measured. This must be planned at the outset [56–58].

Of course, no one strategy will fit all contexts. However, there is increasing agreement that HIV interventions and programs need to move from being either prevention research or service-based to an integrated paradigm in which community engagement based on human rights is at the core. Clearly, lessons learned from CBPR projects, like our own, with diverse settings and populations can help guide this transition.

Acknowledgment The authors would like to acknowledge and thank all members of the Project GRACE Consortium, past and present, for their contributions to the development and implementation of this intervention.

References

1. Collins C, Diallo DD. A prevention response that fits America's epidemic: community perspectives on the status of HIV prevention in the United States. J Acquir Immune Defic Syndr. 2010;55(Suppl 2):S148–50.
2. Kippax S. Effective HIV prevention. The indispensable role of social science. J Int AIDS Soc. 2012;15(2):17357.
3. Kippax S, Stephenson N. Beyond the distinction between biomedical and social dimensions of HIV prevention through the lens of a social public health. Am J Public Health. 2012;102(5):789–99.
4. Bandura A. Social foundations of thought and action: a social cognitive theory. Englewood Cliffs: Prentice-Hall; 1986.
5. Fredriksen-Goldsen KI. Multigenerational health, development, and equality. Gerontologist. 2005;45(1):125–30.
6. Centers for Disease Control and Prevention. HIV Surveillance Report, 2011. Atlanta, GA: US Department of Health and Human Services, 2013. Accessed 21 May 2014.
7. Centers for Disease Control and Prevention. HIV among African Americans. Atlanta: U.S. Department of Health and Human Services; 2013.
8. US Census Bureau. http://www.census.gov/ (2010). Accessed 21 May 2014.
9. Southern AIDS Coalition. Southern States manifesto: update 2012. Policy brief and recommendations. Birmingham, AL: Southern AIDS Coalition; 2012.
10. Southern State Directors Work Group. Southern States manifesto: update 2008. HIV/AIDS and sexually transmitted diseases in the south. Birmingham, AL: southern AIDS coalition; 2008.

11. Rural Center for AIDS/STD Prevention. Tearing down fences: HIV/STD prevention in rural America [Electronic book]. Bloomington, IN; 2009.

12. Adimora AA, Schoenbach VJ, Martinson FE, Donaldson KH, Fullilove RE, Aral SO. Social context of sexual relationships among rural African Americans. Sex Transm Dis. 2001;28(2):69–76.

13. Thomas JC, Clark M, Robinson J, Monnett M, Kilmarx PH, Peterman TA. The social ecology of syphilis. Soc Sci Med. 1999;48(8):1081–94.

14. Akers AY, Muhammad MR, Corbie-Smith G. When you got nothing to do, you do somebody: a community's perceptions of neighborhood effects on adolescent sexual behaviors. Soc Sci Med. 2011;72(1):91–9.

15. Corbie-Smith G, Adimora AA, Youmans S, Muhammad M, Blumenthal C, Ellison A, et al. Project GRACE: a staged approach to development of a community-academic partnership to address HIV in rural African American communities. Health Promot Pract. 2011;12(2):293–302.

16. Corbie-Smith G, Akers A, Blumenthal C, Council B, Wynn M, Muhammad M, et al. Intervention mapping as a participatory approach to developing an HIV prevention intervention in rural African American communities. AIDS Educ Prev. 2010;22(3):184–202.

17. Corbie-Smith G, Odeneye E, Banks B, Shandor Miles M, Roman Isler M. Development of a multilevel intervention to increase HIV clinical trial participation among rural minorities. Health Educ Behav. 2012;40(3)274–85.

18. Rhodes SD, Hergenrather KC, Bloom FR, Leichliter JS, Montaño J. Outcomes from a community-based, participatory lay health advisor HIV/STD prevention intervention for recently arrived immigrant Latino men in rural North Carolina, USA. AIDS Educ Prev. 2009;21(Suppl 1):104–9.

19. Williams M, Bowen A, Ei S. An evaluation of the experiences of rural MSM who accessed an online HIV/AIDS health promotion intervention. Health Promot Pract. 2010;11(4):474–82.

20. Smith MU, DiClemente RJ. STAND: a peer educator training curriculum for sexual risk reduction in the rural South. Students together against negative decisions. Prev Med. 2000;30(6):441–9.

21. US Census Bureau. 2006–2010 American Community Survey 5-year estimates: fast facts for Congress: North Carolina fact sheet. http://www.censusgov/fastfacts/jsp/cws/CWSContentphp?_event=ChangeGeoContext&geo_id=0400000US37&_geoContext=0100000US%3AUnited+States%7C0400000US37s%3ANorth+Carolina&_street=&_county=&_cd=&_state=0400000US37&_zip=&_program=acs&_lang=en&_sse=on&pctxt=fph&pgsl=010&_industry=&currTab=factsheets&_leftNavId=1. Accessed 28 Feb 2012.

22. US Census Bureau. The black population: 2000. Census 2000 brief. http://www.censusgov/prod/2001pubs/c2kbr01-5pdf (2001). Accessed 29 March 2007.

23. Jemmott JB 3rd, Jemmott LS, Fong GT. Reductions in HIV risk-associated sexual behaviors among black male adolescents: effects of an AIDS prevention intervention. Am J Public Health. 1992;82(3):372–7.

24. Marcus MT, Walker T, Swint JM, Smith BP, Brown C, Busen N, et al. Community-based participatory research to prevent substance abuse and HIV/AIDS in African-American adolescents. J Interprof Care. 2004;18(4):347–59.

25. Clark LF, Rhodes SD, Rogers W, Liddon N. The context of sexual risk behavior. In: Raczynski JM, Leviton LC, editors. Handbook of clinical health psychology. Washington, DC: American Psychological Association; 2004. p. 121–46.

26. Clinical and Translational Science Awards Consortium Community Engagement Key Function Committee Task Force on the Principles of Community Engagement. Principles of community engagement. Second edition. ed: Washington Department of Health and Human Services; 2011.

27. Florin P, Mitchell R, Stevenson J. Identifying training and technical assistance needs in community coalitions: a developmental approach. Health Educ Res. 1993;8(3):417–32.

28. VanDevanter N, Hennessy M, Howard JM, Bleakley A, Peake M, Millet S, et al. Developing a collaborative community, academic, health department partnership for STD preven-

tion: the Gonorrhea Community Action Project in Harlem. J Public Health Manag Pract. 2002;8(6):62–8.

29. Cene CW, Akers AY, Lloyd SW, Albritton T, Powell Hammond W, Corbie-Smith G. Understanding social capital and HIV risk in rural African American communities. J Gen Intern Med. 2011;26(7):737–44.

30. Coker-Appiah DS, Akers AY, Banks B, Albritton T, Leniek K, Wynn M, et al. In their own voices: rural African-American youth speak out about community-based HIV prevention interventions. Prog Community Health Partnersh. 2009;3(4):275–6.

31. Bartholomew LK, Parcel GS, Kok G. Intervention mapping: a process for developing theory- and evidence-based health education programs. Health Educ Behav. 1998;25(5):545–63.

32. National Cancer Insitute. Theory at a glance. Washington, D.C.: U.S. Government Printing Office; 2005.

33. Eng E, Rhodes SD, Parker EA. Natural helper models to enhance a community's health and competence. In: DiClemente RJ, Crosby RA, Kegler MC, editors. Emerging theories in health promotion practice and research. San Francisco: Jossey-Bass; 2009. p. 303–30.

34. DeVore ER, Ginsburg KR. The protective effects of good parenting on adolescents. Curr Opin Pediatr. 2005;17(4):460–5.

35. Meschke LL, Bartholomae S, Zentall SR. Adolescent sexuality and parent-adolescent processes: promoting healthy teen choices. Fam Relat. 2000;49(2):143–54.

36. Perrino T, Gonzalez-Soldevilla A, Pantin H, Szapocznik J. The role of families in adolescent HIV prevention: a review. Clin Child Fam Psychol Rev. 2000;3(2):81–96.

37. McLeroy KR, Bibeau D, Steckler A, Glanz K. An ecological perspective on health promotion programs. Health Educ Q. 1988;15(4):351–77.

38. Coyle K, Kirby D, Parcel G, Basen-Engquist K, Banspach S, Rugg D, et al. Safer choices: a multicomponent school-based HIV/STD and pregnancy prevention program for adolescents. J Sch Health. 1996;66(3):89–94.

39. Kirby DB, Baumler E, Coyle KK, Basen-Engquist K, Parcel GS, Harrist R, et al. The "Safer Choices" intervention: its impact on the sexual behaviors of different subgroups of high school students. J Adolesc Health. 2004;35(6):442–52.

40. Semaan S, Lauby J, O'Connell AA, Cohen A. Factors associated with perceptions of, and decisional balance for, condom use with main partner among women at risk for HIV infection. Women Health. 2003;37(3):53–69.

41. St Lawrence JS, Crosby RA, Brasfield TL, O'Bannon RE, 3rd. Reducing STD and HIV risk behavior of substance-dependent adolescents: a randomized controlled trial. J Consult Clin Psychol. 2002;70(4):1010–21.

42. Stanton BF, Li X, Ricardo I, Galbraith J, Feigelman S, Kaljee L. A randomized, controlled effectiveness trial of an AIDS prevention program for low-income African-American youths. Arch Pediatr Adolesc Med. 1996;150(4):363–72.

43. Rhodes SD, Foley KL, Zometa CS, Bloom FR. Lay health advisor interventions among Hispanics/Latinos: a qualitative systematic review. Am J Prev Med. 2007;33(5):418–27.

44. Ferguson YO. Making healthy change happen. [Curriculum]. In press 2010.

45. Higgins DL, Metzler M. Implementing community-based participatory research centers in diverse urban settings. J Urban Health. 2001;78(3):488–94.

46. Israel BA, Schulz AJ, Parker EA, Becker AB. Community-based participatory research: policy recommendations for promoting a partnership approach in health research. Educ Health (Abingdon). 2001;14(2):182–97.

47. Merzel C, Burrus G, Davis J, Moses N, Rumley S, Walters D. Developing and sustaining community-academic partnerships: lessons from downstate New York healthy start. Health Promot Pract. 2007;8(4):375–83.

48. Kim KH, Linnan L, Campbell MK, Brooks C, Koenig HG, Wiesen C. The WORD (wholeness, oneness, righteousness, deliverance): a faith-based weight-loss program utilizing a community-based participatory research approach. Health Educ Behav. 2008;35(5):634–50.

49. Rhodes SD, Hergenrather KC, Montano J, Remnitz IM, Arceo R, Bloom FR, et al. Using community-based participatory research to develop an intervention to reduce HIV and STD infections among Latino men. AIDS Educ Prev. 2006;18(5):375–89.

50. Romero L, Wallerstein N, Lucero J, Fredine HG, Keefe J, O'Connell J. Woman to woman: coming together for positive change-using empowerment and popular education to prevent HIV in women. AIDS Educ Prev. 2006;18(5):390–405.

51. Cashman SB, Adeky S, Allen AJ, Corburn J, Israel BA, Montaño J, et al. The power and the promise: working with communities to analyze data, interpret findings, and get to outcomes. Am J Public Health. 2008;98(8):1407–17.

52. Rhodes SD. Demonstrated effectiveness and potential of CBPR for preventing HIV in Latino populations. In: Organista KC, editor. HIV Prevention with Latinos: theory, research, and practice. New York: Oxford University Press; 2012. p. 83–102.

53. Robinson RG. Community development model for public health applications: overview of a model to eliminate population disparities. Health Promot Pract. 2005;6(3):338–46.

54. King W, Nu'Man J, Fuller TR, Brown M, Smith S, Howell AV, et al. The diffusion of a community-level HIV intervention for women: lessons learned and best practices. J Womens Health (Larchmt). 2008;17(7):1055–66.

55. Thomas JC. From slavery to incarceration: social forces affecting the epidemiology of sexually transmitted diseases in the rural South. Sex Transm Dis. 2006;33(7 Suppl):S6–10.

56. The White Office of National AIDS Policy. National HIV/AIDS strategy for the United States; 2010. p. 60.

57. Centers for Disease Control and Prevention. The care and prevention in the United States (CAPUS) demonstration project. U.S. Department of Health and Human Services; 2012.

58. Centers for Disease Control and Prevention. High impact HIV prevention: CDC's approach to reducing HIV infections in the United States. Atlanta, GA: U.S. Department of Health and Human Services; 2011.

Chapter 3
Preventing HIV among Black Men in College Using a CBPR Approach

Louis F. Graham, Robert E. Aronson, Regina McCoy Pulliam, Lilli Mann and Scott D. Rhodes

The African American/black population is now the second largest racial minority group in the United States and is still disproportionately burdened by HIV and AIDS. Although African Americans/blacks represented 12–14 % of the US population in 2010, they accounted for nearly half of all HIV infections, AIDS diagnoses, people estimated to be living with AIDS, and HIV-related deaths in the United States. Additionally, in 2010, the incidence of HIV among African Americans/blacks was eight times higher than that among whites. Unfortunately, these trends have persisted since the 1990s. For African American/black adolescents, the racial disparity in HIV/AIDS diagnoses is even greater. Almost 70 % of all new HIV infections among 13–19-year-olds were among African Americans/blacks in 2010. In

---

This chapter is dedicated to Dr. Warner McGee, a friend, colleague, and student who devoted his short life to advocating for students and fighting this dreadful disease.

L. F. Graham (✉)
Department of Public Health, University of Massachusetts Amherst, 315 Arnold House, 715 North Pleasant Street, Amherst, MA 01003-9304, USA
e-mail: LFGraham@schoolph.umass.edu

R. E. Aronson
Public Health Program, School of Natural and Applied Sciences, Taylor University, 236 West Reade Avenue, Upland, IN 46989, USA
e-mail: bob_aronson@taylor.edu

R. M. Pulliam
Department of Public Health Education, University of North Carolina Greensboro, PO Box 26170, Greensboro, NC 27402-6170, USA
e-mail: regina_pulliam@uncg.edu

L. Mann · S. D. Rhodes
Department of Social Sciences and Health Policy, Division of Public Health Sciences, Wake Forest University School of Medicine, Medical Center Blvd., Winston-Salem, NC 27157, USA
e-mail: lmann@wakehealth.edu

S. D. Rhodes
e-mail: srhodes@wakehealth.edu

S. D. Rhodes (ed.), *Innovations in HIV Prevention Research and Practice through Community Engagement,* DOI 10.1007/978-1-4939-0900-1_3, © Springer Science+Business Media New York 2014

2008, African American/black men and women ages 25–44 years old had a higher AIDS-related mortality rate than any other racial group [1, 2].

Furthermore, HIV rates in the United States have increased over time among both men and women through heterosexual transmission. It is estimated that more than a quarter of those who are newly infected and more than a quarter of people with HIV acquired the virus through heterosexual transmission. Among African Americans/blacks, 38% of new HIV infections were transmitted through hetero-sexual transmission. Moreover, 87% of African American/black women with HIV acquired the virus through heterosexual transmission. It is estimated that one of 16 African American/black men will be diagnosed with HIV during his lifetime; those infected are more likely than white men to have been infected through heterosexual contact and injection-drug use [1, 2].

The southern part of the United States, in particular, is disproportionately af-fected by the HIV epidemic [1–3]. More than 40% of new AIDS diagnoses and the greatest number of people with HIV and AIDS in 2010 were in the South. Despite this growing epidemic, little is known about innovative intervention approaches that are likely to be successful in this region of the country. Much of what is known about HIV, including prevention, care, and treatment, is based on research con-ducted in early epicenters of the US epidemic. These epicenters have a much longer history of both HIV research and service provision. These epicenters also tend to be large urban cities and do not reflect the unique characteristics of the more rural and resource-poor South [4–7].

Gaps in prevention science

Traditionally, HIV interventions have focused on risk reduction and treatment up-take and adherence among population subgroups such as men, especially sexually marginalized men (e.g., gay, bisexual, same-gender-loving men, and men who have sex with other men [MSM]), injection-drug users, and, more recently, heterosexual women. A paucity of HIV prevention strategies have been demonstrated to be ef-ficacious and effective for African American/black heterosexual men, particularly those of college age [8–13].

To effectively prevent HIV exposure and transmission in the United States, we need to explore, better understand, and more effectively intervene on the complex factors associated with HIV exposure and transmission for African American/black men. This need is important regardless of the race, ethnicity, or gender of African American/black men's sexual partners [48]. We know that HIV risk among African American/black men occurs within multiple social-ecologic contexts. Instead of focusing exclusively on the sexual behaviors of individuals disconnected from cul-ture, gender, and context, we must work, as researchers and practitioners, in more nuanced ways to understand and consider the multidimensional aspects of sexuality, including the complex intersections of identities, roles, and behaviors. Thus, HIV prevention efforts require new, multilevel approaches that reflect culture, gender, and context, to address the distinct and intersecting intrapersonal, interpersonal, institutional, and economic factors influencing black men's risk for HIV exposure and transmission. As has been suggested,

> The relationship between socioeconomic context and sexual networks suggests that continued emphasis solely on individual risk factors and determinants for prevention efforts is unlikely to yield a significant effect on rates of HIV infection among black persons in the United States. [14]

Moreover, HIV prevention efforts among African American/black college and university students have not typically been a priority. However, as HIV infection among African American/black men within colleges and universities continues to increase in less well-resourced regions of the United States, such as the South in general and North Carolina specifically, more formative and intervention research must be conducted to reduce exposure and transmission within this population [10, 11, 15–18]. Sufficient attention must be given to identify beliefs, attitudes, and behaviors related to sexuality, relationships, communication, sexual behavior, and protection (including condom use) that are influenced by culture, gender, and context in order to develop meaningful and successful HIV prevention strategies and interventions.

In this chapter, we define community-based participatory research (CBPR) and describe how members of our collaborative applied CBPR principles in the development of an innovative HIV prevention project designed to fill intervention gaps and reduce HIV exposure and transmission among African American/black heterosexual men attending a predominantly white university in the South. In collaboration with community members, including African American/black men and women, representatives from local community-based organizations, and university staff and faculty, we developed and pilot-tested a novel HIV prevention intervention known as Brothers Leading Healthy Lives (BLHL). We also describe some of the challenges we faced and lessons learned, as well as the strategies we used to target the nature of the community and context within which our project took place.

CBPR and HIV prevention among African American/black college men

CBPR has been defined as a

> ... Collaborative approach to research [that] equitably involves all partners in the research process and recognizes the unique strengths that each brings. CBPR begins with a research topic of importance to the community with the aim of combining knowledge and action for social change to improve community health and eliminate health disparities. [19]

CBPR has been identified as an effective approach to address the ongoing health disparities within vulnerable communities and populations. CBPR results in more informed understandings of underlying factors that contribute to the health and well-being of communities. This more informed understanding, coupled with continued engagement and participation of community members in the application of this improved understanding, yields better actions (e.g., interventions) to meet

Table 3.1 Common principles of CBPR

1. CBPR recognizes community as a unit of identity
2. CBPR builds on strengths and resources within the community
3. CBPR facilitates collaborative, equitable partnership in all phases of the research and involves empowering and power-sharing processes that attend to social, political, and economic inequities
4. CBPR promotes co-learning and capacity building among all partners
5. CBPR integrates and achieves a balance between research and action for the mutual benefit of all partners
6. CBPR emphasizes local relevance of public health problems and ecological perspectives that recognize and attend to multiple determinants of health and disease
7. CBPR involves systems development through an iterative process
8. CBPR disseminates findings and knowledge gained to all partners and involves all partners in the dissemination process
9. CBPR involves a long-term process and commitment

the needs and priorities of community members [19–23]. Furthermore, strategies aligned with CBPR have been effective in the development of culturally congruent, gender-specific, and contextually relevant HIV sexual risk-reduction interventions for predominately racial/ethnic minority heterosexual men, in which community members were fully engaged throughout all phases of the research [24–27].

Our application of CBPR adhered to nine commonly cited guiding principles or characteristics of CBPR (Table 3.1). In this chapter, we do not explore our use of each principle; rather, we provide these principles as a backdrop of how we defined and engaged communities; established and maintained trust with African American/black heterosexual men on a predominately white university campus; and developed, implemented, and evaluated an HIV prevention intervention that was funded by the US Centers for Disease Control and Prevention (CDC).

Our CBPR process

Building trust and history with African American/black men on a university campus

Initially, our CBPR was based on the campus of The University of North Carolina at Greensboro (UNCG), a predominately white university. During the 1999–2000 academic year, an informal student group of African American/black men known as Brother2Brother, led by an African American/black graduate student, began to meet weekly to discuss their struggles as African American/black men on a predominately white campus and in society. Participants were mainly undergraduates and most self-identified as heterosexual. Their discussions about their lives and success at UNCG foregrounded their complex racial and gender identities. They shared stories about navigating the university and how they were perceived and treated. They explored ideas about what it means to be a man, an African American/black man, and an "ideal" African American/black man. Their conversations highlighted the centrality of sexuality in constructions of black masculinities. As a result, they discussed issues related to sexual identity, the importance of sex to a man and his reputation, and their personal sexual risk for HIV.

Brother2Brother meetings were held in a public area at the main entrance of the university cafeteria, a gathering space that attracted many African American/black students after classes in the late afternoon. The rules of the meetings were simple:

- Leave your status at the door
- Respect one another
- Bring your concerns and ideas to the group

As an organization, Brother2Brother emerged organically and remained informal. The group had no official campus recognition, no bylaws or organizational documents, and no officers. Given the members' challenges in navigating institutional policies and practices that were not designed for them and that continued to impede their progress, African American/black men who came to Brother2Brother meetings neither were willing to be governed by campus rules and regulations for official student groups nor were they eager to recreate such structures within their group. They emphasized equitable participation and mutual ownership of the process and its outcomes; thus, Brother2Brother was primed to engage in an authentic CBPR process.

In 2001, two faculty members, one African American/black professor in the Anthropology Department and a white professor in the Department of Public Health Education at UNCG, were invited to meet with the members of Brother2Brother to discuss shared interests and identify ways these faculty and students could be resources to one another. These two professors were academic advisors to and had developed mentoring relationships with some students in the group. The students thought that these faculty could benefit the group by providing guidance and resources, for example. For more than two years, these faculty met weekly with the students during their regularly scheduled meeting times.

Obtaining funding and conducting research together

During the initial two years of collaboration, our emerging student-faculty collaboration, with its origins in Brother2Brother, applied for and obtained funding from the UNCG Center for the Study of Social Issues. We were awarded a small grant to explore issues related to masculinity and adjustment to university life among African American/black men at UNCG. Data collection included interviews and focus groups with African American/black men on campus and observations and notes taken during weekly Brother2Brother meetings.

The Big Man/Little Man framework was used to organize findings [28–31]. This framework suggests that men assert their masculinity through respectability, reputation, or some balance of the two, depending on their economic capacity. Masculine respectability attributes contribute to the maintenance of healthy functioning and social order, whereas attributes of masculine reputation contribute to unhealthy functioning and social disorder. Economic capacity provides higher-income men ready access to respectability attributes, and the lack of economic capacity makes access to respectability difficult for low-income men. As a result, low-income men are left to express reputational attributes in their efforts to achieve a strong sense of the masculine self. Reliance solely on reputational traits—such as sexual prowess, demonstration of toughness, defiance of authority (legal and otherwise), and reputational material goods (e.g., eye-catching jewelry, clothes, and cars)—place lower-income men at greater involvement in illegal activities, violence, incarceration, and death [28–30].

Attributes of being an "ideal" man that emerged in our work with African American/black men at UNCG included the importance of spirituality, values associated with being a family man, and self-determination, attributes commonly associated with respectability. Attributes commonly associated with reputation also emerged. Being an "ideal" man also included characteristics that participants labeled as hustler/pimp (e.g., can handle his liquor, is sexually active, dresses well, is good with women, and drives a nice car); extreme toughness (e.g., is intimidating, is feared by others, and does not need the help of others); and physical strength (e.g., is physically strong, is competitive, and always tries to win) [31].

After completion of this initial study, the collaborative was awarded funding from the TRIAD Center for Health Disparities to further explore constructs of masculinity and issues related to sexual health among African American/black men at UNCG. Some members of Brother2Brother were trained in conducting focus groups, the collection of pile sort data, and the analysis and interpretation of qualitative data. In our findings, men had framed many of their challenges, including institutional, as related to black masculinities, of which sex and sexuality featured prominently.

On completion of this second study, members of our collaborative prepared a report focusing on both our process and our study findings. We presented this report at a forum at Wake Forest University, at the Conference on African American Culture and Experience at UNCG, and at the Annual Meeting of the Society for Applied Anthropology. In addition to the experiences gained during the research process by African American/black men at UNCG and the concrete discovery associated with the research study, personal transformation among partners occurred. For example, African American/black men at UNCG learned new things about themselves, reassessed their current life trajectories, and became change agents in their communities regarding attitudes, beliefs, and expectations about black masculinities. Ultimately, they were more successful in college and sexually safer as a result of participation in this process. They also learned of the power of research and discovery, how knowledge generation can improve their understanding of phenomena, and how this improved understanding can be harnessed to improve their own health and well-being.

Because members of our collaborative also were committed to moving research findings toward action, we used a systematic and equitable process to convene and discuss the possibility of pursuing funding to develop, implement, and evaluate an HIV prevention intervention using CBPR. Thus, together, we pursued and obtained

CDC funding to develop, implement, and evaluate an HIV prevention intervention for African American/black heterosexual men. We also obtained ongoing support from the TRIAD Center for Health Disparities. Over the initial five years of our ongoing student-faculty collaboration, we secured multiple funding awards, using a stepwise approach of starting small and building on successes, and conducted sound research designed to better understand the intersections of culture, gender, and context and their influences on health generally and sexual health specifically. This work represents the development of our community-based collaborative, which in time was called Brothers Leading Healthy Lives (BLHL). The collaborative was formalized to focus on improving the health and opportunities for success among African American/black heterosexual men. Throughout, our values and methods were aligned with CBPR principles (Table 3.1).

The CDC funding allowed members of the BLHL collaborative to develop a culturally congruent, gender-specific, and contextually relevant intervention designed to improve sexual health and reduce HIV-associated sexual risk behaviors among African American/black heterosexual men 18–24 years old, using a peer health education-training model in a university setting. Development of the intervention included sound formative research, with a blending of quantitative brief risk assessment and qualitative data from focus groups and individual in-depth interviews, involving more than 200 African American/black heterosexual college men. We then translated formative findings into a two-component intervention: a five-session curriculum delivered over two days, known as the BLHL Brotherhood Retreat, and a three-month follow-up BLHL Retreat Message Maintenance Phase [11].

Understanding context and identifying the community

CBPR recognizes community as a unit of identity and seeks to strengthen community through engagement [32]. UNCG students come from different regions of the state, the country, and even the world. They bring perspectives, experiences, and expectations that interact with the campus and larger community environments, including the city in which UNCG is located, to shape their college experience. UNCG, which was established in 1891 as a women's college, first admitted black women in 1956 and then opened its doors to men in 1963. UNCG still maintains an enrollment that reflects this history. Currently, UNCG has more than 18,000 students: 35 % are men and 65 % are women. Among the 16 historically white campuses within the University of North Carolina system, UNCG has one of the largest racial/ethnic minority enrollments; 38 % of students identify as a racial/ethnic minority. With the sex and race ratios both at nearly 2 to 1, a premium tends to be placed on black masculinities and heterosexuality. Through our research, we have learned that African American/black men are sometimes preyed on, sexualized, objectified, and eroticized by others, and consequently, their psychosocial and sexual health may be negatively affected.

Moreover, Greensboro, the city in which UNCG is located, is the third largest city in North Carolina and has four historically black colleges and universities

(HBCUs) within a 50-mile radius. Enrollment of an African American/black man at UNCG instead of a neighboring HBCU has unique sociocultural significance. With desegregation occurring just one to two generations ago, some UNCG students have relatives who could not attend UNCG. These relatives may have strong feelings about attending UNCG that affect attitudes and beliefs that African American/black students bring to campus.

African American/black men at UNCG also tend to establish a social network early, initially as freshman. Access to networks and social connections on or near campus has been identified as essential to decreasing the likelihood of African American/black men dropping out. African American/black men have reported that these networks and connections provide various forms of social support (e.g., information on barber shops and local jobs), experiences that contribute to their academic progress (e.g., which majors are more welcoming to African American/black men and which faculty members can be trustworthy allies), and a sense of attachment to the university (e.g., through athletics and step-show contests). Furthermore, African American/black men at UNCG tend to reconnect with hometown friends at nearby HBCUs and take advantage of the social and cultural events on those campuses. This contextual backdrop informed the challenges and opportunities the BLHL collaborative faced in engaging and collaborating with African American/black men. Knowing that research designed to understand and improve sexual health and prevent HIV exposure and transmission must recognize social connections off campus, we welcomed this concept of the expanded community.

Navigating college, masculinity, and sexual identity

It is widely suggested that college students may have better access to information about and resources to prevent HIV and sexually transmitted infections (STIs) than individuals of the same age who do not attend college; however, increased knowledge and resources have not resulted in significant increases in protective sexual behaviors. Although college students have traditionally been considered a low-risk group for HIV, African American/black university students tend to have profound misconceptions about HIV exposure and transmission and may be at risk [8, 16, 33–37].

Moreover, the years that an adolescent spends in college can be an important yet risky time for sexual experimentation. In their transition from adolescence to adulthood during college, students are developing their identities through both crisis-exploration and commitment. Crisis-exploration refers to the period when an adolescent questions goals and values defined by parents and family and examines developmental opportunities and new identities based on their experiences within a larger social context (e.g., beyond one's family). Being away from home and/or attending college can provide opportunities to experiment and gain experiences. Commitment pertains to the extent that an individual expresses allegiance to self-chosen goals, aspirations, values, beliefs, and occupations [38, 39]. Sexual identity and behavior may play an instrumental role in the process of crisis-explora-tion and commitment; however, they also can increase the risk for HIV.

For African American/black men, the passage to adulthood and manhood may be even more complicated than for the typical college student. It may involve a conscious or unconscious negotiation of their masculinity and their intersecting gender, racial, ethnic, cultural, and sexual identities. They may struggle with their masculine identities and expression in a real and perceived racist environment; they face gender-based socialization and societal messages that promote a preoccupation with money.

African American/black men also may struggle with being an independent African American/black man. Despite their challenges on campus, attending college can be seen as a way for African American/black men to make it out of the neighbor-hood and overcome family and personal financial struggles for those of lower SES. As a participant in one of our focus groups noted,

> I'm not here because I want to be here. I'll sit here and tell y'all, I never wanted to go to school. I'm in school because I have to be in school. I'm in school because there's noth-ing… if I do not go to school. I didn't come from a bad neighborhood, but there's nothing to do at home. What am I supposed to do? Just sit home and not do something? I could not take care of myself if I didn't come to school. So I came to school to get an education so I could take care of myself. I do not want to be here.

Furthermore, these young men try to maintain or reclaim those masculine traits as-sociated with a strong African American/black man. These traits may include con-trol and power, respect and influence, reputation, and status. While living in a po-tentially hostile environment, African American/black men also are fighting racial stereotypes. As another participant in one of our studies noted,

> It's not really things you have to do to be a black man, I think it's just the race itself, because no matter how much money you have, how much education you have, no matter how good or bad you're doing, people around you, they're still going to just going to see you as a black man.

African American/black men who struggled academically, came from families of low socioeconomic status, and/or were unable to achieve "ideal" masculinity through respectable attributes often invested their time and effort in building their reputation to achieve an acceptable masculinity. They reported that cultivating their reputation included having concurrent sexual relationships, partying excessively, playing sports, and/or spending a great deal of time in the gym.

To be successful on campus, all students must adjust to managing competing pri-orities such as work, personal relationships, and the academic schedule. Some of the young African American/black men with whom we have engaged secured financial aid to support themselves while taking a full academic load and working a part-time or full-time job in order to send money home to their parents, grandparents, or siblings. Perhaps unique to some groups of college students like these young Afri-can American/black men are expressions of anxiety and discomfort about seeking help for poor grades or for resolving conflicts in their personal lives. Perceptions of professors as intimidating, rude, or uncaring caused some men to avoid interacting with faculty and staff and advocating for better performance reviews or grades.

The establishment and role of a Research and Intervention Advisory Team (RIAT)

An important component of the BLHL collaborative was the establishment and active involvement of a Research and Intervention Advisory Team (RIAT) that identified funding opportunities and guided the development of activities and events to address the needs and priorities of African American/black men at UNCG. Using a snowball recruitment technique, we identified student leaders within and outside of the classroom, on and off campus, and through traditional and unconventional networks. One unique aspect of our approach to CBPR was the engagement of community representatives who may be considered "unsavory" by administrators and faculty and staff mentors, collaborators, and partners. These representatives may include students who seek high status and popularity through reputation (as opposed to respectability) by engaging in risky behaviors (e.g., substance use and risky sexual behaviors). Students with "high numbers of jump-offs" (multiple casual sexual partners) or the "go-to man for smoke" are influential members of the community who have much to contribute to the research process, beyond that of being recruited to provide data or to participate in an intervention. We found that these types of community members can make invaluable contributions to research question conception, study design and conduct, data analysis and interpretation, and the dissemination of findings.

We also identified and recruited representatives from the broader community, including individuals from community-based organizations, businesses, and government agencies, to serve on the RIAT (Table 3.2). Student leaders from the BLHL collaborative were instrumental in the outreach and recruitment effort to invite trusted organizations to serve on the RIAT.

RIAT membership was carefully negotiated, and some groups or individuals requesting membership were, in fact, turned down. For example, an African American/black campus police officer wanted to join the RIAT because of his campus-wide efforts for community engagement and potential resources he thought he could provide students. Members of the RIAT declined the request, however, because of the concern for maintaining student trust and confidentiality. Members wanted to provide a safe place for open dialogue and discussion without the hint of incrimination or reprisal for information shared. We knew that good intentions are not sufficient for successful CBPR.

Members of the RIAT drew on findings from the formative research that had been conducted up to this point [11, 31, 40, 41]; theoretical considerations, including the Big Man/Little Man framework [28–31] and the Information-Motivation-Behavioral (IMB) skills model [42]; and evidence from existing efficacious HIV prevention interventions [43–47] to systematically develop the BLHL intervention,

Table 3.2 RIAT membership

On-campus Organizations and Student Groups	UNCG NAACP
	UNCG Alumni
	UNCG PanHellenic Council and Black Fraternities
Off-campus Organizations Serving Black Men	Winston-Salem Urban League
	Local barbers and barbershops
	Night club owners
	Forsyth County Parks & Recreation
	The Children's Home Society–Family Life Council Division
Student- Focused University Services	North Carolina Agricultural & Technical State University, Student Services
	UNCG Student Health Center
	UNCG Spartan Athletics
	UNCG Office of Multicultural Affairs
Community-based HIV Service Organizations	Guilford County Department of Public Health, Health Education Division
	Guilford County AIDS Coalition
	Piedmont Health Services and Sickle Cell Agency
	Forsyth County Department of Public Health-Health Promotion & Disease Prevention
	Triad Health Project
Other Local Universities and College Campuses and Academic Departments	Department of Social Sciences and Health Policy, Wake Forest University School of Medicine
	Section on Infectious Diseases, Wake Forest University School of Medicine
	North Carolina Central University
	Maya Angelou Center for Health Equity, Wake Forest University School of Medicine
	The Center for Social, Community and Health Research and Evaluation (CSCHRE)
	Winston-Salem State University
Public Health Agencies	NC Division of Public Health
	The Greensboro Health Disparities Collaborative
Students and Community Members	Community advocates
	Winston-Salem community residents
	Greensboro community residents

a culturally congruent, gender-specific, and contextually relevant intervention for African American/black heterosexual men.

All activities of the two primary components of BLHL (the Brotherhood Retreat and the Retreat Message Maintenance Phase) were designed to achieve three primary objectives that were established by the RIAT.

- Support men to identify and develop healthy ways to obtain respect and foster positive reputations.

- Inform, motivate, and provide skills for men to protect themselves, their partners, and the community from HIV.
- Influence social norms and create peer support for men to protect themselves.

The BLHL intervention provides information about sexual health and helps participants assess their own HIV risks, explores and develops personal and social motivations to reduce HIV risk, explores interpretations of "ideal" masculinity, and promotes health protective sexual communication and behaviors. The intervention provides practice and skill training to reduce HIV risk through testing for HIV and other STIs, selection and use of condoms, communication about sexual health and HIV, and maintenance of healthy relationships.

The Brotherhood Retreat includes five consecutive two- to three-hour sessions that were delivered during weekend retreats with up to 20 participants. Each retreat was conducted by two trained peer facilitators and supported by two or three trained peer educators. These facilitators and peer educators were male undergraduate or graduate students 21–30 years old, who identified with the reference group – African American/black men. They were trained and certified as peer health educators in the BLHL intervention by the principal investigators, the project coordinator, and doctoral student graduate assistants.

The BLHL Retreat Message Maintenance Phase was a three-month follow-up to the retreat during which key messages from the intervention as well as prevention messages developed by participants during the Brotherhood Retreat were delivered through a health communication campaign. Messages were delivered by the graduate assistant working on the project using a variety of approaches, including Twitter tweets five times a day (Monday-Friday), with 140-character-long prevention messages created during the Brotherhood Retreat; biweekly postings of key prevention messages from the intervention on the BLHL Facebook page; and biweekly text messages and reminders sent via e-mail (Monday and Thursday) of elements of the group risk-reduction plans developed during the retreats.

Challenges and opportunities of engaging students as CBPR partners

Our CBPR process faced unique challenges and opportunities in accommodating the experiences of African American/black men within a university as CBPR partners. The leadership of students as co-researchers was instrumental to our understanding the characteristics of the community and identify peers and community members to support the project.

One challenge was that our collaborative struggled to balance the involvement of students in meaningful ways without overburdening them and thus contributing to their challenges related to academic performance. Many student members of our BLHL collaborative felt privileged to matriculate into college and considered their matriculation a respectable first step toward employment, a career, and financial freedom. Some struggled with new intellectual challenges (e.g., needing to study instead of just showing up for the exam as in high school), competing priorities (e.g., family, friends, and health) that are often more intense than they are for other students, and conflicts (e.g., racial microaggressions, financial burdens, and addictions) that they were learning to deal with in new contexts, while wanting to exercise leadership on campus as peer educators, student leaders, and academic scholars. Many student members of our BLHL collaborative tended to be natural leaders, accepted by their peers, and called on by campus administration when a representative from a minority group was needed. Thus, they tended to be overcommitted and have tight schedules. One approach to address the issue of potentially overburdening student members was to select students who were doing well academically and who faced few of the aforementioned challenges. The difficulty with this approach was that representation from the most vulnerable students was needed to ensure informed understanding of sexual health and HIV risk and to develop the intervention in ways that addressed the issues of the most vulnerable students. Authentic CBPR includes diverse representatives from the community, not a subset or those who are not truly characteristic of the community.

Furthermore, although students were part of our collaborative, it is safe to assume that members of any collaborative or partnership do not represent *all* community members. By virtue of their participation in a collaborative or partnership, they become different. Members of our collaborative were committed to "staying close" to the community of African American/black heterosexual men by reducing the social distance between the BLHL collaborative and the larger university community. There was much for members of the collaborative to learn about the lived experiences of those who were not part of the collaborative.

Lastly, students' membership in the campus community is temporary and transitory. On a college campus, community members change every four to six years, and students are typically in residence for only nine months of the year. Student leaders are often upperclassmen, further reducing the length of time they can participate in a collaborative. Students come and go and transfer in to and out of the university; every year there is a new cohort of African American/black men. Thus, perhaps different from other CBPR collaboratives and partnerships, we have found that there can be a need for faculty and/or staff mentors, collaborators, and partners who, despite being outsiders from the community of African American/black heterosexual male college students, serve as anchors to provide continuity and develop strategies for true student engagement. Faculty members tend to be on campus throughout the year, providing consistency to an otherwise fluctuating collaborative.

The importance of cultural orientation congruence

Although it may be assumed by some researchers and practitioners, and even preferred by some students, the faculty and staff mentors, collaborators, and partners do not have to share the same ethnic/racial identity, gender, or sexual orientation as the student community collaborators. The key, however, is that the faculty and staff mentors, collaborators, and partners are visible, have demonstrated evidence of being trustworthy and honest, and are connected to students in a meaningful way. This connection is related to "cultural orientation congruence" [40]. In our case, cultural orientation congruence requires that faculty and staff mentors, collaborators, and partners have a knowledge base, a set of experiences, and attitudes that overlap or align well with the students they intend to serve. Their background, commitments, principles, and relationships to other people and institutions must parallel or "square" with those of the students and allow heightened empathy, irrespective of color, race, or any other single characteristic. The experiences of different ethnicities, races, genders, or sexual orientations, as examples, are too diverse and complicated to use pairing as a proxy for cultural orientation congruence.

Constraints on community involvement

A key challenge for our BLHL collaborative generally and for the RIAT more specifically, was balancing what extramural funders required and what our members, as community insiders and those closely attached to the community, wanted and recommended. For example, in our CDC-funded study, representatives from CDC wanted to enroll only "higher-risk" African American/black men who had sex exclusively with multiple female partners and who had never have used injecting drugs. However, given that adolescence is a time of experimentation and identity development, we knew that college-age men, even those who self-identify as heterosexual, may have had same-sex sexual experiences in the not-so-distant past, and, more generally, we know that men who have sex with women may have sex with men. We also know that lower- and higher-risk men interact and are part of one another's social networks. We did not believe that higher risk men are a naturally occurring group or category of men but that they are a part of a larger community of African American/black male students at UNCG. The separation between higher and lower risk that was required by the funding agency had no relevance to the lives of these men, and to separate them and treat them differently reduced the relevance of an intervention. Moreover, rather than build community and harness community assets, this approach did the very opposite of the current understanding of health promotion and health disparities reduction. However, in the end, to maintain funding, the RIAT agreed to the funder's definition of heterosexual and high risk to allow the study to continue. This was a decision that reverberated throughout our BLHL collaborative; it told members that despite our efforts to adhere to CBPR principles, outsiders (the funders), who knew little of the lived experiences of local community members, still held power over us in ways that could potentially jeopardize the health and well-being of our collaborators and members of our community.

Maintaining the engagement of RIAT members was challenging, due to the lengthy process of finalizing administrative procedures: development and approval of the project protocol by the funding institution, two university institutional review boards (IRBs), and ultimately the US Office of Management and Budget (OMB). We managed to maintain RIAT involvement through a combination of meetings, newsletters, e-mails, and telephone check-ins; however, administrative delays stretched from weeks, to months, to approximately one year. During these delays, we continued to discuss options and refine strategies. Some members of the RIAT had worked with external grant agencies and were accustomed to the delays and federally mandated changes to protocols. Others were less familiar with such a process but were committed to the effort, and together we found ways to maintain momentum to support BLHL efforts. However, some students began to distrust the process and see research not as a grand endeavor but a process you endure, strangely familiar to their experiences as African American/black men at a predominately white university.

A flexible research paradigm

The aim of our funding was to conduct formative research leading to the design and piloting of a culturally congruent, gender-specific, and contextually relevant HIV prevention intervention for African American/black heterosexual men. As mentioned, during the formative phase, brief risk assessments, focus groups, and individual in-depth interviews were used to provide empirical data to guide the development of the intervention. When collecting formative data, it was often difficult to adhere to a rigidly defined and detailed research protocol as required by representatives of the funding agency, given that changes could not be made after OMB approval. For example, when a student who was eligible to participate in a focus group arrived at the focus group bringing a friend (who met the eligibility requirements but had not gone through the screening process), the focus group facilitator was faced with a challenge: Should he send the friend away, risking the loss of a participant who was screened and eligible, and jeopardizing the study's reputation? Or, should he allow the friend to participate? The facilitator's decision to permit the friend to attend led to conflict with representatives from the funding agency over what they perceived to be a breach of protocol; they requested that we discard the data from the focus group. At the local level, deviations such as these are reported, and members of a local IRB who understand the local context can make an informed decision; representatives from most funding agencies such as the CDC do not know the local community or understand the local context and thus are less equipped to judge those types of deviations.

Furthermore, we had to defend the suitability, methods, and rigor of qualitative data collection, analysis, and interpretation. The rigidity of highly detailed research protocols did not allow for the flexibility needed in community-based, community-owned research. Flexibility and collaborative decision-making in the community can enhance the quality of the data and their usefulness. In the future, we would caution CBPR collaboratives against including rigid guidelines for data collection,

Table 3.3 Strategies for CPBR on a university campus with African American/Black Men

Understand and build trust with the community

Talk with and get to know formal and informal leaders and nontraditional experts within the community

Inspire community participation by being an engaged member of the community

Engage and value community members as equal partners

Establish history and trust

Safeguard the community members and their interests

Develop a shared language and cultural relativity

Develop a collaborative partnership

Enforce equitable representation of collaborators during all stages of the research

Address the competing needs of collaborative members

Incorporate a flexible pace and timeline

Share power, decision-making, and resources

Buffer collaborators from unnecessary organizational structure barriers

Welcome alternative research paradigms and methodology

"Incite" a RIAT (Research Intervention Advisory Team)

Establish accountability and agreed-on decision-making process with all members

Identify joint research aims and outcomes

Allocate resources for nonacademic student support and life-balance training

Invite the multiple voices from within community

Address conflict with sensitivity and compassion

analysis, and interpretation in protocols for formative research, particularly if these protocols are expected to be followed exactly.

Strategies for CBPR on a college campus with African American/black men

We used several strategies to establish and strengthen the BLHL collaborative (Table 3.3). Central to the process was understanding and building trust with the community. We recognized that establishing a long and ongoing history working in authentic partnership with community members was important for the success of our collaborative and of our BLHL intervention, which included reductions in unprotected sex [11]. Our approach to CBPR did not consist of researchers coming into a community of African American/black students with a research idea or a funded research study. Rather, we talked with and got to know members of the community. We worked to understand community priorities and established mutually beneficial linkages and supportive networks.

The history that we established allowed us to build trust. Building and maintaining trust with communities is *always* integral to CBPR. However, researchers and practitioners often do not invest in communities but rather establish a community advisory board or committee and define the approach as CBPR. Not only is this disingenuous but it also has profound implications for the health and well-being of community members and communities more generally. CBPR is designed to help gain a better understanding of health so that the most informed and promising interventions can be developed. To suggest that a CBPR approach was applied when in fact it had not means that we are not doing everything possible to reduce disparities; we are merely rebranding our approach. We are relying on what we had done in the past, which we know did not promote the health and well-being in the ways that many vulnerable communities needed. CBPR continues to remain innovative because, in fact, it has not been conducted well in many cases; CBPR principles are not easy to follow.

Furthermore, our collaborative was established and structured to ensure equitable project representation at all stages of the research, incorporate a flexible pace and timeline, share resources and power, and consider alternative research paradigms. We have learned that traditional approaches to research that value "gold standards", including strict adherence to reduce bias and threats to validity as examples, may not provide the flexibility that allows more informed understandings of health phenomena to emerge. We know that sharing power, decision-making, and resources is key to buy-in and ownership of research. It is also true to the democratic ideal that communities should have power over their own destinies.

Lastly, we found that establishing a RIAT was vital to our success. It brought the needed persons and their unique perspectives, insights, and experiences to the table. These divergent viewpoints ensured that our decisions and products (e.g., intervention strategies, activities, and materials) were key and innovative to promote sexual health and prevent HIV exposure and transmission among African American/black men.

Discussion and conclusion

We found that using a CBPR approach produced positive outcomes for all collaborators, especially for the students whom we valued as equal partners. Students learned about research, government funding, and community change, while collaborators from universities and other organizations learned about the lived experiences of students, as well as their needs, priorities, and natural "ways of doing things."

Creating opportunities for equitable participation in research and practice can be challenging. In the case of African American/black heterosexual men in college, some common challenges as well as some unique challenges are present. For example, by the very nature of college, university students tend to be a "transitory group"; thus, campus-based communities are apt to have constantly changing memberships. Students may enter or leave the community each semester or year.

Although many students have competing priorities, African American/black men on university campuses may have an even more difficult experience, given their potential obligations to families at home and their expectations to "handle things like a man," particularly given the context of the racially marginalized position of African American/black men on a predominantly white university. Furthermore, we continue to struggle with defining our communities, be they based on location, as in a campus with spatial boundaries; identity, as in racial groups; or some other criteria. Moreover, when thinking about intersecting identities or working with location-based and identity-based definitions of community, we must begin to work with communities rather than a community.

Mutual understanding is a continual process; therefore, researchers and practitioners must be realistic about the amount of time needed to build relationships with community partners (including students). The community of African American/black men is rich in diversity with varied experiences and expectations. To fully understand and engage these men, outside collaborators (including researchers and practitioners) should be open to developing non-research focused relationships that extend beyond the academic classroom and include social networks.

References

1. Centers for Disease Control and Prevention. HIV Surveillance Report, 2011. Atlanta: US Department of Health and Human Services; 2013.
2. Centers for Disease Control and Prevention. HIV among African Americans. Atlanta: U.S. Department of Health and Human Services; 2013.
3. Southern AIDS Coalition. Southern States Manifesto: Update 2012. Policy brief and recommendations. Birmingham: Southern AIDS Coalition; 2012.
4. Rhodes SD, Hergenrather KC, Wilkin AM, Jolly C. Visions and voices: indigent persons living with HIV in the southern United States use photovoice to create knowledge, develop partnerships, and take action. Health Promot Pract. 2008;9(2):159–69.
5. Reif S, Geonnotti KL, Whetten K. HIV Infection and AIDS in the Deep South. Am J Public Health. 2006;96(6):970–3.
6. Rhodes SD, McCoy TP, Hergenrather KC, Vissman AT, Wolfson M, Alonzo J, et al. Prevalence estimates of health risk behaviors of immigrant Latino men who have sex with men. J Rural Health. 2012;28(1):73–83.
7. Ricketts T. Rural Health in the United States. New York: Oxford University Press; 1999.
8. Bowleg L, Teti M, Massie JS, Patel A, Malebranche DJ, Tschann JM. 'What does it take to be a man? What is a real man?': ideologies of masculinity and HIV sexual risk among Black heterosexual men. Cult Health Sex. 2011;13(5):545–59.
9. Centers for Disease Control and Prevention. 2011 Compendium of evidence-based HIV prevention interventions. Available at: http://www.cdcgov/hiv/topics/research/prs/resources/factsheets/hombreshtm. 2011. Accessed Nov. 2011.
10. Bowleg L, Teti M, Malebranche DJ, Tschann JM. "It's an uphill battle everyday": intersectionality, low-Income black heterosexual men, and implications for HIV prevention research and interventions. Psychol Men Masc. 2013;14(1):25–34.
11. Aronson RE, Rulison KL, Graham LF, Pulliam RM, McGee WL, Labban JD, et al. Brothers leading healthy lives: outcomes from the pilot testing of a culturally and contextually congruent HIV prevention intervention for black male college students. AIDS Educ Prev. 2013;25(5):376–93.
12. Frye V, Bonner S, Williams K, Henny K, Bond K, Lucy D, et al. Straight talk: HIV prevention for African-American heterosexual men: theoretical bases and intervention design. AIDS Educ Prev. 2012;24(5):389–407.
13. Henny KD, Crepaz N, Lyles CM, Marshall KJ, Aupont LW, Jacobs ED, et al. Efficacy of HIV/STI behavioral interventions for heterosexual African American men in the United States: a meta-analysis. AIDS Behav. 2012;16(5):1092–114.

14. Adimora AA, Schoenbach VJ. Social context, sexual networks, and racial disparities in rates of sexually transmitted infections. J Infect Dis. 2005;191 (Supplement 1):115–22.

15. Hightow-Weidman LB, Fowler B, Kibe J, McCoy R, Pike E, Calabria M, et al. HealthMpowerment.org: development of a theory-based HIV/STI website for young black MSM. AIDS Educ Prev. 2011;23(1):1–12.

16. Rhodes SD, Hergenrather KC, Vissman AT, Stowers J, Davis AB, Hannah A, et al. Boys must be men, and men must have sex with women: A qualitative CBPR study to explore sexual risk among African American, Latino, and white gay men and MSM. Am J Mens Health. 2011;5(2):140–51.

17. Rhodes SD, Hergenrather KC, Wilkin AM, Alegria-Ortega J, Montaño J. Preventing HIV infection among young immigrant Latino men: results from focus groups using community-based participatory research. J Natl Med Assoc. 2006;98(4):564–73.

18. Reif SS, Whetten K, Wilson ER, McAllaster C, Pence BW, Legrand S, et al. HIV/AIDS in the southern USA: a disproportionate epidemic. AIDS Care. 2013.

19. Minkler M, Wallerstein N. Introduction to community based participatory research. In: Minkler M, Wallerstein N, Editors. Community-based participatory research for health. San Francisco: Jossey-Bass; 2003. p. 3–26.

20. Israel BA, Eng E, Schulz AJ, Parker EA. Introduction to methods in community-based participatory research for health. In: Israel BA, Eng E, Schulz AJ, Parker EA, Editors. Methods in community-based participatory research. San Francisco: Jossey-Bass; 2005. pp. 3–26.

21. Rhodes SD. Community-based participatory research. In Blessing JD, Forister. JG, Editors. Introduction to research and medical literature for health professionals. 3rd Ed. Burlington: Jones & Bartlett; 2013. p. 167–87.

22. Rhodes SD, Duck S, Alonzo J, Daniel J, Aronson RE. Using community-based participatory research to prevent HIV disparities: assumptions and opportunities identified by The Latino Partnership. J Acquir Immune Syndr. 2013;63(Supplement 1):32–5.

23. Rhodes SD, Duck S, Alonzo J, Downs M, Aronson RE. Intervention trials in community-based participatory research. In: Blumenthal D, DiClemente RJ, Braithwaite RL, Smith S, Editors. Community-based participatory research: issues, methods, and translation to practice. New York: Springer 2013. p. 157–80.

24. Rhodes SD, Hergenrather KC, Bloom FR, Leichliter JS, Montaño J. Outcomes from a community-based, participatory lay health advisor HIV/STD prevention intervention for recently arrived immigrant Latino men in rural North Carolina, USA. AIDS Educ Prev. 2009;21(Supplement 1):104–9.

25. Rhodes SD, Hergenrather KC, Griffith D, Yee LJ, Zometa CS, Montaño J, et al. Sexual and alcohol use behaviours of Latino men in the south-eastern USA. Cult Health Sex. 2009;11(1):17–34.

26. Rhodes SD, McCoy TP, Vissman AT, DiClemente RJ, Duck S, Hergenrather KC, et al. A randomized controlled trial of a culturally congruent intervention to increase condom use and HIV testing among heterosexually active immigrant Latino men. AIDS Behav. 2011;15(8):1764–75.

27. Rhodes SD. Demonstrated effectiveness and potential of CBPR for preventing HIV in Latino populations. In: Organista KC, editor. HIV prevention with Latinos: theory, research, and practice. New York: Oxford; 2012. p. 83–102.

28. Whitehead T. Breakdown, resolution and coherence: the fieldwork experiences of a big, brown, pretty-talking man in a West Indian Community. In: Whitehead T, Conawy M, Editors. Self, sex and gender in cross-cultural fieldwork. Urban-Chicago: University of Illinois Press; 1986. p. 213–39.

29. Whitehead T. Urban low-income African American men, HIV/AIDS, and gender identity. Med Anthropol Q. 1997;11(4):411–47.

30. Aronson RE, Whitehead TL, Baber WL. Challenges to masculine transformation among urban low-income African American males. Am J Public Health. 2003;93(5):732–41.

31. Baber WL, Aronson RE, Melton LD. Ideal and stereotypical masculinity and issues of adjustment to college life for men of color. Southern Anthropologist. 2005;31(1 & 2):53–73.

32. Israel BA, Schulz AJ, Parker EA, Becker AB. Review of community-based research: assessing partnership approaches to improve public health. Annu Rev Public Health. 1998;19:173–202.

33. Bogart LM, Thorburn S. Are HIV/AIDS conspiracy beliefs a barrier to HIV prevention among African Americans? J Acquir Immune Defic Syndr. 2005;38(2):213–8.

34. Rhodes SD, McCoy T, Omli MR, Cohen G, Champion H, DuRant RH. Who really uses condoms? Findings from a large internet-recruited random sample of unmarried heterosexual college students in the Southeastern US. J HIV AIDS Prev Child Youth. 2006;7(2):9–27.

35. Duncan C, Miller DM, Borskey EJ, Fomby B, Dawson P, Davis L. Barriers to safer sex practices among African American college students. J Natl Med Assoc. 2002;94(11):944–51.

36. Hou SI. HIV-related behaviors among black students attending Historically Black Colleges and Universities (HBCUs) versus white students attending a traditionally white institution (TWI). AIDS Care. 2009;21(8):1050–7.

37. Essien EJ, Meshack AF, Ross MW. Misperceptions about HIV transmission among heterosexual African-American and Latino men and women. J Natl Med Assoc. 2002;94(5):304–12.

38. Erikson EH. Identity: youth and crisis. New York: Norton; 1968.

39. Clark LF, Rhodes SD, Rogers W, Liddon N. The context of sexual risk behavior. In: Raczynski JM, Leviton LC, Editors. Handbook of Clinical Health Psychology. Washington, DC: American Psychological Association; 2004. p. 121–46.

40. Graham L, Brown-Jeffy S, Aronson R, Stephens C. Critical race theory as framework and analysis tool for population health research. Crit Public Health. 2011;21(1):81–93.

41. Graham LF, Aronson RE, Nichols T, Stephens CF, Rhodes SD. Factors influencing depression and anxiety among black sexual minority men. Depress Res Treat. 2011;2011:587984.

42. Fisher WA, Fisher JD, Harman J. The Information-Motivation-Behavioral skills model: A general social psychological approach to understanding and promoting health behavior social psychological foundations of health and illness. In: Suls J, Wallston KA, Editors. Social Psychological Foundations of Health and Illness. Oxford: Blackwell; 2003. p. 82–106.

43. Lyles CM, Kay LS, Crepaz N, Herbst JH, Passin WF, Kim AS, et al. Best-evidence interventions: findings from a systematic review of HIV behavioral interventions for US populations at high risk, 2000–2004. Am J Public Health. 2007;97(1):133–43.

44. Herbst JH, Beeker C, Mathew A, McNally T, Passin WF, Kay LS, et al. The effectiveness of individual-, group-, and community-level HIV behavioral risk-reduction interventions for adult men who have sex with men: a systematic review. Am J Prev Med. 2007;32(4 Suppl):38–67.

45. Albarracin D, Durantini MR. Are we going to close social gaps in HIV? Likely effects of behavioral HIV-prevention interventions on health disparities. Psychol Health Med. 2010;15(6):694–719.

46. Hemmige V, McFadden R, Cook S, Tang H, Schneider JA. HIV prevention interventions to reduce racial disparities in the United States: a systematic review. J Gen Intern Med. 2012;27(8):1047–67.

47. Romero LM, Galbraith JS, Wilson-Williams L, Gloppen KM. HIV prevention among African American youth: how well have evidence-based interventions addressed key theoretical constructs? AIDS Behav. 2011;15(5):976–91.

48. Graham LF, Treadwell HM, Braithwaite K. Social policy, imperiled communities, and HIV/AIDS in prisons: A call for zero tolerance. J Men Health 2008;5(4):267–73.

Chapter 4
Gay Community Involvement in HIV and STD Prevention: Where We Have Been, Where We Are, and Where We Should be Going

Fred R. Bloom, David K. Whittier and Scott D. Rhodes

Relationships Between Medical and Gay Communities in the USA

In the USA, gay and bisexual men, men who have sex with men (MSM), and transgender persons were initially, and continue to be, profoundly affected by HIV. Despite the substantial impact of the disease, HIV received little attention and support from the media, politicians, or even researchers in the USA early on in the epidemic [1]. There was little political motivation in the larger mainstream community to act against an emerging epidemic that some referred to in a derogatory manner as the "gay plague."

This initial lack of motivation to address HIV and AIDS within gay communities was not surprising. Medical and gay communities have had a turbulent history. The term "homosexuality" appeared in the first edition of the *Diagnostic and Statistical Manual of Mental Disorders* (DSM), published in 1952, and was defined as a

---

Disclosure: The findings and conclusions in this report are those of the authors and do not necessarily represent the official position of the Centers for Disease Control and Prevention.

F. R. Bloom (✉)
Division of STD Prevention, National Center for HIV/AIDS, Viral Hepatitis, STD and TB Prevention, Centers for Disease Control and Prevention, 1600 Clifton Road, Mailstop E-02, Atlanta, GA 30333, USA
e-mail: fcb8@cdc.gov

D. K. Whittier
Division of HIV Prevention, National Center for HIV/AIDS, Viral Hepatitis, STD and TB Prevention, Centers for Disease Control and Prevention, 1600 Clifton Road, Mailstop E-40, Atlanta, GA 30333, USA
e-mail: david.whittier@cdc.hhs.gov

S. D. Rhodes
Department of Social Sciences and Health Policy, Division of Public Health Sciences, Wake Forest University School of Medicine, Medical Center Blvd., Winston-Salem, NC 27157, USA
e-mail: srhodes@wakehealth.edu

S. D. Rhodes (ed.), *Innovations in HIV Prevention Research and Practice through Community Engagement,* DOI 10.1007/978-1-4939-0900-1_4,
© Springer Science+Business Media New York 2014

"sociopathic personality disturbance." This inclusion of homosexuality in the DSM was based in part on a large-scale study that asserted that homosexuality resulted from a pathologic fear of the opposite sex caused by traumatic parent–child relationships [2]. The establishment of homosexuality as an illness had two major consequences. First, for some, homosexuality as an illness meant electroshock therapy, lobotomies, so-called conversion therapy, and commitments to mental hospitals by psychiatrists attempting to cure gay people. Second, the definition provided fuel for antigay hatred, discrimination, harassment, victimization, and violence [3]. These consequences reverberated in the HIV epidemic.

During the 1960s, a nascent gay movement began to challenge both the medicalization and marginalization of homosexuality and sought to demonstrate that "a pseudoscientific ideology had masked the moral strictures that had long dominated Western attitudes towards sexual activity among those of the same sex" [4]. This movement included gay researchers, their allies, and gay rights activists who collected, analyzed, and disseminated data suggesting that no mental health differences existed between heterosexual and gay populations. These researchers, allies, and activists also used community mobilization and organizing and civil disobedience strategies to fight for the removal of homosexuality as an illness from the DSM and the pathologization of homosexuality and marginalization of gay health. The diagnosis of homosexuality as an illness was not included in the revised DSM-III, published in 1987. Despite the removal of homosexuality as an illness from the DSM, the perception of gay communities as being less than other communities lingered and had a profoundly negative affect on initial responses to HIV, the greatest epidemic in modern history.

Given the history between medical and gay communities, gay communities had little outside support as HIV emerged in the USA in the 1980s as a threat to their health and well-being. The values and principles underlying, and methods that are often aligned with, community-based participatory research (CBPR) are reflected within both the initial and current responses by gay communities to the HIV epidemic.

CBPR as an approach to prevention research has received increased attention as academic and public health communities struggle to address persistent health disparities in access to and utilization of health care and the health outcomes among vulnerable populations, including racial/ethnic and sexual minorities [5–12]. Innovative and methodologically robust approaches to prevention research that include authentic community engagement and partnership and CBPR are currently being undertaken within a variety of diverse communities and populations (as shown in other chapters in this book). However, why and how gay communities and their allies came together to respond to the HIV epidemic are important to examine and appreciate given the foundation that these initial responses have provided to the processes and practices of community engagement and partnership and what we now refer to as CBPR.

Gay communities organized and mobilized to identify and meet the needs and priorities of their own communities [13]. Many community leaders, lay community members, advocates, activists, and researchers involved in the earliest

HIV-prevention research and practice efforts were gay themselves [14]; they were members of the community and HIV was their priority. Much of the most innovative and successful HIV prevention and prevention-research efforts sprang from the creativity of gay men and their allies, and these efforts developed by, for, and within gay communities tended to be highly culturally congruent [15]. These naturally emerging community partnerships provided needed care; initiated meaningful community-based educational and prevention programs; advocated for both drug development and expedited drug trials; and developed, implemented, and evaluated prevention strategies in the community. In sum, gay men wanted to provide the much needed support and care to friends, neighbors, and other community members who were infected with and affected by HIV. Still relatively early in the epidemic, friends, neighbors, and other community members were literally dying around these first leaders; gay men and their close allies also strove to raise political awareness of and combat ignorance about both HIV and homosexuality. Too often, individuals with HIV were shunned by families and providers because of their disease and/or because they were gay.

In this chapter, we (1) review the role gay men and their allies have played in HIV-prevention research and practice over time as it relates to CBPR today, (2) review the roots and development of CBPR to identify its relevance and place in the present, and (3) point to new directions or courses for social action, community-based prevention, and applications of CBPR to prevent HIV among gay and bisexual men, MSM, and transgender persons. Although there are important issues regarding HIV for gay men worldwide, our focus in this chapter is on the unique interaction between HIV-prevention research among gay men and the sociopolitical influences in the USA. Importantly, we focus on the response of gay men to provide a context of comparison to explore CBPR for the larger community of gay men in the USA. We note that allies of gay men, including lesbians and heterosexual men and women were important partners in this effort, and we do not intend to minimize the important contributions of those who stood with the gay men who were the earliest casualties in the AIDS epidemic in this country.

CBPR, Gay Men, and HIV

CBPR evolved from action research, participatory action research, and other research paradigms that include community engagement and participation throughout all or many phases of the research process, including research question conception, study design development and conduct, data analysis and interpretation, dissemination of findings, and action. Within a CBPR framework, the process ideally starts with an important issue (based in needs and priorities) as identified by members of a community themselves; includes the participation of the affected community in the design, implementation, and evaluation of the study; and ensures shared ownership of the products of research [16–20]. Thus, communities of gay men identified and implemented interventions and actions attempting to interrupt the spread of HIV.

Gay men, academicians, and health care providers examined these interventions and actions and other data through research and, in some cases, worked to build ongoing research efforts and health care services for gay men in their communities (e.g., Howard Brown Health Center in Chicago, IL, and the Gay Men's Health Crisis [GMHC] in New York City). Taken as a whole, these actions embody many of the principles of CBPR and emerged as a natural bridge between (1) preventing further HIV infections and meeting the needs of and supporting those with HIV and (2) conducting sound science to help guide strategies to prevent infections and support needs.

Early in the HIV epidemic, gay men, along with notable allies, wanted "to do something," because very little was being done outside of gay communities. In fact, it was not until 1987 that then-President Ronald Reagan used the word "AIDS" in public. By that time, more than 36,000 Americans had been diagnosed with AIDS and more than 20,000 had died. Worldwide, it was estimated that there were over 50,000 cases in more than 113 countries. Because of the slow response by the federal government, including the delayed allocation of resources for prevention and treatment innovations and limitations on federal funding for HIV prevention that included sexual health promotion for gay persons [21, 22], much of the initial HIV prevention and care innovations were developed without federal support.

These early HIV-prevention efforts conducted by, for, and within gay communities were congruent with the values and principles underlying CBPR. Gay men and their allies partnered to identify the needs and priorities and develop, implement, and evaluate efforts to prevent exposure and transmission of HIV within their communities—among other gay men just like themselves. Some individuals from marginalized and vulnerable communities tend to become activist leaders in the identification of public health needs and priorities in their communities. This influence on the development, implementation, and evaluation of innovations to a public health challenge like HIV is an important factor in our discussion and a driving force behind CBPR that emerges as community activism focuses on prevention research needs.

As has been suggested, CBPR as an approach to research is not novel [12, 23]. CBPR as we know it today has been conducted in the social sciences and used in approaches such as ethnography and health education at least as early as the 1940s and 1950s [24, 25]. These early versions of CBPR were not conceptualized and categorized as CBPR, yet they employed the underlying values and principles that are now synonymous with CBPR. Furthermore, collaborative partnerships for community health promotion have been documented as early as the 1970s [26], and community–academic partnerships may have been used but are not well documented earlier than that. Community engagement and partnership and CBPR may be under-articulated in earlier prevention research because of the lack of recognition of its methodologic strengths and dominance of claims to science generated by traditional approaches to research (e.g., randomized controlled trials).

Evolution of CBPR in Public Health and Social Science

CBPR can claim philosophical roots to the mid-twentieth century if not before [12, 16, 25]. As with CBPR overall, CBPR within HIV-prevention research for gay men (and other vulnerable, disenfranchised, marginalized, or oppressed groups) has strong ties to the work of Paulo Freire, as is often cited in historical reviews of CBPR [12, 16, 27, 28]. Freire (1973) advocated for the empowerment of vulnerable, disenfranchised, marginalized, and oppressed populations to drive social change from within rather than as advocated from the outside by outside others or by those representing, and having much to maintain by, the status quo. In the tradition exemplified by Freire's work, the importance of gay men's involvement in HIV-prevention research was crucial in maximizing the representation of the self-interests of gay men. This emphasis of empowered communities speaking for themselves and "being heard" crossed multiple disciplines in the social sciences and education [29–31] and provided an accepting environment within which gay men (including those within academic and research communities) could lead a community-driven research agenda and community action.

It is no stretch of the imagination to claim that CBPR is rooted in the long-standing tradition of inquiry known as ethnography, as exemplified by the work of Sol Tax, an anthropologist who conducted ethnographic research with the Fox (Meskwaki) Indian Tribe beginning in the 1930s and, in the following two decades, developed the Fox Project to help the research participants to achieve their own goals [24]. Thus, this collaboration or partnership was at the forefront of action research [32]. Similarly, in the case of HIV-prevention research, some gay men, sometimes with allies, initiated prevention research within their personal and/or professional lives and within the communities in which they lived and worked. They wanted to improve the lives and prevent further exposure and transmission among those within their community who were living with and at risk for HIV [33–37].

Interestingly, as we so often see in CBPR, the ethnography as action research conducted by Tax with the Fox Project depended on an outsider embedding himself within a community to get a greater understanding of insider perceptions, needs, and priorities. In such situations, an outsider may work closely with community insiders in authentic partnership. In contrast, HIV-prevention research within gay communities often was, and in some instances continues to be, characterized by gay men who are more or less insiders in the communities in which they worked. They tended to be friends, lovers, partners/spouses, business associates, health care providers, customers, patients, etc. of those within gay communities [14]. Combining outsider conduct of ethnographic research and insider conduct of community-driven action research has produced the most successful CBPR because together, these two approaches blend diverse perspectives, experiences, and insights to develop more informed understandings of health and health-related phenomena, community needs and priorities, and culturally congruent strategies for action to effect community health [12, 38–42].

Gay Community Involvement in HIV-prevention Research and Practice

Ongoing stigma and related sociopolitical influences played a clear role in further maintaining gay communities as the main drivers of HIV-prevention research and practice among gay men. As HIV emerged as a public health threat in the USA, efforts to focus on gay men as the largest demographic population at risk were hampered by federal restrictions on use of funds for gay men [13, 21]. Thus, communities affected by the emerging pandemic took on the task of intervening without outside support. In so doing, prevention research was conducted as a necessity to provide information for action.

Early in the epidemic, many gay men across the country mobilized and embraced safer sex as a social practice or community norm to reduce exposure to and transmission of HIV [33, 36, 43–47]. For many men, it was a choice between life and death. This response was not engineered or even led by public health; rather, it was indigenous. Perhaps many gay men comprising this indigenous response to HIV had similar values to those extolled by Callen and Berkowitz when they developed and disseminated their historic pamphlet "How to Have Sex in an Epidemic," which outlined strategies to avoid contracting the as-yet-unknown infectious agent through sex [14, 48]. Though not prevention research, the dissemination of this book and other interventions developed by and for gay men at risk for HIV transmission can be seen as an antecedent and a beginning to a structure that facilitated the development of CBPR in gay communities. Gay men developed sensibilities about prevention and mobilized and organized a response to the threat of the disease itself, a disease that had the potential to completely wipe out gay communities, as well as to lead to draconian public health measures (e.g., quarantine), should viable alternatives not be demonstrated.

Thus, the early response to the pandemic within gay communities featured education and support in the form of forums, workshops, small-group support and discussion groups; dissemination of messages through informal social networks; and modeling of safer behaviors. Social support was coordinated informally for affected community members who had challenges with activities of daily living, and case management for care was established where care was extremely expensive and/ or hard to navigate. Informal caregiving was transformed into community-based organizations like the GMHC, the first AIDS-service organization in the country. GMHC formalized and expanded one-on-one support to persons with HIV into what became to be known as "buddy programs"—which probably can be called the core service of early AIDS-service and HIV-focused community-based organizations. Buddy programs were initially community-based programs designed to meet the needs and provide those with HIV social support through telephone calls, home visits, meals, and other support with activities of daily living. The idea of these types of programs came about as some families, friends, coworkers, and even providers were fearful of being close to those with HIV. Many persons with HIV and their caregivers (e.g., lovers, partners/spouses, and friends) were abandoned by some within their social networks, and some feared disclosure.

Some of these congregate programs also have been described as gay community-building through the construction of collective community identities and social support as key components of prevention [49]. Institutions like GMHC were formed by gay men and their allies to support the community in fighting AIDS. These community structures themselves and can be viewed as both agents and outcomes of prevention action.

Advocacy was done by formal organizations like GMHC as well as through informal social movements like ACT UP (the AIDS Coalition to Unleash Power). The role ACT UP played in treatment advocacy is well acknowledged [50]. Furthermore, AIDS Project Los Angeles (APLA), another formal organization that had emerged similarly to GMHC, was perhaps among the first to notice and report, due to its routine client survey process, that persons with AIDS were living longer; this longevity soon was known to be the result of more effective treatments [51].

As mentioned previously, many of the early efforts to respond to the HIV epidemic involved gay men and their close allies. For example, Michael Quadland, who had a master's degree in public health and a doctorate in psychology had strong ties to the gay community in New York City and was a prevention researcher and founder of the GMHC clinical program. Dr. John L. Martin, PhD, a gay man with AIDS working at Columbia University, established a pioneering community sample of gay men in New York City to study the effect of HIV/AIDS longitudinally. He was one of the first to identify successful HIV harm-reduction strategies used among MSM (e.g., cessation of receptive anal intercourse and reduction in number of sexual partners) and the effects of AIDS-related bereavement on psychologic distress among gay men [52, 53]. David Ostrow, MD, PhD, also a gay man living with HIV, was instrumental in initiating the Multicenter AIDS Cohort (MAC) study [54]. Enrollment in MAC began in 1984 and was designed to follow men who were either HIV negative or positive to explore the natural history of HIV, identify risk factors for occurrence and clinical expression of the infection, and establish a repository of biologic specimens for future study [55]. Among his many contributions, Sociologist Martin P. Levine, another gay man with AIDS, consulted with the pharmaceutical company Burroughs Welcome to support HIV-prevention research and advocacy for gay men [56].

These are just a few of perhaps thousands of examples of gay men and their allies who led the charge, and continue to contribute heavily, to HIV prevention and care in the USA (and around the world). They exemplify community insiders who mobilized and organized to take and promote action.

Even we, as authors of this chapter, became involved in the epidemic as gay men who wanted to contribute our talents, perspectives, experiences, and insights to contribute to HIV prevention and care. Although today we are doctoral-level researchers, we came from a place within a community where friends, partners, and family were affected by HIV. Dr. Rhodes (third author of this chapter), for example, was an undergraduate in college when then US Surgeon General C. Everett Koop published and sent to every US household an 8-page brochure about HIV/AIDS transmission, including the role condoms can play to reduce HIV exposure and transmission. When he read the plea on the back page of the brochure for volunteers to provide education and support within their local communities, he felt a sense of duty to support other gay men. He volunteered for a local AIDS service organization in Columbia, South Carolina. It was this initial step that lead him to channel his community activism as an out gay man into work as a health educator at the Whitman Walker Clinic in Washington, DC, after he graduated college. In time, he earned a PhD to meet community-identified research needs and priorities and fill HIV-prevention research knowledge gaps through community engagement and partnership.

Overall, from the beginning of the HIV pandemic, gay men have been at the forefront of prevention and advocacy efforts, with involvement as city, county, state, and federal employees; as those making funding decisions and working on public health prevention efforts at all levels; as leaders in advocacy, AIDS-service and community-based organizations, and coalitions; and as academics and researchers at other types of institutions, which overlap AIDS-service and community-based organizations, in some cases. In addition, gay men also have participated in all levels of prevention research, from scientists to project managers, data collectors, and those whose lives, experiences, mental processes, behaviors, and bodies have been researched. Their involvement continues. As stated earlier, these early efforts were not referred to as CBPR, but in retrospect, met many if not all of the principles of CBPR from community identification of the research question or need through community input on all aspects of research.

The Federal Role, the Availability of Funding, and Intervention Science

Most likely resulting from community mobilization and organization at multiple levels reaching multiple audiences, the earliest federal prevention program funding called for community-based prevention programs and demonstration projects to include collaboration with affected communities (e.g., gay communities) [57]. Early demonstration projects were predicated on public health authorities establishing and using community-based organizations as collaborative partners [58, 59]. Whether the demonstration projects were actually based in collaborations with gay (and other) communities and were participatory is not clear, but there was much emphasis on ethnic and racial minorities and less emphasis on prevention within gay communities [60]. Furthermore, we know that the values and principles of CBPR as currently articulated were not adhered to. In 1989, the US Centers for Disease Control and Prevention (CDC) began to directly support AIDS-service and community-based organizations doing prevention work in the USA [58]. Prior to this, local health authorities had supported such programs as they continue to do today, mostly through funds provided by CDC cooperative agreements to health departments.

As funding became more available through the CDC, the National Institutes of Health, and foundations, prevention research became more academic than community driven and prevention efforts became more top–down. However, by the early 1990s, some researchers were moving toward developing interventions and programs that relied on the structure of the gay community and, in so doing, began moving toward a greater emphasis on engaging community members in the process and intervening at a community level. Community-level interventions and programs were highlighted rather than CPBR; however, some of these efforts would be considered aligned with CBPR values and principles.

For instance, Kelly and colleagues identified key popular opinion leaders within gay communities in several small cities in an intervention study that today would reflect some of the values and principles of CBPR [61]. Although the popular opinion leaders did not participate fully in all facets of the research from beginning to the end, the researchers engaged gay men from the local community to deliver the cognitive behavior-change intervention, which was designed by Kelly and his team of researchers and practitioners. These popular opinion leaders were identified as key community assets that could positively effect behavior change. Thus, there was a growing recognition of the importance of community involvement and buy-in in investigator-initiated research; this recognition reverberated into prevention research within other communities that were and are disproportionately affected by HIV.

The Mpowerment intervention, widely disseminated by the CDC as an intervention for young MSM, is largely the brainchild of a gay man living with AIDS, Robert Hays (working with Susan Kegeles and others) [62, 63]. The Mpowerment intervention, further described in Chap. 11, is perhaps the most clearly community focused of all the interventions included in the Diffusion of Effective Behavioral Interventions (DEBI) Project in terms of its guiding principle of building supportive and healthy communities for young gay men. Mpowerment was developed by researchers, some of whom came from the larger gay community, focused on community health issues for young gay men, and relied heavily on community engagement and mobilization working with community organizations. The DEBI Project, also outlined in Chap. 11, is a CDC initiative that identifies interventions meeting CDC-established criteria for research-based evidence and generates materials intended to support widespread uptake and implementation of these interventions in community-based, programmatic, nonresearch-oriented contexts. These interventions were not widely implemented in the USA until 2004, when the CDC embraced the dissemination of evidenced-based, behavioral risk reduction interventions. Regrettably, this implementation occurred late in the pandemic. Was this CBPR? It certainly meets some criteria for CBPR in retrospect were it presented as such today. It was developed by researchers some of whom came from the larger gay community, focused on community health issues for young gay men, and relied heavily on community engagement and mobilization working with community organizations.

Blurred Boundaries: Gay Community and CBPR

There is always the question of community and community identity. CBPR can focus on gay men in a particular geographic community. At times, gay men might be a predominant demographic category for a community such as West Hollywood,

California, or Wilton Manors, Florida. At other times they may be a minority group in a community, but we can still focus CBPR on a particular community within a larger community. For example, HIV-prevention CBPR with Latino gay and bisexual men and MSM is being conducted in North Carolina [19, 20, 39, 40, 42]; see also Chap. 7. Furthermore, the use of CBPR approaches is influenced by whether the focus of community is on (1) geographic or neighborhood communities characterized as gay communities by virtue of their majority gay-identified demographic, (2) geographic or neighborhood communities where gay men (perhaps including nongay-identified MSM) are a minority component, (3) gay subcommunities (e.g., leather, bear, bareback, online Internet, and app-using men) that may share identity or geographic or virtual space, or (4) a larger gay identity at a regional, national, or international level.

Initial responses to the onslaught of HIV/AIDS by gay communities and gay persons within existing social structures (e.g., politics, medicine, and social and other sciences) preceded the more academic interests of funded HIV/AIDS-prevention research. Then, as now, there were gay men who were politicians, doctors, writers, celebrities, researchers, activists, etc., and some (for instance Randy Shilts [http://www.nndb.com/people/295/000177761/] and Cleve Jones [http://www.clevejones.com/mainmenu.htm] among many others) were able to use their position to bring attention to HIV prevention and care. Intense interest by concerned scientists, politicians, and others regardless of their sexuality was influenced and informed by those gay men who were part of the existing social structure, driving the research agenda from within the community. Early academic interests in HIV prevention and care often ran parallel to community interests or simply documented and explored community responses [45, 64]. Those responses were often untested interventions and programs, which, in time, became natural experiments. Though not CBPR, such responses were community-based intervention and were at times analyzed as prevention research or were further developed as prevention research or evaluation projects. Such interventions and programs included buddy programs (as previously described); peer navigation (use of trained health advisors to help their peers reduce HIV exposure and transmission); outreach and education; advocacy and social action promoting social, political, and structural (environmental) changes; condom-use strategies; small-group support groups; case management for higher-risk individuals; and, more recently, positional harm-reduction or harm-minimization strategies (e.g., anal insertive and oral receptive). Again, though not identified as CBPR, some of these projects would meet some CBPR criteria as research developed with and engaging gay communities in prevention research, action, change, or a combination of the three.

As an example, early in the HIV epidemic, both San Francisco and New York City governments sought to close bathhouses, commercial establishments that promote social and sexual networking among MSM. Eventually, these two city governments took a negotiated approach, working with bathhouse owners, managers, and staff and representatives from local communities to make environmental changes to the actual bathhouse space to limit opportunities for unsafe sex. These sometimes contradictory policies became natural experiments. In San Francisco, doors were removed from private rooms within bathhouses to eliminate privacy and thus limit secluded areas where sex might occur. In New York City, bathhouses eliminated public spaces where unsafe sex might occur [65]. Although neither policy was found to be effective in reducing risk behavior, such community engagement in responding to the threat of HIV created an opportunity for those from academics and public health to collaborate with members of a community who were already heavily engaged in meeting community needs and priorities. Although not CBPR projects, these natural experiments included input and action from the gay community and other principles of CBPR.

Funding Prevention, Politics, and Communities of Identity

As a result of a socially conservative US Congress and its passage of the Helms Amendment in 1987, federal agencies were restricted from funding any research that might be considered as "promoting homosexuality and promiscuity." The Amendment prohibited the CDC from funding AIDS programs that "promote, encourage or condone homosexual activities." The Senate passed it, 96 to 2. Only 47 House members resisted this homophobic action and opposed the Amendment. Unfortunately, the Amendment negatively influenced prevention research and public health through the early 1990s, undeniably resulting in insubstantial funding for HIV prevention specifically within gay communities [66], and thus, reducing prevention efforts among gay men and increasing lives lost to HIV.

Not surprisingly, however, besides the ongoing effort for gay communities to mobilize and meet the prevention needs of their own communities, much funding for HIV prevention initially arose from members of gay communities themselves. Despite socioeconomic status, gay men and their close allies donated large amounts of money to AIDS-service and community-based organizations. Some spent their own money to provide direct prevention services (e.g., purchasing and distributing condoms); fund their own research (e.g., providing incentives for participation); and provide support directly to those with HIV (e.g., purchasing food, clothing, transportation, and drugs). Interestingly, this move toward funding by those who identified as gay may have enhanced a focus of prevention and prevention research on identity-based risk reduction rather than one based solely on behavior [66]. Identity-based risk implies that gay men are at risk for HIV because they self-identify as gay; whereas behavioral risk implies that it is not how someone identifies but rather what they do behaviorally that puts them at risk for HIV.

Thus, prevention research, including that based on the values and principles associated with CBPR, was not immune to the well-documented stigmatization of same-sex behavior—that gay men are at risk simply because of their same-sex sexual practices rather than their exposure to the HIV pathogen [33, 35, 66]. Although early advocates and researchers, including those from the gay community, worked to frame risk around behavior (thus resulting in the emergence of the term MSM), CBPR focuses on community as a unit of identity [27]. The focus on behavior, as opposed to identity, implies that by reducing HIV to behavior, how members of communities identify themselves and their characteristics tied to their identities were not important. However, the pendulum is swinging, as some have found that for some communities, identity as a gay man may be key to HIV prevention and risk reduction [18, 19, 39, 40, 42, 67]. The change in nomenclature from MSM is controversial in some circles, as MSM has itself become a label for identity, even as it was developed to clearly label behavior rather than identity [68]. Overall, CBPR emphasizes local relevance and meaningfulness.

CBPR as an Approach for Action

CBPR is, by its very nature, action oriented; it is research conducted in response to a public health challenge, such as an increase in the rate of disease or health disparities among vulnerable populations. CBPR is not about knowledge generation for its own sake; it is designed to generate knowledge for action [6, 12, 19, 20, 27, 69]. In the case of the emergence of the HIV pandemic, people were dying, and little was being done; there was a health crisis in which gay men were carrying a disproportionate burden yet they were also part of a stigmatized community, facing discrimination, with little "power." Thus, gay men first mobilized, organized, and acted independently setting the stage for prevention research efforts that would follow. It makes sense that members of communities must be fully engaged and broad partnerships with members with diverse perspectives, experiences, and insights must be built, harnessed, and maintained. Furthermore, methods most often associated with CBPR are often geared toward community mobilization, empowerment, and ecologic validity to improve community health. The evolving responses to the epidemic set the stage for prevention research that was enmeshed with gay community action, organization, and engagement.

We have spent a great deal of this chapter describing and discussing the history of community engagement and partnership by gay communities early in the HIV pandemic, and we now turn to a more current example of engagement and partnership. We describe how representatives from federal, state, and local public health programs and community partners, including those from AIDS-service and HIV-focused community-based organizations, gay community centers, and advocacy organizations, among others, mobilized and organized around a national syphilis epidemic. Although this example is not solely HIV focused, the links between syphilis and HIV are clear, and the community described is the community of gay and bisexual men and other MSM.

Syphilis Among Gay and Bisexual Men and MSM

Data show that primary and secondary syphilis rates continue to increase among gay and bisexual men and MSM, who account for more than 70% of all persons with infection [70]. During the 1990s, syphilis primarily occurred among hetero-sexual men and women of racial and ethnic minority groups. However, the tide shifted and cases began to increase among gay and bisexual men and MSM [34]. A growing number of these cases have been reported among young gay and bisexual men and MSM, with the highest rates being found for MSM 20–29-years old [70].

Although the health problems caused by syphilis in adults are serious in their own right, it has been shown that the genital sores caused by syphilis make it easier to transmit and acquire HIV infection sexually. There is an estimated twofold to fivefold increased risk of acquiring HIV if exposed when syphilis is present, and studies have also shown that syphilis will increase the viral load of someone who is already infected with HIV. These facts are especially concerning, as data from several major US cities suggest that about four in ten MSM with syphilis are also infected with HIV [34]. Thus, it is critically important to better understand syphilis exposure and transmission among MSM in order to decrease the rates of subsequent HIV infection.

Rapid Ethnographic Assessments: A Method of Qualitative Data Collection, Analysis, and Interpretation

Rapid ethnographic assessment is a team-based method of rapid qualitative data collection often used to assess program needs, inform intervention develop-ment, and provide feedback to policymakers [71–74]. Based on ethnographic principles of eliciting an understanding or description of the problem from the perspective of community-engaged insiders, rapid assessments are particularly useful to better understand the health and well-being of what are commonly re-ferred as "hidden" or "hard-to-reach" communities and populations. Members of these communities and populations may only be hidden from or hard-to-reach by traditional, outside researchers and practitioners. As a methodology, rapid as-sessments have a long history of success in international public health and have been used in recent years in numerous countries to document and describe the HIV and sexually transmitted disease (STD) prevention needs of sex workers and clients, as examples [75–78]. Methodologies applied to promote community engagement and input at multiple points in ethnographic action research can be synchronous with those of CBPR.

Between 1998 and 2005, CDC scientists conducted one consultation and seven rapid ethnographic assessments to understand a resurgence of syphilis within com-munities of gay and bisexual men and MSM. Particularly concerning was that many of the men infected with syphilis were men with preexisting HIV infection, a find-ing that indicated that these men were not using precautions to reduce HIV exposure and transmission. The ethnographic assessments were conducted in Los Angeles, California; Seattle, Washington; Philadelphia, Pennsylvania; Fort Lauderdale, Flor-ida; suburban Washington, DC; Portland, Oregon; and suburban Chicago, Illinois. Respondents were approached at public venues or interviewed by appointment at agencies providing health or community services to gay men. These assessments used standard research protocols for the collection of scientific ethnographic data [34]. However, the intent of these assessments was based on implementation of a public health response to disease. As such, these investigations were deemed to be public health responses rather than research as defined by federal guidelines for distinguishing between research and nonresearch [79].

All aspects of the rapid ethnographic assessments—from planning through data collection, data analysis and interpretation, report development, recommendations, and implementation—were undertaken as a collaborative effort among representatives from federal, state, and local public health programs and community partners, including those from AIDS-service and community-based organizations, gay community centers, advocacy organizations, and patient advocates, among others. These partners worked together to plan and implement the assessments and collaborated on data analysis and interpretation. Because of the infrastructure that has developed around HIV prevention, the assessments often began through work with existing community planning groups, commonly known as "CPGs." CPGs are composed of representatives from service providers, state and local health departments, and other community members who work cooperatively to develop comprehensive HIV-prevention plans for their regions and/or states. (CPGs are further described in Chap. 9.) Additional representation from community members and agencies was sought; additional leaders, community members, and entities were identified through the process of conducting the assessments; and many of these individuals were engaged in the process as well. Throughout the process, the ethnographic methodologies of working with the data and the public health activities of community engagement matched many of the methods, values, and principles considered to underlie CBPR [27, 34, 80]. As with other examples we present, though meeting criteria for CBPR, this scientific work was conducted without being defined as CBPR.

The rapid ethnographic assessments provided information about gay and bisexual men's and MSM's sexual risk and social responses to HIV, syphilis, STDs, and sexual health overall, and greater understandings of formal and informal community leaders and local public health systems, including government and community agencies. This work resulted in key, concrete actions that were grounded in the needs of the communities affected as determined by the collaborative partnership working on the assessment. These actions were implemented to improve public health prevention services (and thus community health) in each local community. For example, one county health department collaborated with community leaders and a local community-based organization to provide clinical STD services in a designated neighborhood gay men's health clinic that was characterized as a commercial, social, and residential center for gay communities [34]. Furthermore, the Los Angeles County Jail modified its regulations to allow condoms in the holding area for incarcerated gay men when the rapid assessment there showed that a lack of condoms contributed to increases in STDs among the inmate population [80].

Future Directions of CBPR for HIV Prevention Among Gay Men

One of the clear impacts of HIV among gay men on CBPR is the historical legacy of prevention research driven by community members. That legacy encourages us to consider how well our research and practice represent the voices of those we work with and for and whether the result of our work is truly addressing the needs and priorities of community members and populations [35], as opposed to our own needs and priorities. As researchers and practitioners, we often have needs and priorities that compete with authentically engaging with communities. It takes careful reflection to ensure that our work comes from and has meaning for the communities we work with and serve. CBPR is grounded in the voices and experiences of community members and moves away from a more colonial and privileged view of the scientist as the sole generator and proprietor of knowledge and the primary expert on topics that, in reality, are known best by community members. CBPR moves toward engagement, inclusivity, and participation by all, including community members, organization representatives, business owners and staff, and researchers, to bring diverse expertise to promote community health and prevent disease.

However, there is a risk of losing a critical element of CBPR that was clearly exemplified in the gay community's initial mobilization and organization around HIV; this critical element is action. As CBPR becomes more embedded within academic and research institutions, researchers may pursue basic and theoretical research and pay less attention to action to promote positive community change. Although basic research and a strong theoretical framework are valuable and an understanding of best processes (as opposed to practices) of CBPR can be beneficial [81, 82], the loss of a focus on health-promoting action should be considered with attention to all of its ramifications. Early HIV-prevention research within gay communities was action oriented by necessity because members of the community were dying. There was no time to lose; immediate action was called for. At its core, CBPR implies that the research conducted will result in actions to address the needs and priorities of communities and improve their health; however, there seems to be some slippage as CBPR gains in its use and popularity among researchers. We contend that there is a need to ensure that CBPR is synonymous with action, within HIV or other health issues. In fact, at the very foundation of CBPR is maintaining an eye on action and how knowledge gained can be used to reduce and eliminate health disparities explicitly. This explicit action goes beyond HIV. Action is the goal of CBPR when applied to other health issues facing vulnerable populations.

Rationale Underlying CBPR Within HIV Prevention

Besides the inherent values of inclusion, self-determination, and democracy associated with CBPR, a basic reason for the careful use of CBPR, which often resonates with traditional paradigms, is the increased ecologic validity of research and resultant health-promoting and disease-preventing actions (e.g., interventions, programs, and policy changes). Including multiple perspectives and their triangulation are important to this end [12]. It has been suggested that CBPR picks up where traditional outside-expert approaches to research and community health promotion fall short. As has been noted, "The model of prevention science advocated by the Institute of Medicine [83] …fails to consider community and organizational capacity to implement programs, ignores the need for congruence in values between programs and host sites, displays a pro-innovative bias that undervalues indigenous practices and assumes a simplistic model of how community organizations adopt innovations" [38].

The frequently lauded, dominant, and domineering approach to traditional science-based intervention development that relies on controlled lab experiments or statistical and/or physical control through random assignment is increasingly recognized as untenable with dynamic sociocultural phenomena such as human sexual behavior, social change, and human services. These are not relatively inert physical phenomena that are reliably or validly controlled for in an artificial environment, and relevant environmental factors may not be conceptualized and/or incorporated in these studies. A robust method of research is needed to discover highly relevant but otherwise unidentified factors and to develop actions that have higher likelihood of fitting with the lived, highly dynamic sociocultural environment and affecting the most robust and relevant determining factors of these social phenomena, like aspects of human sexuality.

CBPR can address these needs and promises deeper understanding [12, 18, 19]. Community-grounded, and even community-driven, prevention research bears promise to overcome translational problems. If the need for translation and translational research can be reduced through research conducted in the real world in which translation occurs and is necessary to have a significant impact on public health, the so-called time to market can be reduced and that impact can be realized and maximized. Too often, interventions and programs deemed innovative are not really innovative when they arrive to communities, perhaps because the sociocultural environment has changed so much during the time to market that the prescribed actions no longer resonate with the experiences of community members.

Ongoing and structural (not just community-embraced and community-placed, but community-embedded), CBPR is meant to be sustainable and, hence, to build capacity [12, 15]. In addition to promises for greater ecologic validity, translational potential, and capacity building, there are other, not dissimilar, reasons for CBPR, such as its promise in helping (1) to locate members of communities and populations who may be considered hidden and difficult to reach by researchers and other community outsiders; (2) to establish rapport for ongoing engagement, recruitment, and retention; and (3) to motivate community members to feel empowered to be part of the effort to meet their own priorities, build their own and their community's capacity, and access and utilize their unique insider knowledge, etc.

Discussion and Conclusion

The advocacy of gay men and organizations related to HIV prevention and treatment continues to have far-reaching influence for HIV and other health issues, from breast cancer and health care reform [84] to changes in FDA regulations regarding access to investigational drugs [85], and mental health services [86]. Some of these influences are well documented. Boehmer points out the relationship of feminism and women's movements as an influence on AIDS activism, which in turn influenced breast cancer. Lesbians and other women who were AIDS activists brought their experience and expertise to breast cancer activism [87], politicizing breast cancer as ACT UP did with AIDS and modeling the breast cancer quilt after the AIDS quilt, as examples [88]. It is clear that gay men in the USA were responsible for incredible social action and change to better understand the HIV pandemic as it first emerged, and for developing prevention interventions, programs, and strategies to meet the needs and priorities of their own communities. They, and their allies, laid the foundation and have built structures for HIV-prevention programs, prevention research, and evaluation. They have been the subjects of and advisors to still other HIV-prevention programs and prevention research; as has been noted, "They [gay men] have served as researchers, study subjects, community participants, and fundraisers, and have advocated for flexible, rapid, and inclusive study designs and regulatory approaches" [14]. We do not discount the contributions of those from nongay communities; however, the historical example of HIV prevention by, for, and within gay communities exemplifies the values and principles underlying CBPR.

The example of gay men and their close allies engaged in prevention and control of HIV and the direct threat it posed is compelling; however, the implications for CBPR are not entirely transferable. We have illustrated CBPR as an emergent community-driven process and in so doing, added to an understanding of the range of community involvement in CBPR by providing a case in which members from within the community itself engaged in most, if not all, aspects of prevention-research development; financing and fundraising; intervention development, implementation, and evaluation; study participation; and data analysis, interpretation, and dissemination. For the most part and especially early in the pandemic, gay men and their close allies were not partnered with community outsiders. Although community-driven research of the type that we have described has had an important effect addressing HIV exposure and transmission within gay communities, influencing drug development policy, and serving as an example of community activism for other diseases; it raises additional questions as to the role of communities in CBPR and the definition or identification of CBPR.

Other diseases and health concerns have their own unique characteristics that influence the role of communities, scientists, research participants, funders, and others involved in health research and action. What are the optimal roles for these individuals, institutions, and communities? What can we learn by examining the structure of CBPR in terms of those involved in all its aspects from generation of ideas to implementation and beyond? An examination of these and other questions about how CBPR is carried out might help to ensure that such research meaningfully addresses the health concerns of individuals and their communities.

References

1. Curran JW, Jaffe HW. AIDS: the early years and CDC's response. MMWR Surveill Summ. 2011;60(Suppl 4):64–9.
2. Bieber I, Dain HJ, Dince PR, Drellich MG, Grand HG, Gundlach RR, et al. Homosexuality: a psychoanalytic study of male homosexuals. New York: Basic Books; 1962.
3. Andriote JM. Victory deferred: how AIDS changed gay life in America. Chicago: University of Chicago Press; 1999.
4. Bayer R. AIDS and the gay community: between the specter and the promise of medicine. Soc Res: Int Quart. 1985;52(3):581–606.
5. Bowie J, Eng E, Lichtenstein R. A decade of postdoctoral training in CBPR and dedication to Thomas A. Bruce. Prog Community Health Partnersh. 2009;3(4):267–70.
6. Cashman SB, Adeky S, Allen AJ, Corburn J, Israel BA, Montaño J, et al. The power and the promise: working with communities to analyze data, interpret findings, and get to outcomes. Am J Public Health. 2008;98(8):1407–17.
7. Israel BA, Krieger J, Vlahov D, Ciske S, Foley M, Fortin P, et al. Challenges and facilitating factors in sustaining community-based participatory research partnerships: lessons learned from the Detroit, New York City and Seattle Urban Research Centers. J Urban Health. 2006;83(6):1022–40.
8. Minkler M. Community-based research partnerships: challenges and opportunities. J Urban Health. 2005;82(2 Suppl 2):ii3–12.
9. O'Fallon LR, Dearry A. Community-based participatory research as a tool to advance environmental health sciences. Environ Health Perspect. 2002;110(Suppl 2):155–9.
10. Wallerstein NB, Duran B. Using community-based participatory research to address health disparities. Health Promot Pract. 2006;7(3):312–23.
11. Yonas MA, Jones N, Eng E, Vines AI, Aronson R, Griffith DM, et al. The art and science of integrating undoing racism with CBPR: challenges of pursuing NIH funding to investigate cancer care and racial equity. J Urban Health. 2006;83(6):1004–12.
12. Rhodes SD, Malow RM, Jolly C. Community-based participatory research: a new and not-so-new approach to HIV/AIDS prevention, care, and treatment. AIDS Educ Prev. 2010;22(3):173–83.
13. Crimp D. Introduction. In: Crimp D, editor. AIDS: cultural analysis and cultural activism. Cambridge: MIT Press; 1988. p. 3–16.
14. Trapence G, Collins C, Avrett S, Carr R, Sanchez H, Ayala G, et al. From personal survival to public health: community leadership by men who have sex with men in the response to HIV. Lancet. 2012;380(9839):400–10.
15. Altman D. Power and community. Organizational and cultural responses to AIDS. London:Taylor and Francis; 1994.
16. Shalowitz MU, Isacco A, Barquin N, Clark-Kauffman E, Delger P, Nelson D, et al. Community-based participatory research: a review of the literature with strategies for community engagement. J Dev Behav Pediatr. 2009;30(4):350–61.
17. Minkler M, Wallerstein N. Introduction to community-based participatory research. In: Minkler M, Wallerstein N, editors. Community-based participatory research for health: fome processes to outcomes. San Francisco: Jossey-Bass; 2008. p. 5–23.
18. Rhodes SD, Duck S, Alonzo J, Downs M, Aronson RE. Intervention trials in community-based participatory research. In: Blumenthal D, DiClemente RJ, Braithwaite RL, Smith S, editors. Community-based participatory research: issues, methods, and translation to practice. New York: Springer; 2013. p. 157–80.
19. Rhodes SD, Duck S, Alonzo J, Daniel J, Aronson RE. Using community-based participatory research to prevent HIV disparities: assumptions and opportunities identified by The Latino Partnership. J Acquir Immun Defic Syndr. 2013;63(Suppl 1):S32–5.
20. Rhodes SD. Demonstrated effectiveness and potential of CBPR for preventing HIV in Latino populations. In: Organista KC, editor. HIV prevention with Latinos: theory, research, and practice. New York: Oxford; 2012. p. 83–102.

21. Shilts R. And the band played on. Politics, people, and the AIDS epidemic. New York: St. Martin's Press; 1987.
22. Hunter ND. Censorship and identity in the age of AIDS. In: Levine MP, Nardi PM, Gagnon JH, editors. In changing times: gay men and lesbians encounter HIV/AIDS. Chicago: University of Chicago Press; 1997. p. 39–54.
23. Jenkins RA. Challenges in engaging community participation in HIV prevention research. Prog Community Health Partnersh. 2007;1(2):117–9.
24. Tax S. The fox project. Hum Organ. 1958;17(1):17–9.
25. Steckler AB, Dawson L, Israel BA, Eng E. Community health development: an overview of the works of Guy W. Steuart. Health Educ Q. 1993;(Suppl 1):S3–20.
26. Roussos ST, Fawcett SB. A review of collaborative partnerships as a strategy for improving community health. Annu Rev Public Health. 2000;21:369–402.
27. Israel BA, Schulz AJ, Parker EA, Becker AB. Review of community-based research: assessing partnership approaches to improve public health. Annu Rev Public Health. 1998;19:173–202.
28. Rhodes SD. Community-based participatory research. In Blessing JD, Forister JG, editors. Introduction to research and medical literature for health professionals. 3rd ed. Burlington: Jones & Bartlett; 2013. p. 167–87.
29. Freire P. Pedagogy of the oppressed. New York: Herder and Herder; 1970.
30. Freire P. Education for critical consciousness. New York: Seabury Press; 1973.
31. Tierney WG. Self and identity in a postmodern world: a life story. In: McGloughlin D, Tierney WG, editors. Naming silenced lives: personal narratives and processes of educational change. Routledge; 1993.
32. Foley DE. The fox project. A reappraisal. Curr Anthropol. 1999;40(2):171–92.
33. Odets W. AIDS education and harm reduction for gay men: psychological approaches for the 21st century. AIDS Public Policy J. 1994;9(1):2–11.
34. Bloom FR, Leichliter JS, Whittier DK, McGrath JW. Gay men, syphilis, and HIV: the biological impact of social stress. In: Feldman DA, editor. AIDS, culture, and gay men. University Press of Florida; 2010. p. 21–40.
35. Bolton R. AIDS and promiscuity: muddles in the models of HIV prevention. Med Anthropol. 1992;14(2–4):145–223.
36. Martin JL, Dean L, Garcia M, Hall W. Barbara Snell Dohrenwend memorial lecture. The impact of AIDS on a gay community: changes in sexual behavior, substance use, and mental health. Am J Community Psychol. 1989;17(3):269–93.
37. Valdiserri R. Gardening in clay: reflections on AIDS. Ithaca: Cornell University Press; 1994.
38. Miller RL, Shinn M. Learning from communities: overcoming difficulties in dissemination of prevention and promotion efforts. Am J Community Psychol. 2005;35(3–4):169–83.
39. Rhodes SD, Daniel J, Alonzo J, Duck S, Garcia M, Downs M, et al. A systematic community-based participatory approach to refining an evidence-based community-level intervention: the HOLA intervention for Latino men who have sex with men. Health Promot Pract. 2013;14(4):607–16.
40. Rhodes SD, Hergenrather KC, Vissman AT, Stowers J, Davis AB, Hannah A, et al. Boys must be men, and men must have sex with women: a qualitative CBPR study to explore sexual risk among African American, Latino, and white gay men and MSM. Am J Mens Health. 2011;5(2):140–51.
41. Rhodes SD, Vissman AT, Stowers J, Miller C, McCoy TP, Hergenrather KC, et al. A CBPR partnership increases HIV testing among men who have sex with men (MSM): outcome findings from a pilot test of the CyBER/testing internet intervention. Health Educ Behav. 2011;38(3):311–20.
42. Rhodes SD, Hergenrather KC, Aronson RE, Bloom FR, Felizzola J, Wolfson M, et al. Latino men who have sex with men and HIV in the rural south-eastern USA: findings from ethnographic in-depth interviews. Cult Health Sex. 2010;12(7):797–812.
43. Jaffe HW, Valdiserri RO, De Cock KM. The reemerging HIV/AIDS epidemic in men who have sex with men. JAMA. 2007;298(20):2412–4.
44. Centers for Disease Control and Prevention. Self-reported behavioral change among gay and bisexual men—San Francisco. MMWR Morb Mortal Wkly Rep. 1985;34(40):613–5.

45. Martin JL. The impact of AIDS on gay male sexual behavior patterns in New York city. Am J Public Health. 1987;77(5):578–81.
46. Winkelstein W Jr, Samuel M, Padian NS, Wiley JA, Lang W, Anderson RE, et al. The San Francisco men's health study: III. Reduction in human immunodeficiency virus transmission among homosexual/bisexual men, 1982–86. Am J Public Health. 1987;77(6):685–9.
47. Joseph JG, Montgomery SB, Emmons CA, Kessler RC, Ostrow DG, Wortman CB, et al. Magnitude and determinants of behavioral risk reduction: longitudinal analysis of a cohort at risk for AIDS. Psychol Health (London). 1987;1(1):73–96.
48. Berkowitz R. Stayin' alive. The invention of safe sex, a personal history. Boulder: Westview; 2003.
49. Shernoff M, Bloom DJ. Designing effective AIDS prevention workshops for gay and bisexual men. AIDS Educ Prev. 1991;3(1):31–46.
50. Halcli A. AIDS anger andactivism: ACT UP as a social movement organization. In: Freeman JL, Johnson V, editors. Waves of protest: social movements since the sixties. New York, NY:Rowman and Littlefield; 1999. p. 135–50.
51. Klosinski L. PWAs preparing to join work force, survey finds. http://wwwthebodycom/content/art32590html (1998).
52. Martin JL, Dean L. Effects of AIDS-related bereavement and HIV-related illness on psychological distress among gay men: a 7-year longitudinal study, 1985–1991. J Consult Clin Psychol. 1993;61(1):94–103.
53. Martin JL, Garcia MA, Beatrice ST. Sexual behavior changes and HIV antibody in a cohort of New York city gay men. Am J Public Health. 1989;79(4):501–3.
54. Sosin K. AIDS: Dr. David Ostrow: following trajectory of AIDS. Windy City Times. 2012 Feb 12–29.
55. Kaslow RA, Ostrow DG, Detels R, Phair JP, Polk BF, Rinaldo CR Jr. The Multicenter AIDS Cohort Study: rationale, organization, and selected characteristics of the participants. Am J Epidemiol. 1987;126(2):310–8.
56. Kimmel MS, Gagnon JH. http://www2.asanet.org/governance/MartinLevine.html. Accessed 22 March 2005.
57. Valdiserri RO. Achieving an AIDS-free generation: it's the details that matter. Public Health Rep. 2012;127(6):563–4.
58. Bailey ME. Developing a national HIV/AIDS prevention program through state health departments. Public Health Rep. 1991;106(6):695–701.
59. Beyrer C, Wirtz AL, Walker D, Johns B, Sifakis F, Baral SD. The global HIV epidemics among men who have sex with men (MSM). http://elibraryworldbankorg/content/book/9780821387269 (2011).
60. Bailey ME. Community-based organizations and CDC as partners in HIV education and prevention. Public Health Rep. 1991;106(6):702–8.
61. Kelly JA, St Lawrence JS, Stevenson LY, Hauth AC, Kalichman SC, Diaz YE, et al. Community AIDS/HIV risk reduction: the effects of endorsements by popular people in three cities. Am J Public Health. 1992;82(11):1483–9.
62. Kegeles SM, Hays RB, Coates TJ. The mpowerment project: a community-level HIV prevention intervention for young gay men. Am J Public Health. 1996;86(8 Pt 1):1129–36.
63. Kegeles SM. Obituary for Robert B. Hays. Am J Community Psychol. 2003;31(3/4):357.
64. Stall RD, Hays RB, Waldo CR, Ekstrand M, McFarland W. The Gay '90s: a review of research in the 1990s on sexual behavior and HIV risk among men who have sex with men. AIDS. 2000;14(Suppl 3):S101–14.
65. Woods WJ, Binson D. Public health policy and gay bathhouses. J Homosex. 2003;44(3–4):1–21.
66. Sessions KB, Cervero RM. The politics of planning HIV/AIDS education and the disenfranchisement of HIV negative gay men. Stud Contin Educ. 1999;21(1):3–19.
67. Reece M, Dodge B. A study in sexual health applying the principles of community-based participatory research. Arch Sex Behav. 2004;33(3):235–47.
68. Boellstorff T. But do not identify as gay: a proleptic genealogy of the MSM category. Cult Anthropol. 2011;26(2):287–312.

69. Israel BA, Eng E, Schulz AJ, Parker EA. Introduction to methods in community-based participatory research for health. In: Israel BA, Eng E, Schulz AJ, Parker EA, editors. Methods in community-based participatory research. San Francisco: Jossey-Bass; 2005.

70. Centers for Disease Control and Prevention. Sexually transmitted disease surveillance, 2011. Atlanta: U.S. Department of Health and Human Services; 2012.

71. Beebe J. Rapid assessment process: an Introduction. Walnut Creek: AltaMira Press; 2001.

72. Trotter RT, Needle RH, Goosby E, Bates C, Singer M. A methodological model for rapid assessment, response, and evaluation: the RARE program in public health. Field Methods. 2001;13(2):137–59.

73. Bloom F. Research report: rapid assessment and syphilis. Anthropol News. 2001;42(2):56.

74. Scrimshaw SCM, Carballo M, Carael M, Ramos L, Parker RG. HIV/AIDS rapid assessment procedures: rapid anthropological approaches for studying AIDS related beliefs, attitudes, and behaviours. Cambridge: Harvard Center for Population Studies; 1991.

75. Aral SO, St Lawrence JS. The ecology of sex work and drug use in Saratov Oblast, Russia. Sex Transm Dis. 2002;29(12):798–805.

76. Centers for Disease Control and Prevention. International Rapid Assessment Response and Evaluation (I-RARE) training curriculum for field workers. Atlanta: Centers for Disease Control and Prevention; 2005.

77. Needle R, Kroeger K, Belani H, Achrekar A, Parry CD, Dewing S. Sex, drugs, and HIV: rapid assessment of HIV risk behaviors among street-based drug using sex workers in Durban, South Africa. Soc Sci Med. 2008;67(9):1447–55.

78. Parry CD, Dewing S, Petersen P, Carney T, Needle R, Kroeger K, et al. Rapid assessment of HIV risk behavior in drug using sex workers in three cities in South Africa. AIDS Behav. 2009;13(5):849–59.

79. Centers for Disease Control and Prevention. Guidelines for defining public health research and public health non-research. http://wwwcdcgov/od/science/integrity/docs/defining-public-health-research-non-research-1999-pdf (1999).

80. General Accounting Office (GAO). Federal programs: ethnographic studies can inform agencies' actions. GAO-03-455. http://www.gao.gov/cgi-bin/getrpt?GAO-03-455 (2003).

81. Green LW. From research to "best practices" in other settings and populations. Am J Health Behav. 2001;25(3):165–78.

82. Green LW, George MA, Daniel M, Frankish CJ, Herbert CJ. Study of participatory research in health promotion. Vancouver: Royal Society of Canada; 1995.

83. Mrazek PJ, Haggerty RJ. Committee on prevention of mental disorders IoM. Reducing risks for mental disorders: frontiers for prevention research. Wahington, DC: National Academies Press; 1994.

84. Beyrer C. ACT UP!: a history in film. Lancet. 2012;380(9839):329.

85. Pripstein J. When science and passion meet: the impact of AIDS on research. CMAJ. 1993;148(4):638–42.

86. Miller R. Clinicians, researchers and community activism: lessons for mental health services from another field of medicine—HIV/AIDS. Psychiatr Bull. 2013;37(3):81–4.

87. U. B. The personal and the political: women's activism in response to the breast cancer and AIDS epidemics. Albany: State University of New York; 2000.

88. Klawiter M. The biopolitics of breast cancer: changing cultures of disease and activism. Minneapolis: University of Minnesota; 2008.

Chapter 5
HIV Prevention Interventions with Adolescents: Innovations and Challenges in Partnerships across the Integrated Transitions Model

Amanda E. Tanner, Morgan M. Philbin and Alice Ma

The period of adolescence, defined by the Society for Adolescent Health and Medicine as ages 10–25-years old [1], involves immense physical, biologic, and cognitive changes, including rapid maturation, experimentation, and risk [2]. Provision of health care for adolescents remains challenging and complex, as it encompasses general medical needs and factors specific to cognitive and psychosocial developmental phases. Accordingly, adolescent medicine emerged as a subspecialty of pediatrics to address many of the developmental issues and social needs unique to adolescence [3, 4]. A purely physiologic approach is insufficient for comprehensive adolescent health; instead, a psychosocial, holistic orientation that maximizes adolescent development and health is necessary to address the complexities that characterize adolescence [3]. Adolescents must manage new physical and emotional challenges, maintain healthy bodies, and learn skills and responsibilities needed for adulthood (e.g., obtaining jobs).

The physical, emotional, and social changes typical of adolescent development also can heighten their risk of HIV exposure and transmission [2]. For instance, the developing adolescent brain can limit what some may label as responsible decision-making, thereby increasing sexual risk behaviors without the adolescent fully considering longer-term consequences [2, 5]. Thus, HIV-related research and intervention and program development, implementation, and evaluation must consider

A. E. Tanner (✉) · A. Ma
Department of Public Health Education, University of North Carolina Greensboro,
1408 Walker Ave, 437 HHS Building, PO Box 26170, Greensboro, NC 27402, USA
e-mail: aetanner@uncg.edu

A. Ma
e-mail: f_ma@uncg.edu

M. M. Philbin
Department of Health, Behavior & Society, Johns Hopkins University School of Public Health,
Baltimore, MD, USA
e-mail: mp3243@columbia.edu

HIV Center for Clinical & Behavioral Studies, Columbia University and New York State
Psychiatric Institute, 1051 Riverside Drive, Unit 15, New York, NY 10032, USA

S. D. Rhodes (ed.), *Innovations in HIV Prevention Research and Practice*
through Community Engagement, DOI 10.1007/978-1-4939-0900-1_5,
© Springer Science+Business Media New York 2014

adolescent-specific issues such as brain development (e.g., abstract thinking skills), assent and consent (e.g., being under 18-years old and parental consent), insurance (e.g., public and parents'), and disclosure (e.g., to parents and to current and potential sexual partners) [6, 7]. Interventions and programs must further be tailored to the contexts and communities in which adolescents live.

In the USA, the incidence of HIV is rapidly increasing among adolescents and young adults 15–24-years old [2]. Approximately 56,300 Americans become HIV-positive each year; of these, 34%—or approximately 19,000—are 13–29-years old [8]. In 2009, an estimated 8,294 adolescents and young adults between 13- and 24-years old were diagnosed with HIV infection in the 40 states with long-term HIV reporting [9].

High rates of HIV among adolescents, coupled with the typical developmental processes of adolescence, suggest that HIV-prevention efforts are essential for both adolescents at risk for HIV acquisition and those who have HIV [2]. Primary prevention interventions focus on preventing HIV exposure and transmission to uninfected adolescents to keep them negative and increase their self-protective behaviors and skills [10, 11]. These types of interventions can take various forms, including biomedical approaches such as clinical trials to evaluate HIV-preventive vaccines, microbicides, and preexposure prophylaxis and behavioral methods to increase condom use and reduce numbers of partners [10]. Secondary prevention serves to minimize, alleviate, or prevent health and psychologic consequences among adolescents with HIV [11] and examine behavioral and therapeutic interventions, ideally at earlier stages of infection, to prevent disease progression [10]. Secondary prevention can also be designed to preserve both the health of adolescents with HIV and the health of their potential sexual partners, including test-and-treat initiatives [12] and disease management strategies such as earlier initiation of antiretroviral therapy (ART) [10].

Both primary and secondary HIV-prevention and -care efforts for adolescents should consist of interdisciplinary collaborations that address the complexity of the population and comorbidities, as well as mental, psychiatric, and neurocognitive disorders [10]. Partnerships among academic researchers; representatives from educational and testing organizations, health departments, clinics, and other community-based organizations (including youth-serving organizations); and adolescents themselves are essential. These partnerships can encourage innovative strategies that address adolescent-specific issues related to HIV prevention, diagnosis, and care, as well as cultural norms and gender role expectations particular to adolescents, their developmental stage, and their local communities. Such collaborations can increase understanding during exploratory and formative evaluation phases, inform the development of interventions and programs that are most relevant to adolescents, and increase the likelihood that interventions and programs will be implemented, found to be effective, and sustained (if warranted) by communities. Prevention programs may benefit from partnerships between academic researchers, clinicians, and other providers and youth-serving organizations to address the substantial adolescent-specific barriers that they may experience, including their feeling invincible to HIV (or perhaps more precisely a willingness to "play the odds"), discomfort communicating about sexual issues, unfamiliarity with care systems, and limitations with transportation [13–15]. Some academic researchers, clinicians, and other providers partner directly with adolescents, whereas others partner with youth-serving organizations.

In this chapter, we use the *integrated model of continuities and transition in adolescent/youth HIV prevention, diagnosis and treatment* [16], and the care continuum [17] to illustrate innovative adolescent HIV-prevention interventions and programs that engage adolescents and representatives from community organizations, incorporate partnerships, and promote community participation along a continuum. Specifically, we explore two types of partnership strategies—youth- and organization-engaged—throughout this chapter. First, we provide an overview of the model's phases and associated programs with (and without) partnerships with adolescents and community organizations. We conclude with lessons learned and directions for future community-engaged research, interventions, and programs for primary and secondary HIV prevention with adolescents [11].

Integrated Model and Care Continuum: An Overview

The *integrated model of continuities and transition in adolescent/youth HIV prevention, diagnosis, and treatment* (referred to as the integrated model; [16]) provides a framework for understanding the relationships between adolescents and HIV infection and highlights the importance of partnerships across networks. This model moves from primary HIV-prevention services through testing and care, and promotes consideration of the specific needs of adolescents both before and, if necessary, after HIV exposure and transmission (Fig. 5.1). The progression of adolescents through the integrated model is used within this chapter to highlight their unique vulnerability to HIV and potentially reduced access to services, factors that are particularly important, given that adolescents comprise a significant proportion of those with HIV in the USA.

Furthermore, the ongoing narrative in the USA regarding gaps in addressing the HIV and AIDS epidemic needs to consider the care continuum [17]. Generally, the steps in the care continuum include [1] the identification of HIV status, [2] active linkage in care, [3] initiation of ART, [4] retention in care, and [5] eventual suppression of viral load [17]. The care continuum also offers a way to visualize the number of individuals with HIV throughout the country and their rates of attrition as they move from being identified to getting therapy to having stable undetectable viral loads. In 2011, CDC scientists analyzed HIV surveillance datasets and laboratory reports to estimate the number of HIV-positive people at each step of the care continuum (Fig. 5.2; [18]). CDC scientists concluded that for every 100 individuals living with HIV, 80 were aware of their status, 62 had been linked to HIV care, 41 were engaged in HIV care, 36 received ART, and of those, 28 had acheived viral suppression (beneficial for both improved health quality and decreased transmission capability; [17]).

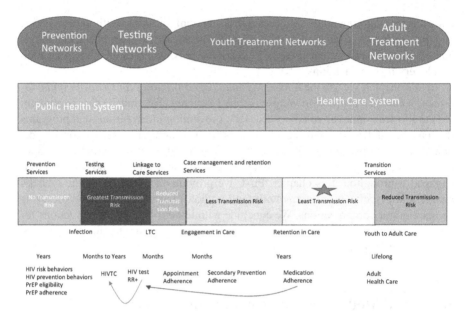

Fig. 5.1 An integrated model of continuities in transition in adolescent/youth HIV prevention, diagnosis, and treatment. *PrEP* Pre-exposure prophylaxis, *HIVTC* HIV testing and counseling, and RR+ Rapid results are positive

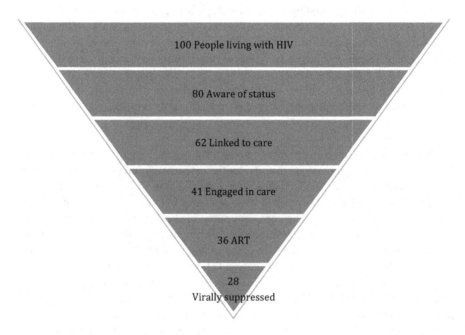

Fig. 5.2 Care continuum. (Adapted from Garnder et al. 2011)

Providers, policymakers, and representatives from organizations across all levels—federal, state, and local—use the care continuum to identify gaps in service delivery across the continuum of HIV testing and care, and thus identify opportunities for well-designed and focused interventions and programs. The care continuum also highlights the work that needs to be done for retention in care to improve quality of life for individuals living with HIV and for population-level reductions in the incidence of HIV.

Together, the integrated model and care continuum provide an innovative, useful, and comprehensive framework for considering the challenges of identifying and treating adolescents with HIV. Rates of infection and attrition are partially due to both developmental and structural barriers that exist for adolescents across all the phases of the integrated model and, if positive, the care continuum.

For primary prevention services, adolescents may not feel at risk for HIV acquisition, in part because of their developmental stage (e.g., feeling invincible or "playing the odds;" [2]). Similarly, adolescents with HIV may find it difficult to acknowledge their disease because they do not feel sick and thus do not seek out testing to confirm their status [14]. Attending medical appointments may be perceived as a reminder of their serostatus, which adolescents may choose to avoid [14]. Adolescents with associated comorbidities (e.g., substance use, mental health issues, and housing instability) are especially unlikely to be linked to needed HIV care [9]. Other barriers to HIV testing and care include the following [19–25]:

- Individual characteristics (e.g., stigma, shame, and denial regarding HIV and risk behavior, low educational attainment, and psychiatric disorders)
- Family characteristics (e.g., lack of financial resources and/or medical/health insurance, family dysfunction, and past and current neglect/abuse)
- Health care system characteristics (e.g., costs to patients, services available, access, mistrust of health-care professionals, concerns about confidentiality, and difficulty negotiating complex health-care systems)
- Provider and treatment characteristics (e.g., shortage of providers with expertise in both HIV and adolescent medicine, the extent of adolescent-friendly staff and services, and complexity of medical regimens, although regimens are becoming simpler).

These potential barriers differ from those for adults because adolescents are often still in school and tend to be dependent on others for resources, insurance, transportation, and access to clinics and pharmacies [26]. This dependence on others such as family members, for example, requires disclosure of HIV risks and/or status, which may have potential benefits (e.g., social support), but disclosure also can place adolescents at risk for backlash and ostracism [27]. The rates of retention, medication adherence, and health outcomes are poor for adolescents diagnosed with HIV, making it especially important to keep them from being exposed to HIV and becoming positive.

Prevention, testing, and care networks must collaborate in order for adolescents to avoid HIV infection or, if infected, to move seamlessly across each stage of the integrated model (Fig. 5.1) and through the care continuum (Fig. 5.2). Although adolescents have been successfully engaged in multiple types of research, intervention, and programmatic efforts—for instance, education [28], physical activity and healthy eating [29], and violence [30]—adolescent engagement in HIV prevention is more limited [31, 32]. The available HIV-prevention efforts have demonstrated two types of partnerships that have been most successful: academic researchers, clinicians, and other providers partnering directly with adolescents or partnering with community- and faith-based organizations that serve youth (e.g., churches and organizations working with lesbian, gay, bisexual, and transgender [LGBT] adolescents and homeless adolescents). We explore these two types of partnership strategies—youth- and organization-engaged—throughout this chapter.

Integrated Model: Phases and Programs

The integrated model describes the different points of transition for adolescents' needs related to primary prevention, testing, and care that emphasizes secondary prevention (e.g., treatment as prevention; [16]). These phases of the integrated model and interventions and programs associated with each phase are described here. Some of these programs involve youth and/or organizational engagement; the programs presented also provide an overview of adolescent HIV prevention across a range of needs, highlight the importance and challenges of working with adolescents, and provide strategies for developing engagement and partnership.

Preventing HIV Among Adolescents

Overview Prevention often takes the form of outreach and education to identify and increase awareness among adolescents at higher risk for HIV acquisition. Adolescents at elevated risk for HIV include ethnic and sexual minorities [8, 9]. In 2010, African–American/black adolescents accounted for 69 % of HIV diagnoses reported among individuals 13–19-years old, and Latino/Hispanic and white adolescents accounted for 15 % and 14 %, respectively [33]. Among male adolescents 13–19-years old, approximately 91 % of all diagnosed HIV infections stem from male-to-male sexual contact [8]. Indeed, adolescent men who have sex with men (MSM) between the ages of 13–24 were the only age-group to have an increase in new infections between 2001 and 2006 [2]. In 2009, adolescent MSM accounted for 27 % of total incident cases, and MSM 13–29-years old accounted for 69 % of new HIV infections [9]. There is also an interaction between race and sexual orientation; 63 % of all adolescent MSM 13–24-years old with HIV infection in 2009 were African–American/black, followed by white (18 %) and Latino/Hispanic (16 %; [8]).

Although any adolescent can acquire HIV, particular attention should be given to these so-called hidden or hard-to-reach adolescents [34, 35, 36] to ensure that efforts have an impact and address the needs of those at higher risk of HIV exposure and transmission. Of course, being considered hidden or hard-to-reach is purely subjective; most often these terms describe being difficult to reach by community outsiders (e.g., academic researchers, clinicians, and other providers).

Primary prevention for adolescents who are at higher risk for HIV acquisition is also increasingly complex due to a range of factors, including comorbidities, such as substance use and mental-health issues, that increase the risk of HIV exposure and transmission [36]. Such complexities reinforce the importance of meaningful prevention. The integration of substance use and mental health services into HIV prevention can be an important step in reaching those adolescents at elevated risk [37].

As illustrated, HIV disproportionately affects specific adolescent population subgroups, which implies that prevention programs must address their unique issues, needs, and priorities, including perceptions of risk and substance use and abuse [38]. This need emphasizes the importance of research and programmatic partnerships (e.g., a social service organization that provides counseling services). Accordingly, a variety of partnership strategies have been employed to prevent HIV exposure and transmission among higher risk adolescents. Again, these include working directly with adolescents or indirectly through youth-serving organizations.

Youth-engaged Partnerships A variety of primary prevention programs involve adolescents, sometimes as full partners. Adolescents participate in these programs by recruiting other adolescents, developing suitable materials, assessing the cultural appropriateness of the programming, and implementing the program.

Within these youth-engaged partnerships that include academic researchers; representatives from educational and testing organizations, health departments, clinics, and other community-based organizations (including youth-serving organizations); and adolescents, different strategies have been employed in HIV prevention. For example, a rural HIV-prevention study used participant-driven recruitment to reach and recruit adolescents living in rural upstate New York [32]. The study used peers who built trust and recruited their adolescent peers to participate in an intervention. An important component of peer recruitment, in rural and urban areas, is the inclusion of adolescents from varied and diverse population subgroups [39]. Partnering with adolescents from different backgrounds can be more effective for reaching a broad spectrum of higher-risk adolescents. This inclusivity can also serve to sustain and further partnership efforts [32, 39].

Adolescent partners also inform the development and design of appropriate methods and materials. In the HIV-prevention study just noted, a pilot group of nine adolescents developed the educational sessions and modified the research protocols and questionnaire to reflect the context and language of local adolescents [32]. Their involvement in the design and implementation of the study enhanced their familiarity with, and commitment to, the research and its process and success. Their engagement was further validated by posters presenting the themes garnered from design and implementation discussions that illustrated for adolescent partners' concrete contributions to the study. Two members of the pilot group were later involved as paid research assistants to plan and facilitate survey and educational sessions, assist with data interpretation, and coauthor a journal article about the study. These varying levels of research opportunities and involvement contributed to the success of the study, given that adolescents were treated as significant and nontoken partners. This involvement may have motivated them to recruit other young people to participate. The inclusion of adolescent partners in this study helped reach segments of the rural adolescent population that would not have been reached and engaged otherwise, thereby contributing to its success [32].

Organization-engaged Partnerships Another strategy academic researchers, clinicians, and other providers apply to engage adolescents, especially those at higher risk for HIV, is the formation of partnerships with youth-serving organizations, including community-based organizations working with LGBT or minority racial/ethnic communities and faith-based organizations. Prevention efforts that are delivered in partnership with specific organizations can be important vehicles to disseminate sensitive but accurate information. For example, faith-based organizations have helped reach African–American/black adolescents, which is essential given the disproportionate impact of HIV on this population [33]. Similar to youth-engaged programs, organization-engaged partnerships can facilitate successful recruitment, development and implementation of culturally congruent interventions and programs, and intervention sustainability. Providing sexual health training to organizational leaders, as part of the co-learning within partnerships, can enhance sustainability through building the capacity of community- and faith-based organizations to address HIV in their own communities, particularly with the support of trusted community partners [13, 40–43].

For some minority populations, community-based organizations have played an important role in the delivery of HIV-prevention services [44]. One prevention intervention, SHERO (a female-gendered version of the word "hero"), was developed, implemented, and evaluated by a collaboration of academic researchers and representatives of a Latino-serving organization. This intervention addressed the gender- and culture-specific psychosocial and ecologic factors that influence HIV risk and protection for Mexican–American female adolescents [44]. SHERO demonstrates that collaborating with community organizations to implement HIV interventions and programs can assist in ensuring a high level of cultural congruence and a realistic potential of sustainability, if warranted [44]. Safer sexual behaviors and beliefs among Mexican–American female adolescents increased after participating in the 9-session SHERO intervention, compared with a single information-only HIV-prevention control session, demonstrating the value of tailoring an intervention to reflect cultural factors [44]. The quality of these community-based partnerships and the care taken by academic researchers to maintain them was essential for the recruitment and retention of adolescent participants and for the participation of additional community-based organizations to widen the reach of the program [42, 44, 45]. It is important to note that each community and community-based organization is unique, so interventions and programs that involve partnerships among academic researchers, clinicians, and other providers are more likely to be successful [43]. For instance, a diverse coalition that worked to implement Project Bold, Ready, Intelligent, Dedicated, Guided, & Equipped (Project BRIDGE) generated initial ideas to develop a meaningful and context-appropriate HIV curriculum with experiential activities tailored to African–American/black middle-school students attending evening church sessions. The combined skills and active participation of the partners enhanced the likelihood that the HIV–prevention materials were meaningful and appropriate for, and thus respectful of, the unique culture and values of community members and the missions of partner organizations [40, 42, 43]. Further, the success of Project BRIDGE led to program growth and sustainability, with plans for continued collaborative activities and possible expansion to other churches and to schools. Part of the program's success may be attributed to its original goals, which sought to harness religious affiliation as a protective benefit, while also reducing risk behaviors related to adolescence. Moreover, the faith community's values and concerns were aligned and congruent with those of the academic researchers for the common goal of reducing HIV exposure and transmission [42].

The engagement and participation of adolescents in programs can be facilitated by organizational staff (e.g., youth pastors and outreach workers), whose intimate involvement in the study design can convey confidence and trust in the process to adolescents and parents [42, 43]. For example, the high level of engagement among adolescents in Project BRIDGE was attributed to the active involvement of organizational partners in the design and implementation of the program and to the building on existing strengths and resources of community partners [40, 43].

The YOUR Blessed Health intervention provides another example of the capacity of faith leaders and faith-based organizations to mobilize around prevention of HIV and other sexually transmitted infections (STIs) among adolescents in predominately African–American/black communities. The YOUR Blessed Health intervention was developed in collaboration among the Faith Access to Community Economic Development, Flint Odyssey House Health Awareness Center, Pastors' Spouses of Genesee County, the University of Michigan School of Public Health, and the YOUR Center. After careful networking and trust building and ongoing relationship maintenance, this partnership developed a multilevel HIV- and STI-prevention intervention that respected church doctrine and built on faith-based institutional capacity to effectively promote HIV prevention. To date, more than 350 faith leaders from 55 churches across nine different dominations have trained over 15,000 congregants. Faith leaders' involvement in the YOUR Blessed Health program enhanced the credibility of the intervention and the participating faith-based organizations' capacity to address HIV with their congregants and in their communities [40, 46], and resulted in sustainability, further uptake, and broad reach of the intervention. The increased trust as a result of this intervention helped to increase HIV/AIDS awareness and reduce HIV-related stigma among the African–American/black faith community and among vulnerable adolescents.

Summary A partnership approach to the development and implementation of each of these interventions and programs has helped to cultivate trust among academic researchers; representatives from community and youth-serving organizations, health departments, clinics, and adolescents. Without a doubt, trust is necessary for the engagement and participation of adolescents in, and the success of, HIV prevention interventions [43]. The partnerships highlighted established trust among the partners. The high level of collaboration inherent in community-engaged prevention allowed each partner, including adolescents, to contribute to all phases of planning and implementation processes. Issues such as cultural congruence can be addressed as needed, thereby creating and ensuring a common foundation of understanding in each phase of the project [41, 42]. The highlighted interventions and programs underscore the value of culturally grounded HIV primary prevention services that are created in collaboration with adolescents and other partners to address ecologic factors affecting adolescents' HIV-related risk.

Identifying HIV-Positive Adolescents

Overview The middle section of the integrated model focuses on testing and counseling services for adolescents. These services are essential to identify adolescents with HIV and prevent secondary infections. Furthermore, efforts to reach higher risk adolescents are important, as comorbidities (e.g., substance use and abuse and mental health issues) and frequent double stigma (i.e., race and sexual orientation) faced by adolescents may make it more challenging for them to seek testing services. These efforts help promote HIV testing by increasing accessibility and also by changing attitudes and beliefs to "normalize" testing [47, 48]. The hidden nature of higher risk adolescents has challenged academic researchers, clinicians, and other providers to develop and implement interventions and programs that have a community presence and can overcome the reluctance of adolescents to get tested and subsequently treated [34, 35]. Several interventions and programs have focused on innovative efforts to reach adolescents and increase HIV counseling and testing, including peer outreach workers to overcome barriers (e.g., insurance accessibility and mistrust of health-care professionals), mobile testing units, and venue-based testing programs (e.g., bars and clubs; [47]). In this section, we describe some of these types of intervention and programs; however, we do not describe venue-based testing programs, as they tend to be ubiquitous.

Youth-engaged Partnerships Programs engaging adolescents have utilized a variety of strategies to increase HIV counseling and testing, including peer outreach workers from local communities and mobile testing units. The Teen Outreach Project University of Miami (TOP-UM), the Adolescent HIV/AIDS Project at the New Jersey Medical School, and the Chicago HIV Risk Reduction Partnership for Youth (CHRRPY) all used peer outreach to expand HIV testing services to higher risk adolescents [34, 39, 49]. Adolescents with HIV were involved as peer outreach workers who partnered with testing program staff to conduct pretest counseling, distribute educational materials, and facilitate follow-up appointments with higher risk adolescents [34, 39]. The incorporation of peer outreach workers in these programs helped overcome adolescents' mistrust of traditional health-care professionals and reluctance to approach clinics. Using peer outreach workers also increased the acceptability of HIV testing and counseling [34, 39,

49]. The results from these programs suggest that peer partners recruited from the community and representative of the diversity of affected adolescent subgroups are able to best reach and engage other adolescents. For instance, peer partners from particular subgroups and/or subcultures were familiar with where adolescents congregated. Thus, they operated comfortably and easily within these settings [39]. Furthermore, they were more familiar with the way language was used and with the subtleties of language, which facilitated communication with adolescents, and, as a result, HIV testing [39].

In conjunction with peer outreach workers, mobile testing units staffed by peer educators, social workers, and counselors delivered HIV testing as a way to connect with adolescents who were resistant and/or reluctant to access and utilize traditional testing services [34, 49]. The mobile unit traveled to community settings where adolescents congregated "on-the-street," thus serving to increase accessibility of testing services and reduce transportation barriers by going to adolescents rather than having adolescents come to them [49]. Inside the mobile units, adolescents received confidential screening for HIV infection, STIs, and mental health issues; were given appropriate referrals; and were offered prevention materials and risk-reduction counseling [49]. In addition, the mobile units provided HIV medical care and support services, such as case management, counseling, and peer advocacy [34] to ensure that adolescents who tested positive returned for posttest counseling and linkage to HIV treatment [49].

Organization-engaged Partnerships Academic researchers, clinicians, and other providers have also often developed partnerships with youth-serving organizations to help identify HIV-positive adolescents in different settings and transition them into care [39]. Some HIV-counseling and -testing programs have partnered with agencies providing services to homeless adolescents, gay youth, youth detainees, and gang members [34]. For instance, staff from CHRRPY partnered with a large variety of youth-serving organizations to link clinical and program services. This partnership increased the number of adolescents receiving HIV counseling and testing, reduced adolescent risk behaviors, and, among adolescents who tested HIV-positive, increased the number that entered into comprehensive health-care clinics for early intervention and care [34, 39].

The Boston HIV Adolescent Provider and Peer Education Network for Services Program partnered with a network of youth-serving organizations, including multiservice outreach agencies, community health centers, and hospitals, to reach adolescents who were HIV-positive, homeless, and/or considered by community outsiders as hard-to-reach [50]. This collaboration served to provide a coordinated network of care for adolescents unable to access consistent care. The Division of Adolescent Medicine at Children's Hospital Boston was the lead agency and primary site of HIV clinical care [50], and collaborative organizations covered a wide gamut of services, including case management, case coordination across sites, adolescent and HIV clinical care, and HIV education and training.

Social media/marketing campaigns have also formed partnerships with advertising and health communications agencies, adolescents, health-care providers, academic researchers, community-based organizations (e.g., Boys and Girls Club), and community advisory boards to promote HIV testing through adolescent-focused efforts [47, 51, 52]. These types of innovative partnerships can maximize the reach of the campaign and enhance its relevance to adolescents—both important aspects in connecting with difficult-to-reach adolescents. Particular methods that can be used in forming effective messages to reach adolescent population subgroups include identifying competing narratives [51] that support healthy sexual behaviors while rejecting perceived norms of risk behaviors, consulting adolescents themselves to ensure their opinions are included in the development of intervention and program materials [47, 51, 52], and using culturally congruent messages to enhance protective health beliefs and behaviors [51, 52]. For instance, HIV-prevention campaigns with messages targeted to African–American/black adolescents presented messages that reflected African–American/black oral culture (e.g., skilled and expressive speech; [51]), included African–American/black adolescent actors [52], and partnered with advertising agencies that had experience in reaching this population [51].

By using social marketing to promote HIV testing through adolescent-focused efforts, such campaigns can normalize and reduce the stigma of HIV testing among adolescents and thus change their attitudes about such testing, while at the same time promote more routine testing among health providers [47, 53]. The relevance and quality of partnerships involved in these campaigns is a vital component to success in promoting the visibility of HIV infection and testing among adolescents, thus, increasing the number of higher risk adolescents participating in HIV counseling and testing.

Summary Partnerships among academic researchers; representatives from educational and testing organizations, health departments, clinics, and other community-based organizations; and adolescents themselves can help to locate adolescents considered by community outsiders as hidden and hard-to-reach and to increase uptake of HIV counseling and testing. Adolescents in particular may be more comfortable and more likely to receive HIV testing in community-based (e.g., mobile testing units) rather than clinic-based venues, in part because of relatively low rates of adolescents seeking routine health care and low rates of providers and other staff offering testing to adolescents in clinical settings [54]. However, rates of successful linkage to care are lower in community-based settings compared with clinic-based settings [55]. Thus, better linkage to care in these venues is clearly needed to overcome adolescents' potential difficulty navigating fragmented care systems [e.g., separate testing and care sites; [56]).

Linking, Engaging, and Retaining HIV-Positive Adolescents in Care

Overview The final phase of the integrated model is care services, which includes linkage to, and engagement and retention in, care for adolescents with HIV. Care services for secondary prevention refer to a systematic process of initiation of, and maintenance in, medical, psychologic, and social services. Care linkage refers to the systematic process of initiating HIV-related medical, psychologic, and social services for persons with newly diagnosed HIV [57]. Linkages that result in sustained engagement improve health outcomes among those with HIV and are important for community-level reduction in HIV exposure and transmission [58–60]. It remains a challenge for many providers to establish adolescents with HIV in care in a way that will preserve their health and prevent further disease transmission [10, 47]. Linkage to care is particularly relevant for adolescents with HIV, who encounter more obstacles and challenges compared with adults (e.g., insurance, disclosure, and transportation; [61]) and are living with an often asymptomatic chronic illness [49].

Not being linked to and engaged in care is associated with delayed initiation of medication and poorer long-term clinical outcomes [59, 61]. Younger adolescents with HIV, in particular, have more difficulty establishing linkages with, and being retained in, care [61], which increases their risk of morbidity and mortality [62, 63]. Indeed, younger age is associated with worse retention to care in the first 2 years following an HIV diagnosis [60], and those with HIV who are younger than 35 years have more difficulty establishing, and being retained in, care [61]. This difficulty may be due in part to the relatively few HIV-related health services specifically designed for adolescents. Interventions and programs that aim to identify, engage, and retain adolescents with HIV ideally offer, or arrange for, medical care, case management, psychosocial support, and secondary prevention counseling [64].

Living with a chronic illness, adolescents with HIV face a lifetime of clinical care as they transition into adulthood. Routine health maintenance, ART adherence, and care retention across the life course are paramount as adolescents move through the integrated model [2, 65]. Tailoring services to their unique needs can serve to keep them engaged and retained in routine care [64] including during the transition from adolescent to adult care. This is a crucial period that hinges on the availability and accessibility of clinics specialized to address and welcome transitioning adolescents who may be hesitant to move from a youth-tailored clinic [15, 48].

Youth-engaged Partnerships Several interventions and programs have worked to address the barriers to linking and keeping adolescents in care through youth-engaged research and programming to create a seamless transition from diagnosis to care [66, 67].

The peer-run organization known as Bay Area Young Positives (BAY Positives) was designed to decrease isolation, reduce risk behaviors, and promote advocacy skills among adolescents with HIV. Among its services, the program provides care linkage through its peer-based support and mentorship model [68, 69]. The organization has found that when young people are brought together to support each other, living with HIV becomes more manageable. The program also serves as a link to the clinical care system, empowering infected young people to gain information about and access to available services [68].

The Mobile SafeSpace program in New York City also used a peer education model to enhance program acceptability and help transition adolescents into care [49]. A fully equipped motor home served as an outreach unit and provided a comprehensive continuum of supportive services for street youth, including HIV testing, transport to safe and secure shelter, and connection to other necessary services. The program connected youth into care by traveling twice per day to areas where street youth congregated so that they could access these services [49].

Similarly, some of the Adolescent Medical Trials Network (ATN) clinics have used peer advocates (other adolescents with HIV) in its clinics. When they meet with peer advocates, adolescents with newly diagnosed HIV are able to see someone living successfully with HIV and can ask questions that they may not feel comfortable discussing with their providers. These advocates help improve the relationships between adolescents with newly diagnosed HIV and clinic staff.

Community-based organizations have also more recently begun establishing HIV-specific youth advisory boards or committees in which adolescents are partners in program development and implementation. For instance, youth advisory boards at ATN clinics inform clinical policy (e.g., appointment protocols) and programs (e.g., "open mic night") [24]. The adolescents provide insights into their needs and priorities and offer suggestions to make the clinic a place that is welcoming to adolescents with HIV. In addition, at several ATN sites, staff (e.g., child life specialists) collaborate directly with the youth advisory boards and other adolescents to develop and obtain resources for adolescent-specific programs designed to enhance adolescent engagement with the clinic [24].

Adolescent involvement in interventions and programs aimed at linkage, engagement, and retention in care is essential given that adolescents with newly diagnosed HIV face barriers at clinics because of their potential lack of experience with the health-care system. Adolescents with HIV may be more likely to engage in care services if they have support from other adolescents, who may reduce their perceived fear and distrust of clinics, while also providing social support [49, 68].

Organization-engaged Partnerships In conjunction with direct youth engagement, academic researchers, clinicians, and other providers partner with youth-serving organizations to support care linkage and engagement. One ATN program, the Strategic, Multisite Initiative for the Identification, Linkage and Engagement in Care of Youth with Undiagnosed HIV Infection (the Care Initiative), was designed to facilitate care linkages and engagement processes for adolescents with newly diagnosed HIV through formal partnerships between the ATN clinical sites, local health departments, and community-based organizations. A memorandum of understanding between partners was developed to describe linkage-to-care processes, specify public health authority (if any) granted to the program, and specify sharing (if any) of patient-related data. These partnerships allowed for a more streamlined process from diagnosis to care across testing and treatment networks [15]. The program also assisted with care engagement through relationship development between adolescents and staff and increased connections of adolescents to clinics [24].

Another ATN-specific strategy is the development of community coalitions through Connect2Protect [70]. The Connect2Protect coalitions are designed to address structural issues related to HIV-prevention strategies, including facilitating adolescents' engagement in HIV-related services [70].

After an adolescent is linked to care, the primary goals become supporting this adolescent's retention in care and medication adherence, once prescribed. These activities typically occur within the clinic, limiting the utilization of partnership models. One useful strategy for maintaining adolescents in care is active case management and the provision of integrated, comprehensive services [37, 71]. The Division of Adolescent Medicine at Children's Hospital Los Angeles implemented an integrated care model for adolescents with HIV that included HIV care plus psychosocial services such as case management, counseling, and related ancillary services [71]. A key aim of this project was to ensure the privacy and confidentiality of HIV status for adolescents in the waiting room to decrease passive disclosure and increase comfort with and confidence in the clinic [71]. Other work has addressed the role of adolescent-friendly clinics in facilitating engagement in HIV care among adolescents [24]. Through these adolescent-focused efforts, adolescents with HIV may be more likely to remain in care because of increased trust of health-care professionals and acceptability of care settings and services [24].

After being engaged in care and prescribed medical therapies, HIV medication adherence becomes of utmost importance for adolescents, especially within the treatment as prevention model [12, 92]. Research illustrates that adolescents' perceptions of, and experiences with, ART is largely negative, indicating that adolescents may need support for managing their care and treatment regimens [72]. Accordingly, adolescents have low rates of reported adherence [76] and of achievement and maintenance of undetectable viral loads [77]. There is interest in improving adolescent adherence to medication regimens through the use of directly observed therapy [73], support group networks [74], and social media (e.g., Facebook and MSM networking sites [75]). Although existing research has supported the feasibility of a modified directly observed therapy among adults in particular, few studies have determined feasibility with adolescents. Community-based modified directly observed therapy programs tailored to the unique needs of adolescents with HIV can improve adherence to medication regimens and provide psychosocial, public health, and other medical benefits, particularly social and emotional support gained from relationships with program staff [72, 73] or peers [74]. For example, to promote adolescent adherence to ART, the Therapeutic Regimens Enhancing Adherence in Teens (TREAT) Program used adolescents' perspectives to develop and implement an evidence-based clinical intervention to promote optimal, long-term adherence to medication among adolescents with HIV [76].

Increasing adolescents' comfort with care-seeking behaviors can also be enhanced through the connection to "place" (e.g., clinic and community-based organization) and/or "people" (e.g., peer educators and program staff), in addition to the provision of appropriate and needed services. Adolescents with HIV, particularly those who are difficult to engage in care, have a unique set of needs and motivations affecting their care behaviors. These potential issues may be alleviated as comfort increases with the specific clinic space and/or as relationships develop with a peer or program staff [24, 35, 37, 49]. Connection to place and people who are trained in adolescent-specific issues and contexts can facilitate progression through the integrated model, especially at the crucial moments of care linkage and transition to adult care [24].

Summary Overall, care linkage programs have benefited from partnerships across diagnostic and care networks (Fig. 5.1); engagement in care programs have relied more exclusively on clinic resources. Improvements in retention in care could be made through engaging adolescents and youth-serving organizations in the programming process.

Lessons Learned

Benefits and Challenges of Youth-Engaged Partnerships

The integrated model provides a variety of lessons related to HIV prevention and care among adolescents. Creating interventions and programs that address the specific needs, interests, and priorities of adolescents requires their engagement and participation. In partnering with adolescents, academic researchers and representatives from educational and testing organizations, health departments, clinics, and other community-based organizations, for example, should ensure that adolescents are engaged in effective and meaningful participation [32].

First and foremost, adolescents' knowledge and experience make them important partners in HIV-prevention research and programs. The value of including adolescents lies in the insights they can provide in understanding contextual issues, perceptions, and areas of need. These insights can help to enhance intervention relevance and sustainability [73, 78]. Many existing programs involve adolescents but do not engage them as full partners. Although it can be challenging to partner with adolescents, as they may have unpredictable schedules, conflicting views, and other responsibilities, efforts must focus on helping adolescents understand that they (and their input) are crucial for programming. Perhaps more important, however, program staff must be flexible and patient to make partnership possible for adolescents and also be open to the differing perspectives and insights provided. A high level of creativity is often needed, and program staff often assume that they know the answers or have the insights based on their ongoing service provision. However, HIV-prevention interventions and programs may particularly benefit from partnerships with local adolescents, as these adolescents (in comparison to program staff) may be able to better identify, and reach out to, marginalized and higher risk adolescents to educate, get tested, and facilitate care linkage if positive.

Adolescent partners partnering can provide vital input on intervention and program components, such as whom to employ as study recruiters and facilitators, intervention strategies and format, relevant content and delivery options, acceptable recruitment and intervention locations, and incentive structures. For instance, the researchers involved with Choosing Life: Empowerment! Action! Results! (CLEAR), a client-centered intervention, improved on their previous iteration by better tailoring to the concerns and life situations of adolescents: providing one-on-one counseling sessions rather than small groups to protect HIV disclosure, providing telephone sessions to increase accessibility, and updating the delivery modalities to make them specific to each adolescent's unique situational context [79].

Furthermore, adolescents can contextualize the barriers and context of adolescents' behavioral decisions [2, 13]. Thus, a wide range of adolescents—not just adolescents who are popular community leaders, more proactive, and/or easier to reach and work with—should be engaged, and have an opportunity to adapt their level of participation to their changing developmental needs. Adolescent participation should also take place in the context of a realistic time frame that can foster the development of new skills. Adolescents can be engaged on short-term projects that they can successfully finish, although some adolescents may be willing and available for full project engagement from start to completion.

Adolescents should be given increasingly complex responsibilities that match both the needs of the intervention and/or program and the adolescents' stage of development. Adolescents benefit through engagement and participation and increased roles and responsibilities (e.g., increased research skills and helping others); however, their work needs to be supported with appropriate human, financial, and logistical resources. It is important to note that adolescents must be informed about the rights and responsibilities involved in human subjects research; human subjects training can contribute substantially to ensuring that confidentiality concerns are addressed in an effective, context-specific manner [32] and at the same time develop adolescents' understanding of, and ongoing contribution to, research. Adolescents should also receive incentives to encourage their participation. Compensation for adolescents' involvement in research aids in shared power in the research process [80], while ensuring the ethical engagement of adolescents as partners [81].

The population of adolescents at risk for, and infected with, HIV is not a homogenous group. Academic researchers, clinicians, and other providers must pay attention to similarities and differences (e.g., gender, sexual orientation, race/ethnicity, and geography), as these factors affect the ways in which adolescents conceptualize their risk for HIV exposure and transmission and also affect the availability and accessibility of services. Although HIV disproportionately affects young sexual minority adolescents (e.g., gay and bisexual), especially young African–American/black and Latino/Hispanic gay and bisexual men, MSM, and transgender persons, other sexual orientations, races, and ethnicities must also be included in prevention research [9]. Female adolescents, including lesbians and other women who have sex with women (WSW), may be marginalized or ignored, given that many programs are specific to MSM [82]. Furthermore, racial/ethnic minority female adolescents may have specific individual and dyadic needs shaped by cultural values and beliefs that affect HIV-prevention and -care efforts. Contextual issues that are specific to women, such as violence and gendered power dynamics in heterosexual relationships, must also be considered [83]. Thus, partnering with adolescents representing diverse experiences and backgrounds can help interventions and programs meet the unique needs of adolescents with respect to demographics, context, culture, values, and beliefs [25, 34, 40, 49, 84].

Benefits and Challenges of Organization-Engaged Partnerships

As adolescents at risk for and with HIV are often considered by community outsiders as hidden or hard-to-reach, additional time and effort may be needed [34, 35], thus highlighting the utility of partnering with youth-serving organizations. Therefore, the importance of other community partners cannot be underestimated. For example, youth-serving and faith-based organizations can be involved in HIV-prevention efforts for adolescents. In line with community-based participatory research (CBPR), partnering with community-based organizations shows promise for academic researchers, clinicians, and other providers, in particular, to tap into the expertise and community-level knowledge of these organizations, allowing a "blending of lived experiences" [85]. Interventions and programs using community engagement to support adolescents with HIV have explored collaborations with youth-serving organizations to develop comprehensive culturally and ecologically tailored interventions and programs. Youth-serving organizations have played a unique role in prevention and health promotion efforts because of their position as frontline service providers. They offer an intimate and essential perspective to the factors influencing HIV risk, exposure, and transmission within communities and insights for the development and implementation of culturally congruent HIV-prevention interventions and for formulation of partnerships with adolescents [86]. Additionally, engaging organizational partners aids in recruitment and retention of adolescent participants and additional organizational partners [43].

Forming community–academic partnerships when designing programs can be helpful in ensuring that adolescent perspectives are integrated into the process of intervention and program development [13]. Compared with academic researchers, clinicians, and other providers, youth-serving organizations are able to develop different relationships with adolescents that may or may not be related to HIV and serve in a different capacity to meet the needs of adolescents. As many youth-serving organizations focus on specific issues and populations (e.g., racial/ethnic minorities, sexual orientation, and geography [urban/rural]), these partnerships have been particularly useful for engaging adolescents epidemiologically at risk for HIV acquisition. Organizational partners' roles can be expanded to include health education through activities that correspond with institutional beliefs, doctrines, and culture [41]. Engaging community partners, including nonhealth community institutions (e.g., community- and faith-based organizations) with existing relationships with adolescents, in HIV-prevention and -care efforts is helpful. Specifically, these partnerships can assist: in facilitating adolescents in accessing a diverse array of services, in coordinating care across agencies and institutions, in mobilizing communities around the issue, in enhancing community capacity, and in changing community norms to better integrate and fully consider the social-ecologic context of local adolescents [37, 45].

When collaborating with youth-serving organizations, it is important to develop and harness their capacity, strengths, and resources by accommodating each organization's individuality and culture [40–42, 45, 85]. To ensure cultural congruence, ecologic factors should be addressed, such as community and cultural norms, community priorities, acculturation, familial norms/expectations, gender role expectations, and ethnic pride [42, 44, 85]. For example, to navigate the sensitivity of HIV discussions in faith-based settings, it may be helpful to ensure that the program is congruent with the values, beliefs, and comfort levels of adolescents, their parents, and faith leaders. It is also important to frame the program in a way that addresses members' perceptions of HIV and frames HIV as a public health and medical issue rather than a sexual or moral issue [40, 41, 46, 87]. Although a certain level of stigma may exist for faith-based organizations (e.g., discomfort with being "out" at church due to homophobia or homo-negativity), these faith-based partnerships can help diminish the stigma because of the trust that parents and local community members have for these institutions [40, 42].

Organizational partnerships serve to enhance community capacity and intervention sustainability and to foster mutual learning, understanding, and trust. Community coalitions can be especially useful in formalizing partnerships, attending to diverse perspectives, and promoting resource sharing and sustainability [70, 88]. As funding policies are beginning to require partnerships (e.g., HIV-testing programs must have linkage partners), a more collaborative approach is imperative. This approach is helpful; as has been noted, "Collective actions can be strengthened by bringing together partners that share similar vision or services…it is also the people who bring the resources to the common community table, along with the combination of personalities, agency dynamics, and political agendas involved that can move a coalition to either success or failure" [70].

Lastly, maintaining access and connection to services across the transition points within the integrated model is important to keep adolescents involved in research, interventions, and programs and is especially important for secondary prevention efforts. Integrating adolescents' perspectives to enhance accessibility and acceptability of prevention and care services may help establish trust and comfort among adolescents. This, in turn, may help adolescents disclose to particular persons (e.g., staff and providers) and use particular places (e.g., organizations and clinics). Traditional client-provider relationships may not be sufficient for developing these trusting relationships. Instead, partnerships in which adolescents can be true partners may allow for a flexible and adjustable system of relationships and services [37, 84]. Programs can serve as a bridge or mediator between adolescents with HIV who are considered by community outsiders to be hidden or hard-to-reach and healthcare delivery systems; a program's presence can motivate adolescents to be tested or engaged in care through institutional referrals or word-of-mouth [34]. For counseling and testing efforts conducted within institutional settings, accessibility and acceptability may mean being as unobtrusive as possible and normalizing HIV testing as nonthreatening. Within community settings, this may mean establishing a distinct, consistent presence to build both individual and community acceptance. In all settings, risks to privacy and confidentiality must be considered to ensure acceptability and comfort with the program and to respect and protect adolescents [37, 73].

Research Needs and Priorities

Partnerships among academic researchers; representatives from educational and testing organizations, health departments, clinics, other community-based organizations, and adolescents are needed and should be established across the spectrum of the integrated model to create a seamless transition from HIV prevention, testing, and diagnosis to HIV-related care [15, 89, 90]. Thus, research should continue to use innovative strategies to develop and sustain direct partnerships with adolescents and consider the role that community-based youth-serving organizations can play in HIV prevention and care. Ongoing community collaborations to address structural level changes are useful in decreasing the incidence of HIV and keeping adolescents with HIV healthy [70, 88].

The implementation of enhanced testing initiatives has heightened the need for a more developed set of tools for HIV prevention and care. These tools could include an assessment of best practices, development of models for better integration of screening/testing and care organizations, individual-focused tools for assessment of readiness for care engagement, and provide education to improve retention in care. At the federal level, grantors, including the US Centers for Disease Control and Prevention (CDC) and the National Institutes of Health (NIH), can play an important role in facilitating the collaboration among academic researchers; representatives from educational and testing organizations, health departments, clinics, other community-based organizations, and adolescents through grant requirements [24]. These approaches will be a vital foundation to effectively realizing goals outlined in the *National HIV/AIDS Strategy* [66, 67].

Studies show that strong partnerships and networks aid in structuring efficient HIV-prevention and -care models that avoid service duplication and promote the health of adolescents [15, 70]. The integrated model demonstrates that HIV prevention and care are lifelong issues, especially for adolescents with HIV. Thus, it is important not only to get adolescents engaged in the clinic but to acknowledge that adolescents must eventually transition to adult care and away from the clinics and providers that are safe and known to them [24].

Future research should explore adolescents' attrition along the HIV-care continuum (e.g., diagnosis to care and transitions from adolescent to adult care) through adolescent partner insights and ethnographic and qualitative research methodologies to obtain deeper understandings of the perspectives of adolescents with HIV. For intervention and program planning to be successful, it is essential to gain a better understanding of adolescents' views on HIV risk reduction behaviors (e.g., whose responsibility is it to use condoms and factors associated with retention and attrition in care), the motivations for these behaviors (e.g., altruism, fear of infecting others, and fear of legal reprisal), and other insights and underlying emotions.

Discussion and Conclusion

The ongoing HIV epidemic among adolescents in the USA highlights a profound and immediate need for innovative approaches to primary and secondary prevention that engage adolescents as equal partners [55, 91]. The *integrated model of continuities in transition in adolescent HIV prevention, diagnosis, and care* [16] provides a helpful framework to depict the variety and stages of community-engaged scholarship that have emerged and examples of partnerships with adolescents and youth-serving organizations. Although academic researchers, clinicians, and other providers have created interventions and programs that receive input from adolescents, adolescent partnerships are rarely utilized to the fullest extent possible. It is imperative that research programs partner with adolescents so they can improve the relevance of intervention and program planning, implementation, and evaluation. Engaging adolescents and youth-serving organizations in participatory research and practice requires listening to adolescents' voices and acting on their recommendations with the same rigor as adult voices in the reflection and decision-making process [32]. This process is essential for the development and implementation of culturally relevant HIV-prevention programs.

In this chapter, we demonstrated how engaging and partnering with adolescents and hearing their voices has multiple benefits, such as better recruitment of adolescents in HIV-prevention and -care interventions and programs, decreased fear and distrust of health services, reduced barriers to testing and care, and improved identification of needs and priorities. Although each of these benefits can be useful throughout the integrated model, particular benefits are salient in each of the integrated model's phases.

In addition, engaging adolescents in program planning can lead to the development of more appropriate materials and more culturally congruent interventions and programs overall [32]. This overall enhancement can be accomplished through stronger adolescent-tailored language in educational sessions and questionnaires, potentially increasing the strength and quality of the collected data [32]. Trusted community- (e.g., SHERO; [44]) and faith-based organizations (e.g., Project BRIDGE; [42, 43]) can be powerful partners in addressing HIV among adolescents, reducing fear of involvement and/or increasing comfort in using prevention services, as well as improving overall community acceptance.

Interventions and programs promoting HIV testing and counseling may benefit from adolescent partners who aid in overcoming barriers to reach higher risk adolescents and positively influencing attitudes and beliefs related to testing. The involvement of peer workers in various aspects of program implementation has helped to increase acceptability of HIV testing and counseling among adolescents considered to be hard to reach as some of these adolescents have not otherwise been to a clinic [34, 39, 49]. Engaging adolescents can also help in the identification of better communication channels and optimal locations to reach adolescents, such as in the use of mobile testing units to deliver on-the-street testing, thereby increasing accessibility of services and reducing transportation barriers [49]. The particularly vulnerable nature of adolescents at higher risk for, or currently living with, HIV who may also be experiencing comorbidities makes it essential to include youth-serving organizations. Social marketing campaigns [47] and community-based, rather than clinic-based, settings for intervention or program delivery [54] can assuage the stigma and misconceptions among adolescents regarding using health-care services.

Lastly, interventions and programs related to care services have benefited from adolescent partnerships by identifying specific needs and priorities of particular subgroups. Such partnerships aid in the identification of important characteristics of key staff members, such as the need to hire peer educators with experience living on the streets for an intervention recruiting street youth [49]. Involving adolescents in programs related to care linkage, engagement, and retention can also build social support among adolescents and between adolescents and program staff [72, 73]. Indeed, adolescents with HIV may be more likely to stay in care if they receive support from peers. In successful programs such as BAY Positives [68], Mobile SafeSpace [49], and TREAT [76], positive intervention and program outcomes and sustainability would have been more difficult to achieve without the involvement of adolescents in the implementation process.

In summary, adolescents represent a unique population in terms of behavioral risk factors, cognitive and psychosocial development, and potential length of HIV disease trajectory. Thus, both primary and secondary HIV-prevention and -care efforts are essential. The ultimate goal of HIV prevention among adolescents is to keep them negative, or if they become positive, to keep them healthy as they navigate their disease status while maturing into adults. For adolescents who become positive, it is imperative to create programs that will help them overcome barriers to health-care access and increase their involvement in their own care. Including other adolescents and youth-serving organizations in the linkage-to-care process can help adolescents communicate with health-care providers and locate clinics that best meet their own needs. Working closely to keep adolescents engaged in care and adherent to medication will improve both individual and community/population health by reducing secondary transmission. As we further explore biomedical (e.g., vaccines, microbicides, and PrEP) and behavioral (e.g., test and treat and treatment as prevention) interventions and programs, partnering with adolescents and community-based youth-serving organizations to improve HIV prevention will only become more important in the future.

Acknowledgment J. Dennis Fortenberry provided valuable insight into the construction of this chapter through the conceptualization and development of the integrated model of continuities in transition in adolescent/youth HIV prevention, diagnosis, and care.

References

1. English A, Park MJ, Shafer M-A, Kreipe RE, D'Angelo LJ. Health care reform and adolescents—an agenda for the lifespan: a position paper of the Society for Adolescent Medicine. J Adolesc Health. 2009;45(3):310–5.

2. Mascolini M. Finding solutions for HIV's lost generation: adolescents and young adults [Internet]. Houston (TX): AIDS Research Consortium of Houston dba; 2010 Fall [cited 2012 Jun 18]. http://www.centerforaids.org/pdfs/dec2010rita.pdf. Accessed 22 May 2013.
3. Goldenring JM, Rosen DS. Getting into adolescent heads: an essential update. Contemp Pediatr. 2004;21(1):64–90.
4. Alderman EM, Rieder J, Cohen MI. The history of adolescent medicine. Pediatr Res. 2003;54(1):137–47.
5. Ferrell K. Teen: ages and stages [Internet]. Elk Grove Village: American Academy of Pediatrics; 2011 May [cited 2012 Jun 18]. http://www.healthychildren.org/English/ages-stages/teen/pages/Whats-Going-On-in-the-Teenage-Brain.aspx.
6. Steinberg L. Adolescence, 7th ed., Chap. 2: Cognitive Transitions. McGraw Hill; 2005. pp. 63–94.
7. Tanner AE, Short MB, Zimet GD, Rosenthal SR. Research on adolescents and microbicides: a review. J Pediatr Adolesc Gynecol. 2009;22(5):285–91.
8. Centers for Disease Control and Prevention (US). HIV and young men who have sex with men [Internet]. Atlanta (GA): National Center for HIV/AIDS, Viral Hepatitis, STD, and TB Prevention, Division of Adolescent and School Health; 2012 Jun [cited 2012 Jun 18]. http://www.cdc.gov/HealthyYouth/sexualbehaviors/pdf/hiv_factsheet_ymsm.pdf.
9. Centers for Disease Control and Prevention (US). HIV Among Youth [Internet]. Atlanta (GA): National Center for HIV/AIDS, Viral Hepatitis, STD, and TB Prevention, Division of HIV/AIDS Prevention; 2011 Dec [cited 2012 Jun 18]. http://www.cdc.gov/hiv/youth/pdf/youth.pdf.
10. Adolescent Trials Network for HIV/AIDS Interventions. Purpose [Internet]. Bethesda (MD): Adolescent Trials Network for HIV/AIDS Interventions; 2012 [cited 2012 Jun 18]. https://www.atnonline.org/public/purpose.asp.
11. Kelly JA, Kalichman SC. Behavioral research in HIV/AIDS primary and secondary prevention: recent advances and future directions. J Consult Clin Psychol. 2002 Jun;70(3):626–39.
12. Dodd PJ, Garnett GP, Hallett TB. Examining the promise of HIV elimination by 'test and treat' in hyperendemic settings. AIDS. 2010;24(5):729–35.
13. Coker-Appiah DS, Akers AY, Banks B, Albritton T, Leniek K, Wynn M, et al. In their own voices: rural African American youth speak out about community-based HIV prevention interventions. Prog Community Health Partnersh. 2009;3(4):301–12.
14. Philbin MM, Tanner AE, Duval A, Ellen J, Kapogiannis B, Fortenberry JD. Linking HIV-positive adolescents to care in 15 different clinics across the United States: creating solutions to address structural barriers for linkage to care. AIDS Care. 2014;26(1):12–9.
15. Tanner AE, Philbin MM, Ott MA, Duval A, Ellen J, Kapogiannis B, et al. Linking HIV+ adolescents into care: the effects of relationships between local health departments and adolescent medicine clinics. J HIV AIDS & Soc Serv. 2013;12(3–4).
16. Fortenberry JD. An integrated model of continuities in transition in adolescent/youth HIV prevention, diagnosis & treatment [Internet]. Message to: Amanda E. Tanner. 2012 Jul 10 [cited 2012 Jul 14].
17. Gardner EM, McLees MP, Burman WJ, Steiner JF, Del RC. The spectrum of engagement in HIV care and its relevance to test-and-treat strategies for prevention of HIV infection. Clin Infect Dis. 2011;52(6):793–800.
18. Valdiserri R. (2012). HIV/AIDS treatment cascade helps identify gaps in care retention [Internet]. Washington, DC: AIDS.gov; 2012 Jul [cited 2013 Jan 17]. http://blog.aids.gov/2012/07/hivaids-treatment-cascade-helps-identify-gaps-in-care-retention.html?utm_source=feedburner&utm_medium=feed&utm_campaign=Feed%3A+aids%2Fgov+%28Blog.AIDS.gov%29.
19. Hosek SG, Harper GW, Rocco D. Psychological and social difficulties of adolescents living with HIV: a qualitative analysis. J Sex Educ Ther. 2000;25(4):269–76.

20. Hosek SG, Harper GW, Lemos D. Martinez J; Adolescent Medicine Trials Network for HIV. An ecological model of stressors experienced by youth newly diagnosed with HIV. J HIV AIDS Prev Child Youth. 2008;9(2):192–218.

21. Kang SY, Goldstein MF, Deren S. Health care utilization and risk behaviors among HIV positive minority drug users. J Health Care Poor Underserved. 2006;17(2):265–75.

22. Mallinson RK, Relf MV, Dekker D, Dolan K, Darcy A, Ford A. Maintaining normalcy: a grounded theory of engaging in HIV-oriented primary medical care. ANS Adv Nurs Sci. 2005;28(3):265–77.

23. Mill JE, Jackson RC, Worthington CA, Archibald CP, Wong T, Myers T, et al. HIV testing and care in Canadian Aboriginal youth: a community based mixed methods study. BMC Infect Dis. 2008;8(1):132–44.

24. Tanner AE, Philbin MM, Duval A, Ellen J, Kapogiannis B, Fortenberry JD. 'Youth friendly' clinics: considerations for engaging HIV+ adolescents into care. 2014;26(2):199–205.

25. Augustine J. Serving HIV-Positive Youth [Internet]. Washington, DC: Advocates for Youth; 2002 November [cited 2012 Jun 18]. http://www.naccho.org/toolbox/_toolbox/Serving_HIV_Positive_Youth_1.pdf.

26. Sales JM, DiClemente RJ. Adolescent STI/HIV prevention programs: What works for teens? [Internet]. Ithaca (NY): Assets Coming Together (ACT) for Youth Center of Excellence (US); 2010 May [cited 2012 Jun 18]. http://www.actforyouth.net/resources/rf/rf_sti_0510.pdf.

27. Lam PK, Naar-King S, Wright K. Social support and disclosure as predictors of mental health in HIV-positive youth. AIDS Patient Care STDS. 2007;21(1):20–9.

28. Ruglis J. Mapping the biopolitics of school dropout and youth resistance. Int J Qual Stud Educ. 2011;24(5):627–37.

29. Goh Y-Y, Bogart LM, Sipple-Asher BK, Uyeda K, Hawes-Dawson J, Olarita-Dhungana J, et al. Using community-based participatory research to identify potential interventions to overcome barriers to adolescents' healthy eating and physical activity. J Behav Med. 2009;32(5):491–502.

30. Yonas MA, Burke JG, Rak K, Bennett A, Kelly V, Gielen AC. A picture's worth a thousand words: engaging youth in CBPR using the creative arts. Prog Community Health Partnersh. 2010;3(4):349–58.

31. Reed SJ, Miller RL. The benefits of youth engagement in HIV-preventive structural change interventions. Youth Soc. 2012. doi: 10.1177/0044118X12443372

32. Powers JL, Tiffany JS. Engaging youth in participatory research and evaluation. J Public Health Manag Pract. 2006;12 Suppl:79–87.

33. Centers for Disease Control and Prevention (US). Child Development: Teenagers (15–17 Years of Age) [Internet]. Atlanta (GA): National Center on Birth Defects and Developmental Disabilities, Division of Human Development and Disabilities; 2012 Mar [cited 2012 Jun 18]. http://www.cdc.gov/ncbddd/childdevelopment/positiveparenting/adolescence2.html.

34. Bell DN, Martinez J, Botwinick G, Shaw K, Walker LE, Dodds S, et al. Case finding for HIV-positive youth: a special type of hidden population. J Adolesc Health. 2003;33(2 Suppl):10–22.

35. Jenkins RA. Challenges in engaging community participation in HIV prevention research. Prog Community Health Partnersh. 2007;1(2):117–9.

36. Wilson CM, Houser J, Partlow C, Rudy BJ, Futterman DC. Friedman LB; Adolescent Medicine HIV/AIDS Research Network. The REACH (Reaching for Excellence in Adolescent Care and Health) project: study design, methods, and population profile. J Adolesc Health. 2001;29(3 Suppl):8–18.

37. Woods ER, Samples CL, Singer B, Peters NP, Trevithick LA, Schneir A, et al. Young people and HIV/AIDS: the need for a continuum of care: findings and policy recommendations from nine adolescent-focused projects. AIDS Public Policy J. 2002;17(3):90–111.

38. Peralta L, Deeds BG, Hipszer S, Ghalib K. Barriers and facilitators to adolescent HIV testing. AIDS Patient Care STDS. 2007;21(6):400–8.

39. Martinez J, Bell D, Sell R. HIV/AIDS Bureau, editors. Lessons learned: innovations in the delivery of HIV/AIDS services. Rockville (MD): Human Resources and Services Adminis-

tration (HRSA), The Special Projects of National Significance Program (SPNS); 2001. Identifying HIV-positive youth and transitioning them into the health care system: Chicagoland HIV Risk Reduction Partnership for Youth (CHRRPY), Cook County Hospital.

40. Griffith DM, Pichon LC, Allen JO, Campbell B. YOUR Blessed Health: a faith-based CBPR approach to addressing HIV/AIDS among African Americans. AIDS Educ Prev. 2010;22(3):203–17.

41. Griffith DM, Campbell B, Allen JO, Robinson KJ, Stewart SK. YOUR Blessed Health: an HIV-prevention program bridging faith and public health communities. Public Health Rep. 2010;125(1 Suppl):4–11.

42. Marcus M, Walker T, Swint JM, Smith BP, Brown C, Busen N, et al. Community-based participatory research to prevent substance abuse and HIV/AIDS in African-American adolescents. J Interprof Care. 2004;18(4):347–59.

43. Williams TT, Griffith DM, Pichon LC, Campbell B, Allen JO, Sanchez JC. Involving faith-based organizations in adolescent HIV prevention. Prog Community Health Partnersh. 2011;5(4):425–31.

44. Harper GW, Bangi AK, Sanchez B, Doll M, Pedraza A. A quasi-experimental evaluation of a community-based HIV prevention intervention for Mexican American female adolescents: the SHERO's program. AIDS Educ Prev. 2009;21(5):109–23.

45. Griffith DM, Allen JO, DeLoney EH, Robinson K, Lewis EY, B Campbell, et al. Community-based organizational capacity building as a strategy to reduce racial health disparities. J Prim Prev. 2010;31(1–2):31–9.

46. Pichon LC, Griffith DM, Campbell B, Allen JO, Williams TT, Addo AY. Faith leaders' comfort implementing an HIV prevention curriculum in a faith setting. J Health Care Poor Underserved. 2012;23(3):1253–65.

47. Futterman DC, Peralta L, Rudy BJ, Wolfson S, Guttmacher S, Rogers AS. Project ACCESS Team of the Adolescent Medicine HIV/AIDS Research Network. The ACCESS (Adolescents Connected to Care, Evaluation, and Special Services) project: social marketing to promote HIV testing to adolescents, methods and first year results from a six city campaign. J Adolesc Health. 2001;29(3 Suppl):19–29.

48. Fischer S, Reynolds H, Yacobson I, Barnett B, Schueller J. HIV counseling and testing for youth: a manual for providers [Internet]. Arlington (VA): Family Health International; 2007 [cited 2012 Aug 11]. http://www.fhi360.org/NR/rdonlyres/eolxm36ulklpmcihmalj5ljyv5iqj-f243ody56rh55pqtu6vjxam2koffrj2wo723im6syphvna7dm/YouthVCTmanual.pdf.

49. Johnson RL, Martinez J, Botwinick G, Bell D, Sell RL, Friedman LB, et al. Introduction: what youth need – adapting HIV care models to meet the lifestyles and special needs of adolescents and young adults. J Adolesc Health. 2003;33(2 Suppl):4–9.

50. Woods ER, Samples CL, Melchiono MW. Harris SK; Boston HAPPENS Program Collaborators. Boston HAPPENS Program: HIV-positive, homeless, and at-risk youth can access care through youth-oriented HIV services. Semin Pediatr Infect Dis. 2003;14(1):43–53.

51. Horner JR, Romer D, Vanable PA, Salazar LF, Carey MP, Juzang I, et al. Using culture-centered qualitative formative research to design broadcast messages for HIV prevention for African American adolescents. J Health Commun. 2008;13(4): 309–25.

52. Romer D, Sznitman S, DiClemente R, Salazar LF, Vanable PA, Carey MP, et al. Mass media as an HIV-prevention strategy: using culturally sensitive messages to reduce HIV-associated sexual behavior of at-risk African American youth. Am J Public Health. 2009;99(12): 2150–9.

53. Joint United Nations Programme on HIV/AIDS. Social marketing: an effective tool in the global response to HIV/AIDS [Internet]. Geneva (Switzerland): Joint United Nations Programme on HIV/AIDS; 1998 [cited 2012 Aug 26]. http://www.unaids.org/en/media/unaids/contentassets/dataimport/publications/irc-pub01/jc167-socmarketing_en.pdf.

54. Swenson RR, Hadley WS, Houck CD, Dance SK, Brown LK. Who accepts a rapid HIV antibody test? The role of race/ethnicity and HIV risk behavior among community adolescents. J Adolesc Health. 2011;48(5):527–9.

55. Centers for Disease Control and Prevention (US). Results of the Expanded HIV Testing Initiative—25 Jurisdictions, United States, 2007–2010 [Internet]. Atlanta (GA): Morbidity and Mortality Weekly Report; 2011 Jun [cited 2012 Jun 18]. http://www.cdc.gov/mmwr/preview/mmwrhtml/mm6024a2.htm.

56. Mugavero MJ, Norton WE, Saag MS. Health care system and policy factors influencing engagement in HIV medical care: piecing together the fragments of a fractured health care delivery system. Clin Infect Dis. 2011;52(2 Suppl):S238–46.

57. Mayer KH. Introduction: linkage, engagement, and retention in HIV care: essential for optimal individual- and community-level outcomes in the era of highly active antiretroviral therapy. Clin Infect Dis. 2011;52(2 Suppl):S205–7.

58. McCoy SI, Miller WC, MacDonald PD, Hurt CB, Leone PA, Eron JJ, et al. Barriers and facilitators to HIV testing and linkage to primary care: narratives of people with advanced HIV in the Southeast. AIDS Care. 2009;21(10):1313–20.

59. Mugavero MJ, Amico KR, Westfall AO, Crane HM, Zinski A, Willig JH, et al. Early retention in HIV care and viral load suppression: implications for a test and treat approach to HIV prevention. J Acquir Immune Defic Syndr. 2012;59(1):86–93.

60. Ulett KB, Willig JH, Lin HY, Routman JS, Abroms S, Allison J, et al. The therapeutic implications of timely linkage and early retention in HIV care. AIDS Patient Care STDs. 2009;23(1):41–9.

61. Giordano TP, Visnegarwala F, White AC Jr, Troisi CL, Frankowski RF, Hartman CM, et al. Patients referred to an urban HIV clinic frequently fail to establish care: factors predicting failure. AIDS Care. 2005;17(6):773–83.

62. Giordano TP, Gifford AL, White AC Jr, Suarez-Almazor ME, Rabeneck L, Hartman C, et al. Retention in care: a challenge to survival with HIV infection. Clin Infect Dis. 2007;44(11):1493–9.

63. Metsch L, Pereyra M, Messinger S, del Rio C, Strathdee S, Anderson-Mahoney P, et al. HIV transmission risk behaviors among HIV-infected persons who are successfully linked to care. Clin Infect Dis. 2008;47(4):577–84.

64. AIDS Alliance for Children, Youth & Families. Finding HIV-positive youth and bringing them into care [Internet]. Washington: AIDS Alliance for Children, Youth & Families; 2005 [cited 2012 Aug 11]. http://www.aids-alliance.org/resources/publications/youthcasefinding-english.pdf.

65. Reiter, GS. Comprehensive clinical care: managing HIV as a chronic illness. AIDS Clin Care. 2000;12(2):13–9.

66. Office of National AIDS Policy. National HIV/AIDS strategy for the United States. 2010. www.whitehouse.gov/sites/default/files/uploads/NHAS.pdf.

67. Office of National AIDS Policy. National HIV/AIDS strategy: Update of 2011–2012 federal efforts to implement the national HIV/AIDS strategy. 2012. http://aids.gov/federal-resources/national-hiv-aids-strategy/overview/.

68. Bettencourt T, Hodgins A, Huba GJ, Pickett G. Bay Area Young Positives: a model of a youth-based approach to HIV/AIDS services. J Adolesc Health. 1998;23(2 Suppl):28–36.

69. Moore, Curtis. HIV + youth book chapter – recent papers on Bay Positives? [Internet]. Message to: Alice Ma. 2012 Jul 10 [cited 2012 Jul 14]. [1 paragraph].

70. Straub DM, Deeds BG, Willard N, Caster J, Peralta L, Francisco VT, et al. Partnership selection and formation: a case study of developing adolescent health community-researcher partnerships in fifteen U.S. communities. J Adolesc Health. 2007;40(6):489–98.

71. Schneir A, Kipke MD, Melchior LA, Huba GJ. Childrens Hospital Los Angeles: a model of integrated care for HIV-positive and very high-risk youth. J Adolesc Health. 1998;23(2 Suppl):59–70.

72. Veinot TC, Flicker SE, Skinner HA, McClelland A, Saulnier P, Read SE, et al. "Supposed to make you better but it doesn't really": HIV-positive youths' perceptions of HIV treatment. J Adolesc Health. 2006;38(3):261–7.

73. Garvie PA, Lawford J, Flynn PM, Gaur AH, Belzer M, McSherry GD, et al. Development of a directly observed therapy adherence intervention for adolescents with human immunode-

ficiency virus–1: application of focus group methodology to inform design, feasibility, and acceptability. J Adolesc Health. 2009;44(2):124–32.

74. Hightow-Weidman LB, Smith JC, Valera E, Matthews DD, Lyons P. Keeping them in "STYLE": finding, linking, and retaining young HIV-positive black and Latino men who have sex with men in care. AIDS Patient Care STDS. 2011;25(1):37–45.

75. Health Resources and Services Administration (US). Social Media and HIV [Internet]. Rockville (MD): U.S. Department of Health and Human Services, HIV/AIDS Bureau; 2011 Jun [cited 2012 Aug 26]. http://hab.hrsa.gov/newspublications/careactionnewsletter/june2011.pdf.

76. Rogers AS, Miller S, Murphy DA, Tanney M, Fortune T. The TREAT (Therapeutic Regimens Enhancing Adherence in Teens) program: theory and preliminary results. J Adolesc Health. 2001;29(3 Suppl):30–8.

77. Flynn PM, Rudy BJ, Lindsey JC, Douglas SD, Lathey J, Spector SA, et al. Long-term observation of adolescents initiating HAART therapy: three-year follow-up. AIDS Res Hum Retrovir. 2007;23(10):1208–14.

78. Rosenfeld SL, Keenan PM, Fox DJ, Chase LH, Melchiono MW, Woods ER. Youth perceptions of comprehensive adolescent health services through the Boston HAPPENS program. J Pediatr Health Care. 2000;14(2):60–7.

79. Rotheram-Borus MJ, Swendeman D, Comulada WS, Weiss RE, Lee M, Lightfoot M. Prevention for substance-using HIV-positive young people: telephone and in-person delivery. J Acquir Immune Defic Syndr. 2004;37(2 Suppl):S68–77.

80. Cahill C. Doing research with young people: participatory research and the rituals of collective work. Child Geogr. 2007;5(3):297–312.

81. Ritterbusch A. Bridging guidelines and practice: toward a grounded care ethics in youth participatory action research. Prof Geogr. 2012;64(1):16–24.

82. Deol AK, Heath-Toby A. HIV risk for lesbians, bisexuals & other women who have sex with women [Internet]. New York (NY): Gay Men's Health Crisis, Women's Institute; 2009 Jun [cited 2012 Aug 11]. http://www.gmhc.org/files/editor/file/GMHC_lap_whitepaper_0609.pdf.

83. Amaro H, Raj A, Vega RR, Mangione TW, Perez LN. Racial/ethnic disparities in the HIV and substance abuse epidemics: communities responding to the need. Public Health Rep. 2001;116(5):434–48.

84. Hymel MS, Greenberg BL. The Walden House Young Adult HIV Project: meeting the needs of multidiagnosed youth. J Adolesc Health. 1998;23(2):122–31.

85. Rhodes SD, Malow RM, Jolly C. Community-based participatory research: a new and not-so-new approach to HIV/AIDS prevention, care, and treatment. AIDS Educ Prev. 2010;22(3):173–83.

86. Painter TM, Ngalame PM, Lucas B, Lauby JL, Herbst JH. Strategies used by community-based organizations to evaluate their locally developed HIV prevention interventions: lessons learned from the CDC's Innovative Interventions project. AIDS Educ Prev. 2010;22(5):387–401.

87. Williams PL, Leister E, Chernoff M, Nachman S, Morse E, Di Paolo V, et al. Substance use and its association with psychiatric symptoms in perinatally HIV-infected and HIV-affected adolescents. AIDS Behav. 2010;14(5):1072–82.

88. Deeds BG, Straub DM, Willard N, Castor J, Ellen J, Peralta L. Adolescent Medicine Trials Network for HIV/AIDS Interventions. The role of community resource assessments in the development of 15 adolescent health community-researcher partnerships. Prog Community Health Partnersh. 2008;2(1):31–9.

89. Craw JA, Gardner LI, Marks G, Rapp RC, Bosshart J, Duffus WA, et al. Brief strengths-based case management promotes entry into HIV medical care. J Acquir Immune Defic Syndr. 2008;47(5):597–606.

90. Penner M, Leone PA. Integration of testing for, prevention of, and access to treatment for HIV infection: state and local perspectives. Clin Infect Dis. 2007;45(4 Suppl):S281–6.

91. Centers for Disease Control and Prevention (US). HIV Surveillance in Adolescents and Young Adults [Internet]. Atlanta (GA): National Center for HIV/AIDS, Viral Hepatitis, STD, and TB Prevention, Division of HIV/AIDS Prevention; 2012 Jun [cited 2012 Jun 18]. http://www.cdc.gov/hiv/topics/surveillance/resources/slides/adolescents/index.htm.

92. Cohen MS, Chen YQ, McCauley M, et al. Prevention of HIV-1 Infection with early antiretroviral therapy. N Engl J Med 2011;365:493–505.

Chapter 6
Community Engagement and HIV Prevention with American Indian/Alaska Native Communities: Working with the Whole Person

Flavio F. Marsiglia, John Gallagher, Deborah Secakuku Baker and Jaime M. Booth

Colonization of the new world, which took the form of conquest and conversion, has had significant impacts on American Indian/Alaska Native (AI/AN) communities. The process of colonization restricted the ability of members of AI/AN communities to use their land and practice their customs and imposed Western values on them [1]. In the dominant narrative, the conquest and conversion of native people was framed as an altruistic mission to save AI/ANs from their "savage" behaviors [2]. Unfortunately, this narrative has persisted throughout the centuries, creating disempowering stereotypes. This narrative of salvation, which also implies a less capable "other," can easily and unconsciously be reflected in HIV prevention efforts if paternalistic "top-down" approaches to prevention are used when designing, implementing, and evaluating interventions and programs.

However, a postcolonial perspective of public health aims to address stereotypical narratives by honoring both indigenous and Western scientific knowledge and empowering communities to identify and address health priorities within their unique historical and cultural frames. Because indigenous and Western scientific values and ways of knowing and ascribing meaning are not always congruent, approaching HIV prevention from these sometimes divergent perspectives can be challenging. In this chapter, we examine how postcolonial perspectives are being

F. F. Marsiglia (✉) · J. Gallagher · D. Secakuku Baker
Southwest Interdisciplinary Research Center, Arizona State University School of Social Work, ASU Downtown Campus 411 N. Central Ave., Suite 720, Phoenix, AZ 85004-0693, USA
e-mail: marsiglia@asu.edu

J. Gallagher
e-mail: jmgallag@asu.edu

D. Secakuku Baker
e-mail: debuwp8183@yahoo.com

J. M. Booth
School of Social Work, University of Pittsburgh, 2117 Cathedral of Learning, 4200 Fifth Avenue, Pittsburgh, PA 15260, USA
e-mail: jmbooth2@outlook.com

S. D. Rhodes (ed.), *Innovations in HIV Prevention Research and Practice*
through Community Engagement, DOI 10.1007/978-1-4939-0900-1_6,
© Springer Science+Business Media New York 2014

used in community-based HIV prevention efforts within AI/AN communities. We detail the importance of authentic community engagement and partnership.

Epidemiology

In the 520 years since the first Europeans started the long process of invasion, colonization, and genocide in the Americas, AI/ANs have been affected disproportionately by a wide variety of physical and mental health challenges [3]. In 2008, the US Centers for Disease Control and Prevention (CDC) recognized HIV as an emerging public health issue for AI/AN communities [4, 5]. The AI/AN population makes up only 1 % of the total US population living with the disease; however, when the size of the AI/AN population is taken into account, it ranks third in rates of infection, behind African American/black and Hispanic/Latino populations. The rate of AIDS diagnoses for this group has been higher than that for the white population since 1995; in fact, the rate of HIV infection is 30 % higher for the AI/AN population than for the white population [5, 6]. The disparity is even greater within certain states and communities [7, 9]. Moreover, there are reasons to conclude that the HIV burden borne by AI/AN communities is underestimated because of a failure to properly document the race/ethnicity of those screened and to provide HIV screening as recommended. For instance, the race/ethnicity of 30 % of AI/ANs was incorrectly classified in the HIV/AIDS reporting systems of several US states [10]. Furthermore, an evaluation of the accuracy of prenatal electronic health records across a random sample of Indian Health Service facilities found that 40 % of prenatal women had not been screened for HIV according to standardized Indian Health Service guidelines [11]. In addition, some AI/ANs do not access HIV testing because of a lack of real and/or perceived confidentiality in rural tribal areas. This worry about confidentiality may further significantly affect the known rates of infection within AI/AN communities [12, 13].

HIV Risk and Protection Within AI/AN Communities

The prevalence of known risk factors among AI/ANs, including high rates of substance use and sexual risk behaviors, raises concerns about the potential of HIV becoming another devastating disease within AI/AN communities [14, 15]. Some have argued that the disproportionate rates of many risk factors within AI/ANs are directly or indirectly linked to the process of colonization through experiences of trauma and ongoing discrimination [16, 17]. On the surface, these risk factors appear to be similar to those observed in the general population, but distinct contexts and unique underlying mechanisms suggest that different approaches to HIV prevention are needed. Because effective HIV prevention interventions and programs are typically guided by understanding both the risk and protective factors of a given population, we offer a brief review of factors that increase and decrease HIV risk in AI/AN communities. Taking a postcolonial perspective, we consider these factors in conjunction with the strengths of indigenous ways of understanding health in order to advance a holistic approach to HIV prevention.

Substance Use and Abuse

Rates of alcohol and other drug abuse, consistently identified as risk factors for HIV infection, are disproportionately high in AI/AN communities [18, 19]. Although, AI/ANs only comprised 1.2 % of all admissions for treatment for injection-drug use in 2009, injection-drug use was the route of HIV transmission for 15 % of new HIV/AIDS infections among AI/AN men and 29 % of new infections among AI/AN women [20]. This percentage of injection-drug use associated with HIV infection is much higher than that in other populations in which infection through injection-drug use has been reduced substantially [5]. Despite the low number of injection-drug users in AI/AN communities, the potentially rapid spread of HIV through sharing needles and other paraphernalia puts this population at particularly high risk [21].

In addition to the direct risk posed by injection-drug use, alcohol abuse and non-injection-drug abuse may also affect HIV risk among AI/ANs [15, 21–23]. In 2011, 16.8 % of AI/ANs reported alcohol-use behaviors characterized as abuse (defined as meeting at least one of the four criteria outlined in the *Diagnostic and Statistical Manual of Mental Disorders*, DSM-IV), or dependence (defined as meeting three out of the seven dependency criteria outlined in the DSM-IV). This rate was the highest among all racial/ethnic groups; in fact, this rate of alcohol-use disorders was 6% higher than the rate among Native Hawaiian and other Pacific Islanders, a community with the second highest rate [24].

In 2011, the rates of illicit drug use were highest in the AI/AN population than in any other racial group in the three time periods measured: lifetime (58.4%), past year (24.4%), and past month (13.4%) [22]. Although the rates of infection among AI/AN noninjection-drug users are not known, data from other populations suggest that rates may be comparable to injection-drug users. For example, 17 % of noninjection-drug users in New York City were found to have HIV; this rate is comparable to that of injection-drug users [21].

By definition, substance abuse and dependence disorders indicate risk. Individuals meet the criteria for substance use disorders when they continue to use substances despite serious health consequences. Engaging in risk behaviors, such as alcohol and drug abuse, despite consequences is highly correlated with sexual risk, including decreased condom use and an increase in an individual's average number of sex partners[15, 21–23, 25]. Similar to substance users in the general population, AI/ANs who engage in sex under the influence of drugs and alcohol are much less likely to practice safer sex (e.g., they are less likely to use condoms consistently) because of decreased inhibitions and impaired judgment, increasing their risk of HIV exposure and transmission [22]. In an urban sample of AI/ANs, those who engaged in sexual activity while drunk or high were 14 times more likely to engage in sexual risk behaviors than those who were not drunk or high [18]. Lastly, substance users are more likely to engage in sexual contact within networks of other substance users, again increasing their risk for HIV exposure and transmission [21].

Sexually Transmitted Infections

Although sexual risk is often described within the context of substance use and abuse, rates of infection with other sexually transmitted infections (STIs) in AI/AN communities must be considered as well. The rates of chlamydia, gonorrhea, and syphilis are disproportionately high among AI/ANs [25]. An active STI increases the risk of HIV transmission physiologically [26], and current and/or past STIs clearly suggest engagement in sexual risk behaviors also associated with HIV exposure and transmission.

Condom Use

Condom use during sex is a well-established and effective strategy for reducing transmission of HIV and other STIs; however, evidence suggests that condom use among AI/AN men tends to be inconsistent [26, 27]. For example, 73 % of AI/AN men reported having vaginal or anal sex without a condom in the past 6 months and 52 % reported never having used a condom when engaging in vaginal or anal sex in the same time frame [16]. Similarly, in a sample of AI/AN men who have sex with men (MSM), 49 % reported having unprotected anal sex during the past 12 months. The levels of other types of sexual risk are high among AI/AN MSM as well; for example, 45 % of that same sample reported some type of current or previous engagement in sex work [27]. Overall, high rates of STIs among AI/ANs, coupled with low rates of condom use, indicate that sexual risk is a prevalent risk factor for HIV exposure and transmission in this population.

The Context of Colonialism

In order to gain a fuller and more complete understanding of typical HIV risk behaviors (i.e., substance use and sexual risk), the history of colonialism and its impact on the contexts in which AI/ANs live must be considered. Although rates of substance use and sexual risk are clear, attempts to identify overarching cultural factors that have an impact on HIV exposure and transmission are challenging because of the diversity among and within AI/AN communities. The US federal government recognizes 566 AI/AN tribes and villages in the USA [28], each with cultural, political, geographic, and economic differences. One key distinction among tribes, in addition to differences in history, traditions, and beliefs, is the degree to which communities have acculturated to Anglo-American norms and values [29]. Tribes had varying experiences and responses to the early years of colonization and later to the implementation of policies that promoted forced assimilation (e.g., boarding schools). For example, despite active efforts to discourage the use of native language among children in the 1950s, some AI/AN communities have maintained precolonial languages and ways of life, but in many other AI/AN communities, the rates of assimilation are higher.

Migration Colonization has had an impact on sexual risk among AI/ANs through the intersection of assimilation and migration from tribal land to city centers. Some tribal communities (reservations) are within the boundaries of tribal ancestral lands whereas other communities were forcibly removed from their ancestral lands and relocated. Some reservations are located within, or contiguous to, large metropolitan areas, and others are geographically isolated [30]. Although tribal land remains central to the identity of many AI/ANs, most AI/ANs (70%) do not live on tribal lands and instead live in major urban centers; this shift can be traced back to the forced and voluntary relocation efforts that took place in the 1950s [31]. During that time period, AI/AN adults were recruited to cities to participate in vocational training [32], and many AI/AN children were taken from their homes and placed in boarding schools in urban centers [33]. The migration from tribal lands to urban centers has been associated with increases in health disparities in general and in HIV infection rates more specifically [22]. For example, urban drug users are more likely to be exposed to and transmit HIV than their counterparts living on the reservation because of the co-occurrence of drug use and sexual risk and higher rates of trading sex for money, drugs, alcohol, shelter, and food [33, 34]. Furthermore, the challenges faced in urban spaces (e.g., discrimination, disconnection with land, and the loss of tribal connectedness) further contribute to risk.

Homophobia The frequent migration to and from urban centers coupled with the adaptation of homophobic attitudes has created risky conditions for some AI/AN gay and bisexual men, MSM, and transgender persons both on and off reservations. Among AI/AN men with HIV, 61% contracted HIV through sexual contact with another man [16].

During the precolonial era, homophobia was nonexistent in most AI/AN cultures; in fact, individuals with different gender identities tended to be incorporated into communities without discrimination [35]. In contemporary times, however, many AI/AN gay and bisexual men and MSM face bias and vulnerability in their communities of origin, in the larger society, and within majority communities of gay and bisexual men and MSM due to their multiple minority status. Stigma, both on and off the reservation, coupled with a strong collective orientation, forces some AI/AN gay and bisexual men and MSM to hide or deny their identities, increasing their risk. As has been documented, some AI/AN gay and bisexual men and MSM who live in tribal communities—some of whom may be married to women—make brief trips into border communities adjacent to tribal lands and engage in risky sexual encounters with non-AI/AN gay and bisexual men and MSM and then return to their own communities [16, 36]. This, in conjunction with the circular nature of migration between reservations and urban centers in which the rates of HIV are higher is a unique risk for AI/AN communities [10, 11, 31, 34].

Trauma Historical trauma and individual experiences with trauma among AI/ANs are interrelated and also increase HIV risk [16, 17, 35, 37]. The AI/AN population as a whole has suffered significant historical trauma, including massacres, forced relocation, forced enrollment in boarding schools, and forced removal of cultural and spiritual practices [16, 38]. The pain carried from these abuses has been transmitted from generation to generation through cycles of violence and victimization

[17, 38, 39]. It has been suggested that historical trauma is a root cause of the disproportionately high rates of substance abuse, intimate partner violence, and sexual assault within AI/AN communities, although empirical evidence is limited because of methodological challenges [17, 31, 38–42]. However, it makes sense that the powerlessness and hopelessness associated with historical trauma contribute to high rates of risk.

Individual trauma also is an important predictor of sexual risk in general [42] and for urban AI/AN women in particular [29, 42–44]. In fact, trauma is a greater predictor of engaging in sexual risk than social cognitions or knowledge and beliefs about HIV [22]. Although studies of prevalence rates of intimate partner violence among AI/ANs are rare, studies that do exist indicate lifetime rates of intimate partner violence that range from 46–92 %; these rates are dramatically higher than in non-AI/AN samples [41, 42, 45]. In a large sample of AI/AN female adolescents, 19 % reported a history of sexual abuse and 17 % reported physical abuse [45]. Furthermore, AI/ANs who had experienced intimate partner violence were nine times more likely to engage in sexual risk behaviors then those who had not, and those who had been victims of nonpartner sexual assault were also more likely to use condoms inconsistently [18], Among AI/ANs living off a reservation, those who had experienced physical abuse were more likely to use a condom, whereas those who reported a history of sexual abuse were less likely to use protection [30].

Substance abuse is linked to both physical and sexual abuse, with 60 % of injection-drug users reporting a history of sexual abuse and 55 % reporting physical abuse [46]. It has also been found that drug use leads to more exposure to sexual and physical assault, increasing the need for drugs and alcohol to self-medicate and perpetuating a vicious cycle of risk [47]. This cycle illustrates how trauma, sexual risk, and substance use are interrelated and may converge to create increased risk for HIV infection among AI/ANs [42].

Overall, experiences of trauma linked to a history of violence against AI/AN communities (and individuals) that occurred during colonization may be drivers of sexual risk and substance abuse and are therefore crucial to consider and include within HIV prevention interventions and programs designed for AI/AN communities.

History with Western Medicine The intentional spread of disease during colonization and the unethical medical practices that followed have created mistrust of Western medicine and research within AI/AN communities, potentially exacerbating HIV risk. Historically, the spread of disease played a large role in the conquest of AI/AN communities [43]. Three hundred years after Europeans first arrived in the "new world," the AI/AN population decreased from between 2.1 and 18 million people to 250,000 people; this decline in population is primarily due to the spread of diseases and epidemics [48]. More than violence, disease facilitated colonial expansion, decimating entire AI/AN communities. The detrimental impact of colonization on health did not stop with disease transmission. In the early part of the nineteenth century, many medical experiments were conducted in Indian Country with deleterious side effects [49], and as recently as the 1970s, 40 % of all sterilization procedures performed by Indian Health Service were done without adequate informed consent [50].

This history of exploitation has led to an understandable mistrust of Western medicine, inhibiting the effectiveness of medical prevention efforts and deterring individuals from seeking care when needed [2, 49, 50]. In fact, AI/ANs often are suspicious of prevention initiated by individuals outside of their community; they often are not willing to engage and participate in "outsider"-led prevention initiatives. Thus, HIV prevention interventions and programs may benefit from authentic engagement and participation of local AI/ANs.

Rates of migration, homophobia, the impact of historical trauma, violence experienced by AI/ANs, and mistrust of public health officials directly and/or indirectly affect substance use and sexual risk within this population, putting AI/ANs at high risk for HIV exposure and transmission. Prevention efforts may address the primary risk factors, but intervening on the cultural, historical, and contextual factors in addition to typical intervention and program components may have greater impact. It is well acknowledged that HIV prevention interventions and programs tend to focus on promoting individual-level change rather than changes that intervene "upstream" [51–59]. They focus on proximal antecedents to HIV risk, often including knowledge, attitudes, and skills to increase condom use and/or HIV testing, or to reduce the number of sex partners. However, there is a profound need for interventions and programs to address the contexts in which individuals live. Although there has been recognition of the importance of, and movement toward, understanding the contexts in which risk behavior occurs in order to design interventions and programs that are culturally congruent, much still must be done to intervene on these contextual factors to bolster strengths and reduce weaknesses [54, 56, 58, 60, 61].

AI/AN-Specific Protective Factors Against HIV

Taking a postcolonial perspective, prevention efforts should honor and build on indigenous knowledge about health and wellness, which have been identified as strengths, community assets, and protective factors within AI/AN communities. Specifically, spirituality, traditional health beliefs and practices, and ethnic identity have been identified as protective factors against a variety of negative health outcomes among AI/ANs [62, 63].

Like other aspects of culture, spirituality varies greatly by tribe and is typically a blend of traditional beliefs and postcolonial Christianity [62]. Spiritual rituals and ceremonies have supported AI/AN communities forced to adapt to change. Rituals and ceremonies provide supports and strategies to promote healing, connections to tradition, and systems for coping with both individual- and community-level stressors [53, 64]. Although the impact of spirituality on sexual risk generally, and HIV specifically, has not been well tested, spirituality among AI/AN adolescents has been found to be protective against substance use [36]. In fact, affiliation with traditional spirituality (but not Christianity) predicts less substance use among AI/AN adolescents [53]. Thus, identification with traditional belief systems and participation in traditional rites and rituals may also protect against sexual risk, but research is needed to further test these connections.

Fig. 6.1 Medicine wheel

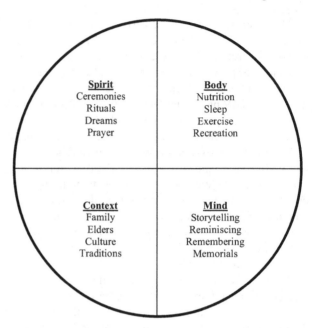

Within an AI/AN world view, traditional health and wellness center around spirituality [52, 65]. From the traditional AI/AN perspective, the body is understood to be a vessel for the spirit as it moves through human experiences [51, 65]; this is an important perception to consider when constructing interventions and programs. It also may be important to understand that physical health is perceived to be only one of four parts of wellness that must be in balance in order for an individual to be healthy [51, 68]. This concept of balance among different systems in life is traditionally represented by the medicine wheel. According to this wheel, traditional health consists of (1) the spirit that is maintained through ceremonies, rituals, dreams, and prayer; (2) the body that is cared for with proper nutrition, sleep, exercise, and recreation; (3) context that includes connection to community through family, elders, culture, and tradition; and (4) the mind that is kept healthy by storytelling and remembering and respecting the past (Fig. 6.1). In this holistic concept of health, all facets of the wheel are interconnected. When one aspect is not healthy, the entire system is at risk; the individual, or community for that matter, may have compromised health. These relationships among facets of health are not linear but rather circular, with each having an impact on the other.

During illness, a traditional AI/AN response is to acknowledge that a part within this system is out of balance and to identify what must be attended to [66, 67]. If the illness is physical, the explanation and treatment may be physical but may also incorporate ceremonies, storytelling, or other cultural traditions. Although balance is believed to be a natural state of functioning, actively pursuing harmony requires effort [69]. This means that the whole individual must be attended to when conducting health promotion and disease prevention efforts in general and HIV prevention specifically. This holistic orientation is a strength that can be used to encourage health behaviors and protect AI/ANs from HIV.

In addition to spirituality and traditional health, other community assets have been identified as strengths among AI/ANs. Across many tribes, a sense of strong ethnic identity has been maintained and serves as a protective factor. This sense of identity is evident in the frequent gathering of family, tribe, clan, and nation [67, 69, 70]. One aspect of this ethnic identity and collective orientation is the importance of tribal survivability and sovereignty [69–71]. The value of survivability can be built upon to motivate AI/ANs to take protective measures for the benefit of their larger community [72]. Furthermore, the Cherokee commitment to self-reliance has been shown to promote community health [52, 53, 65].

The central role of elders and the respect they are given in communities is yet another cultural asset that can be used in the prevention of HIV [18, 52, 53, 68, 71]. Drawing on existing AI/AN community assets such as the wisdom inherent in the community and harnessing it to promote health may be essential to successful HIV prevention. In addition, research with urban AI/AN adolescents in the Southwest USA identified family communication as offering protection against sexual risk [69]. Although unique challenges face AI/AN communities, rich community assets (e.g., strong collective bonds, commitment to tribal survivability, respect for elders, history and community-based wisdom, and family communication) may serve as protective factors that can be harnessed and/or enhanced in HIV prevention interventions and programs.

Community-Driven HIV Prevention and Research

Approaches that have been developed for and implemented within the dominant culture to reduce HIV risk may not work within AI/AN communities, and there remains a need for authentic, culturally grounded HIV prevention interventions and programs developed by and for AI/AN communities. To illustrate, based on ethnographic work with AI/AN prevention workers and community members in the western part of the USA, conceptions of shame in AI/AN communities require more discrete approaches to condom distribution in tribal settings [73]. Thus, although condom distribution has been a common strategy used to curb both the HIV and STI epidemics within other populations and communities [74], such an approach many not be appropriate within AI/AN communities. Within AI/AN communities, each member of the family is responsible for maintaining the reputation of the entire family; thereby, family members may be discouraged from behaviors that are perceived to be contrary to social norms and values. Distributing and accepting condoms may conflict with these social norms and values and thus are often discouraged. Moreover, discussing sexuality in public spaces is not acceptable in most tribes and to do so may be perceived as bringing shame to oneself and one's family. However, unlike in many other communities, cultural norms also may endorse the discussion of sexuality across genders and generational status [72]. Understanding this dynamic within tribal communities is crucial to harnessing community assets and strengths and implementing HIV prevention interventions and programs that will have a positive impact. These examples also illustrate why community engagement and partnership are critical to the success of HIV prevention interventions and programs.

The individual focus of most HIV prevention interventions and programs is often a poor fit in more collectively organized communities, including AI/AN communities. A variety of things—artifacts of popular culture or HIV prevention approaches—often need to be translated and/or substantially refined in order to "make sense" in traditional AI/AN communities. For example, prevention interventions and programs that emphasize the importance of taking responsibility for oneself may fail in AI/AN communities, whereas discussing safer sex as a method to fulfill individual responsibility to one's family, community, and tribe may be more meaningful and therefore more effective. When safer sex is communicated in the context of maintaining cultural traditions and health for future generations, the narrative is more likely to be in harmony with values that are already embedded in tribal histories and practices [75, 76].

Of course, other barriers to successful HIV prevention exist. The small, insular nature of many rural AI/AN communities may deter testing and accessing prevention resources because of concerns about confidentiality [9, 10], necessitating strategies that ensure confidence in confidentiality. Such strategies may include having nontribal members conduct testing, carrying out testing in regular health clinics so the purpose of the visit is not clear, and distributing testing materials in packaging that disguises the contents.

Furthermore, several barriers to successful HIV prevention efforts have been identified: the use of disease as a tool of conquest; racism, discrimination, marginalization, and ongoing profound socioeconomic disparities; slow and/or coercive public health responses; and distrust of Western medicine and the public health system [12, 36, 52, 65]. Even Western stereotypes of AI/ANs have created mistrust between AI/AN communities and "outside" prevention professionals (including non-AI/AN community members, organization representatives, and academic researchers), limiting the acceptability, meaningfulness, and effectiveness of their HIV prevention efforts within tribal communities [75].

Duran et al. drew attention to the disconnect between the emphasis placed on evidence-based interventions (EBIs) and the importance of using culturally oriented interventions [36]. They noted that although the federal and state agencies that fund HIV prevention strongly encourage the use of EBIs that have been found to be efficacious and "endorsed" by the CDC (see Chap. 11, which outlines community engagement within the DEBI Project), none of the current CDC-disseminated interventions were developed by, for, or tested with, AI/AN communities [36].

More broadly, distance between AI/AN communities and the state-level agencies and groups (including academic researchers) involved in HIV prevention planning, development, implementation, and evaluation is problematic. The different realities and obligations of community leaders and academic researchers have resulted in compromises on the design of interventions [75–78]. Formal and informal community leaders who live with the daily challenges facing their family, friends, neighbors, colleagues, and constituencies are primarily concerned with meeting the needs of their community and protecting individuals from undue burden, whereas academic researchers are often more detached and may be primarily more concerned with research methodology [78, 79]. Meeting the needs of the communities to provide efficient services may require the use of research designs with no control/comparison groups, smaller sample sizes, and shortened measurement tools. Additionally, academic researchers may need to move quickly in order to fulfill funding requirements, inhibiting their ability to take the time to develop, nurture, and maintain authentic relationships and power sharing with community members and conduct truly engaged and participatory research.

Challenges, such as changes in federal funding priorities and research design compromises, are certainly not circumscribed to working with AI/AN communities. However, because these challenges occur against a backdrop of historical and ongoing colonialism and stark poverty, the stakes are higher and the complications may be magnified. Historical mistrust makes community–university partnerships more prone to misunderstandings and frustrations when expectations are not met and interests are not fully explained or understood. The high level of need in the community, coupled with rigorous methodological requirements and strict timetables imposed by funding agencies, exacerbate the gaps between community interests and academic researcher interests, challenging partners' intentions of establishing an evidence base of culturally grounded HIV prevention efforts.

Community Engagement

Sound HIV prevention science and practice conducted with AI/AN communities must be rooted in collaborative, equitable, and authentic partnerships. The aims of prevention should be identified by community members within the context of their knowledge and beliefs, priorities, strengths, and assets. Once identified, and in the absence of the requisite expertise within the local community, trusted research partners can be engaged to provide assistance in the development, implementation, and evaluation of the prevention interventions and programs. In order for these community–academic partnerships to be successful, there must be trust, mutual respect, and a common conceptualization of the issue. It takes time for these partnerships to develop and extensive listening on the part of the academic researchers is required. Within HIV prevention practice and research specifically, there is a need for frank conversations about intimate and often stigmatized transmission routes as well as which community members are at greatest risk. There is profound need to develop trust and discuss and identify the different priorities among stakeholders (including tribal elders and agencies providing services to an AI/AN community). Moreover, as partners engage in the development of HIV prevention interventions and programs, the geographic, social, and cultural distances should be acknowledged [10, 48, 71, 80]. Honesty, recognition of differences, and humility among all partners are key; however, academic researchers have a history of being less humble and not recognizing that what they assume to be generalizable may in fact be stereotyping.

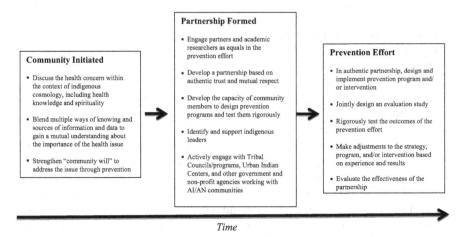

Fig. 6.2 American Indian/Alaska Native community-driven prevention research proces

One of AI/AN communities partnering with practitioners and academic researchers to develop and test HIV prevention interventions and programs is promising (Fig. 6.2). One key aspect of this process is the development of tribal capacity to design, implement, and rigorously evaluate prevention interventions and programs [81]. It is crucial that AI/AN community partners participate in all aspects of the research process, again to ensure the most grounded and promising interventions and programs possible. The concept is simple: Engagement and partnership ensure that phenomena are better understood and make it more likely that developed interventions and programs will be successful [58, 59, 79]. Moreover, besides having the best HIV prevention interventions and programs possible, participating in the process as equal partners builds community members' capacity to solve problems; conduct research; and create, implement, and evaluate evidence-based interventions and programs themselves. These skills reach far beyond HIV and are transferrable to other health issues. In fact, it has been noted that the skills developed through engaged research (including what is commonly referred to as community-based participatory research, CBPR) may have an impact on the health and well-being of communities more broadly through the development of skills that can be applied to reduce other health disparities experienced by vulnerable communities [58, 59, 79, 82, 83].

Specific Promising and Evidence-Based HIV Prevention Interventions

Tribal governments and nonprofits are working in tribal communities and making an appreciable impact on HIV at some level; however, few HIV prevention interventions and programs have been implemented and rigorously tested with AI/

ANs. This lack of evidence may in part be explained by the cultural mismatch of preexisting prevention interventions and programs and the history of mistrust between AI/AN communities and "outsiders." Although the criteria for scientific rigor (as is often defined by Western-trained academic researchers) are important, we discourage an analysis of the state of prevention efforts among AI/AN communities based solely on rigorous methodological standards, because such limited perspective places value solely on Western knowledge and ways of knowing without acknowledging the value of indigenous knowledge and ways of knowing. For many of these interventions and programs, what they often lack in traditional scientific rigor is made up for in creative partnerships and the incorporation of unique AI/AN-specific cultural and contextual factors. In other words, it is important to recognize the continuum between evidence-based practice and practice-based evidence. Thus, we reviewed six current prevention interventions and programs within AI/AN communities to highlight some of the successes, challenges, and opportunities, as well as the importance of cultivating and maintaining relationships among community members, community leaders, organization representatives (including tribal structures), and academic researchers, while acknowledging the existence of multiple ways of knowledge generation and knowing and of defining health and illness. We take a postcolonial perspective by considering both the quality of the community partnership as well as the scientific rigor of the available evidence.

In our review of these interventions and programs, we outlined the population that the intervention or program is designed to reach and affect, the research design, aspects of community engagement and partnership, outcomes, and whether the program or intervention is promising (Table 6.1). We also identified whether a holistic view of health (Fig. 6.1) was incorporated. Because the reviewed interventions all have significant methodological limitations and some do not measure or report outcomes, we do not focus on these aspects; these types of challenges are clear. Rather, we highlight the ways community engagement and partnerships are used and harnessed to attune them to the local cultural context.

Native American Prevention Project Against AIDS and Substance Abuse (NAPPASA)

NAPPASA is a school-based curriculum designed to reduce HIV and other sexual risks as well as alcohol and drug use. NAPPASA is listed as a promising intervention by the US Department of Justice, Office of Juvenile Justice and Delinquency Prevention, and reports have been published on its development [72] and positive outcomes [84]. This intervention was the result of a partnership among members from several AI/AN communities in the southwestern part of the USA, health care professionals, and researchers. Early in the development process, interviews and focus groups were conducted to identify community knowledge of and attitudes about HIV, HIV risk, and alcohol and drug use. These interviews and focus groups also were used to help identify culturally congruent prevention messages. Baldwin and

Table 6.1 Identified HIV/AIDS prevention interventions, results, and level of available evidence

Intervention title or description	Target population	Research design	Community engagement and partnership	Holistic view of health	Outcomes	Status of intervention
Native American Prevention Project Against AIDS and Substance Abuse (NAPPASA) [73, 85]	8th and 9th grade students	Quasi-experimental with comparison group	The community was consulted through interviews and focus groups	Yes	⇑ abstinence and ⇓ in sex while using substances	Promising
Circle of Life (COL) [88]	Middle-school students	Longitudinal with waitlist control group	A community advisory board was created and extensive community outreach took place	Yes	No significant difference between groups	Results unclear
Gathering of Native Americans (GONA) [90]	Adolescents	Single group with pre/posttest	Developed, implemented, and tested by the community	Yes	⇑ in knowledge and self-efficacy; no change in ethnic identity or behaviors	Promising
Intervention with motivational interviewing and transtheoretical changes [81]	Adults in substance abuse treatment	Single group with pretest and posttest	Limited, implemented in partnership with organizations serving the community	No	⇑ Knowledge and ⇑ in rate of testing	Unclear due to significant limitations in research design
HIV prevention in Maine [95]	Entire community	Posttest only	Partnered with a community agency and conducted a needs assessment, and community members developed the intervention based on the findings	Unclear	Behavior change not measured	Unclear due to significant limitations in research design
Women's Circle: toward healthier relationships [77]	Adult women	Outcomes not measured	Collaboration between a community health educator and social scientist; focus groups were conducted with the community to identify important topics to address in the intervention	Yes	Outcomes not measured	Outcomes not measured

colleagues offered a thorough description of their theoretical model and emphasized that it incorporated both Western, biomedical conceptions of health and behavior, and holistic views of health rooted in AI/AN communities and cultures [72, 85].

NAPPASA was tested with eighth and ninth grade students in 14 schools located on reservations or in adjacent communities. Almost 80 % of the 2,704 participants identified as AI/AN or AI/AN and another racial/ethnic identity, and male and female students were represented equally. The study design was quasi-experimental with pre, post, and follow-up assessments; the intervention was used for 2,038 participants, and 666 drawn from the same grades served as the nonintervention control group. Some students received the intervention curriculum for 1 year and others for 2 years. Outcomes included reduced sexual risk and alcohol and drug use. Specific to HIV risk, individuals in the intervention group maintained abstinence longer and among those who were sexually active, the rate of having sex while drunk or high was lower.

The intervention was identified as having a rigorous design in a comprehensive systematic review of the literature of culturally sensitive interventions for AI/AN adolescents [84]. Because it is one of the only evidence-based interventions for AI/AN adolescents to reduce HIV risk, it was subsequently adapted for urban AI/AN adolescents [86].

Circle of Life (COL)

The COL intervention encompasses two HIV prevention curricula for AI/AN adolescents. Developed in the late 1990s and early 2000s and implemented without peer-reviewed evaluation, COL intervention had discrete versions for elementary and middle-school students. More recently, however, researchers have begun adapting the intervention and evaluating the middle-school curriculum [87]. Researchers partnered with tribal governments and school districts in the Northern Plains to conduct a longitudinal evaluation of the COL intervention for middle-school students [88]. When originally approached about partnering to implement an intervention, the tribe was interested and had a high level of awareness of challenges and risks facing adolescents. This "readiness" was attributed to the success of highly active community health organizers who had laid the groundwork by raising awareness within the tribe about HIV and substance use among adolescents. Furthermore, these community health organizers used a holistic conceptualization of health.

As a result of community awareness and readiness and the culturally congruent (thus acceptable and meaningful) approach, staff from all 13 middle schools provided letters of support for a grant application to fund the project. A community advisory board was formed to foster clear and transparent communication among all partners, including community members, parents, tribal groups, schools, and researchers. Additionally, there was impressive community outreach, often conducted by community members, to explain the study to parents and obtain informed consent. For example, the research team established a field office in the community, hired community members, and met individually with each parent or guardian to explain the project and what they were consenting to. When parent contact information was not provided or was not accurate, parents were contacted through community meetings and local media or outreach workers who attended community events. In addition, memorandums of understanding (MOUs) were established with each school, outlining clear roles and expectations. MOU, for example, included data-sharing plans prior to data collection, given that a common value of community engagement includes the notion that data from the community are, in fact, owned by the community. Furthermore, community members reviewed all measurement items before implementation, and they suggested additional items that added to the measurement tool.

Similar to NAPPASA, the COL intervention used a hybrid of standard Western HIV prevention approaches, behavior change theories, and AI/AN conceptualizations of health. It built on the traditional medicine wheel, which includes mental, spiritual, physical, and emotional facets of health (a version of which is presented in Fig. 6.1), and also on social cognitive theory, theory of reasoned action, and theory of planned behavior. This balance is a good example of the implementation of post-colonial perspectives in HIV prevention. The intervention was developed by staff of an AI/AN-controlled organization with extensive input from other community members as well. The intervention was pilot tested and modifications were made on the basis of input from focus groups and preliminary results.

To test the final intervention, schools were randomly assigned to two conditions. As a compromise with tribal and school leaders, the design used a wait-list control; this design has been identified as more appealing within many communities that want all community members to benefit from a potentially health-promoting and disease-preventing innovation [59, 79, 88]. Recognizing that from the perspective of a longitudinal study they lacked a true control group because they randomized at the school level when they were interested in outcomes at the individual level, Kaufman et al. noted a plan to examine how baseline differences affected long-term efficacy of the COL intervention. Although community engagement and participation were high, cultural congruence and meaningfulness were clear, theoretical foundations were solid, and community ownership and outreach were impressive; initial findings showed no significant differences between intervention assignments (i.e., intervention versus wait-list control).

Adaptations of the COL intervention have been explored. Because of the great variability with the AI/AN communities, the developers of the intervention designed and included topic areas that could be adapted depending on characteristics of the community. They included instructions on how to effectively and efficiently adapt the intervention.

Although they did not report outcomes, Kaufman and colleagues discussed an adaptation of the COL intervention for use in Native Boys and Girls Clubs after-school programs, shifting the content to fit an after-school program rather than a school setting. They concluded that the adaptation was generally well received, but they noted that many of the local clubs refused to include the chapters on homosexuality and condom use. Drawing on qualitative interviews, they identified a need to develop regional variations of the intervention to better reflect the cultural diversity among AI/AN communities and the settings in which the intervention may be implemented. Despite some methodological limitations and a lack of strong statistical findings to date, the COL intervention remains one of the more rigorously designed and tested HIV prevention interventions for AI/AN communities.

Gathering of Native Americans (GONA)

The GONA intervention was developed by tribal leaders through a grant funded by the Center for Substance Abuse Prevention (CSAP). GONA intervention was primarily designed as a substance abuse prevention intervention. This intervention is rooted in an explicit discussion of colonialism and historical trauma and focuses on AI/AN conceptualizations of holistic health and wellness. The 4-day curriculum embraces traditional values such as belonging, mastery, interdependence, and generosity and includes empowerment and skills development [89, 90].

Although not originally designed to have an impact on sexual risk and prevent HIV exposure and transmission, the GONA intervention has been implemented and tested by The Native American Health Clinic (NAHC) in Oakland, CA. The initial study used participant satisfaction surveys and found the majority of participants reported that (1) their refusal skills improved, (2) their knowledge of and connection to AI/AN culture increased, (3) their communication skills improved, and (4) their community involvement tended to increase. Staff from NAHC conducted another study of the GONA intervention and tested its impact on knowledge, perception of risk, sexual self-efficacy, and sexual risk. In this second study, attempts were made to increase the sample size conducted at pretest and posttest. The sampling process, however, was responsive more to the needs of participating agencies than study design, and 46 % of participants were lost at follow-up. This study found increased HIV knowledge and self-efficacy. Unfortunately, behavior (e.g., increased consistent condom use) did not change significantly [91]. Despite the challenges and methodological limits, overall the programs implemented by NAHC are promising. The ongoing efforts made by researchers and a tribal entity to engage and partner to design and rigorously test an HIV intervention are also impressive.

Intervention with Motivational Interviewing and Transtheoretical Stages of Change

An intervention that used both motivational interviewing [92] and the transtheoretical stages of change [93] was designed and implemented through a broad-based partnership among substance abuse counseling providers, an AI/AN-focused AIDS service organization (ASO), the Indian Health Service, and academic researchers.

The two-part intervention designed for and implemented in a residential substance abuse treatment program consisted of one 60-min group information session followed by a 30-min one-on-one session. Acknowledging that the lack of a control group limits the strength of the findings, the partnership documented an increase in HIV knowledge and a high rate (78 %) of HIV testing [80]. The choice of setting is an important response to the elevated rates of alcohol and other drug abuse within AI/AN communities and the ways in which substance abuse can elevate HIV risk. Similarly, the approach of motivational interviewing and the use of stages of change seem an appropriate fit for the population and setting—one where seeds of change are routinely planted for future growth.

HIV Prevention in Maine

Working with a rural AI/AN community in Maine, a social work educator and a service provider in an agency that serves AI/AN communities, developed, nurtured, and maintained a partnership and conducted research to explore the HIV prevention needs in the community. Based on formative data from a needs assessment, they identified three key strategies that could be employed to reduce risk. They partnered with members of the community to develop an intervention to increase awareness and reduce risk. Because they knew that some community members had attitudes that discouraged condom use and they found low rates of actual use, they drew on culturally relevant approaches to craft their intervention. Primarily, they (1) trained respected elders to provide HIV education and discuss safer sex with younger community members, (2) used a theater troupe to put on plays telling stories about HIV, and (3) distributed AI/AN-made jewelry featuring condoms in the design. Their evaluation did not measure change in behavior; rather, they documented that the intervention was memorable, and high-risk community members reported that the approach was appropriate. Despite limitations, the partners demonstrated authentic academic and agency partnership to develop a promising and culturally grounded intervention [94].

Women's Circle: Toward Healthier Relationships

Klein et al. reported on a unique collaboration between an urban AI/AN health clinic and researchers to develop an HIV prevention program for AI/AN women in the San Francisco Bay area. The intervention was known as Women's Circle: Toward Healthier Relationships. The partnership was established early during the grant preparation phase, the intervention was developed; it was not established "after the fact" or in response to a need for participant recruitment. Each partner brought unique talents that complemented one another, and the process included ongoing communication and negotiation among partners. Discussions about resource allocation were conducted upfront, when the grant was being written, in order to reduce possible subsequent conflicts. The development of the intervention included input from potential participants through focus groups, who offered input on topics of importance as well as the structure of the intervention. Reflecting a broad view of health, the topics were diverse, including HIV/AIDS, intimate partner violence, parenting, substance abuse, and welfare reform. Furthermore, although both the intervention and other agency services were available to AI/ANs and non-AI/ANs, the intervention was developed with AI/AN cultural values in mind, including a holistic view of health and an emphasis on the connection between individual and community health. The resulting intervention had 11 sessions (a mix of small groups and individual sessions) and videos [76].

Klein et al. described key lessons learned from their partnership process. They reported that the team had difficulty identifying specific outcomes that should be included in the evaluation instrument because the intervention covered a wide array of topics, spanning from parenting to substance abuse. Time limitations and respect for participant burden required that the survey length be reasonable (e.g., short); thus, the team had to carefully select what was necessary to measure in order to create a parsimonious survey. This problem occurs often in community–academic research partnerships; academic researchers want to ensure they can adequately measure outcomes and community partners are concerned with feasibility. In addition to tension about which measures to include in the evaluation instrument, at one point a community provider questioned the value of research. Potential misunderstandings during the evaluation were averted because the strong personal relationship developed between the community provider and the academic researcher prior to the implementation of the intervention allowed them to express and address skeptical attitudes and other potential challenges through open dialogue. Members of the team reported that, overall, the relationship built during the intensity of the grant writing process facilitated their ease to work through issues when they faced challenges during implementation and evaluation of the intervention [76].

Emerging Common Themes in HIV Prevention with AI/AN Communities

Importance of Community Perception and Readiness

The issue of community perception was present throughout many of the studies we explored. Some researchers have suggested that HIV is sometimes seen by community members as an external issue; HIV infection may be perceived as happening only to "others," not to oneself [61]. Even when identified as a community priority, knowledge, attitudes, and resources greatly shape how a particular community responds. For example, given the stigma around sex, sexuality, and substance use, communities may struggle over how, when, where, and with whom to discuss sex and substance use. Other concerns and questions emerge as well, including the following examples:

- Should a community with stark immediate needs and a history of mistreatment from academic research and medical communities accept the use of a control group, which increases design validity but—at least in the short-term—serves fewer individuals?
- How much time and resources can community "insiders" (e.g., members) and providers be expected to spend going to research meetings, helping to secure informed consent, and capturing outcome data?
- Should a resource-poor community divert talent and resources from clearly established epidemics such as alcoholism and diabetes, which are often perceived as more immediate, to prevent the worsening of the impact of HIV locally?

Clearly, such questions can have an impact on a community's readiness to act to reduce HIV risk among its members. The Community Readiness Model has been suggested as helpful for building support for interventions and programs in AI/AN communities [15, 95, 96]. The Community Readiness Model assesses a community's awareness of an issue and readiness for change with nine stages, ranging from no awareness to complete community ownership (Fig. 6.3). This assessment is followed by the development of a "readiness action plan" that suggests next steps in response to current community priorities and climate. This approach has proved successful in helping multiple AI/AN communities prepare to implement behavioral HIV prevention interventions specially approved and disseminated by the CDC [95].

Areas for Expansion

Two broad themes that emerge from the literature on the prevention of HIV in AI/AN communities warrant further elaboration. First, significant and insightful attempts have been made to bridge the divide between indigenous communities and the medical and research communities through community engagement and partnership. However, authentic partnerships that include an equitable distribution of power are rare. Second, there are few published studies of approaches to HIV prevention with AI/AN communities that can be considered methodologically rigorous by Western standards.

Characteristics of Effective Partnerships

Despite the fact that we have often focused on the challenges of partnerships, the literature offers examples of how effective partnerships can be cultivated and maintained. From the perspective of the academic researcher, seeing research as a relationship to cultivate and maintain is essential. Indigenous communities have made it clear that "drive-by research" is not helpful or welcome. Discussing capacity building in AI/AN communities, Chino and DeBruyn emphasized the importance of a cyclical and iterative approach to the development and testing of interventions [90]. Baldwin and colleagues focused on the value of using CBPR to help build partnerships that include members of AI/AN communities, organization representatives, and academic researchers [96]. Consistent with a CBPR approach, they argue for early collaboration during design of the project and development of the intervention and program, the use of a very involved and nontoken community advisory body, and the employment of community members in the effort.

An optimal way to bridge the chasms is to increase the number of indigenous individuals involved in academic research; however, it is important not to assume that an academic researcher from the community understands current priorities and needs; "assumed understanding" can have its own pitfalls. After someone has "left" a community, interacted with "others" and nontribal systems through school and work, for instance, and earned an advanced degree, they may not represent the community from which they came. Reflexivity, as discussed in Chap. 10, is one approach to reduce the reliance on assumed understanding, knowledge, and tokenism. Cultural humility, as described in Chap. 1, also is a good approach for both insiders and outsiders to reduce assumptions.

Adaptation Issues

The literature on adapting prevention interventions for use with communities in which they were not tested is limited [97–100]. However, the process of adapting HIV prevention interventions for new contexts has been explored [101, 102]. There is an inherent trade-off when the decision is made to use an intervention developed in another context and with another population. It is important to note that the CDC and state health departments continue to set a priority for the use of previously tested and evidence-based interventions. In fact, use or adaptation of evidence-based interventions increases the likelihood of receiving government funding. Unfortunately, none of these evidence-based interventions was developed with or for AI/AN communities.

From 2009–2012, the CDC worked in partnership with the Arizona Intertribal Council and three tribes in that state to adapt the intervention known as Sisters Informing Sisters On Topics about AIDS (SISTAS). SISTAS is an evidence-based intervention initially developed to prevent HIV exposure and transmission among female African American/black adolescents [103]. The adaptation process has recently been completed and included the incorporation of AI/AN symbols and iconography, use of storytelling, and other culturally specific content throughout the intervention. Moreover, the CDC has encouraged each tribal community to further adapt the intervention to its specific tribal context, such as language and symbolism [104]. Although the AI/AN-adapted version has not yet been evaluated through a

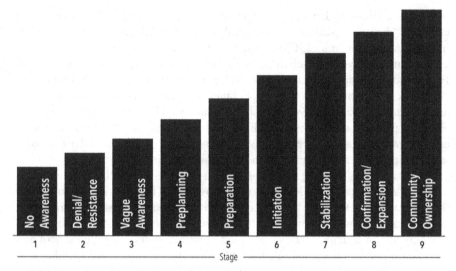

Fig. 6.3 Nine stages of readiness adapted for HIV/AIDS

randomized control trial, focus groups conducted with participants identified high levels of satisfaction with the adapted version. On the other hand, evaluators have reported difficulties with what they define as "appropriate" implementation and fidelity. Another potential problem is that the original intervention was developed nearly 20 years ago, which means that, in addition to the different context and population, the intervention may be outdated and its relevance may be limited.

Moreover, there are concerns when an intervention or program that has worked within one community or population is adapted for another; an error can occur in multiple places. As examples, the theoretical foundation of an efficacious intervention or program may not make sense for the community or population for whom adaptation is taking place; formative data collection can be rushed; translation of formative data into adapted intervention or program components can be inaccurate; and program components themselves may not even make sense. When adaptation is planned to make an intervention or program "fit" another community or population, the necessary steps may not be taken or taken with enough rigor to ensure its appropriateness and its potential to promote health and prevent disease. Indeed, not giving the same focus and attention to the entire development and efficacy-testing process that has been given to interventions and programs for other racial/ethnic communities may be a vestige of colonialism.

Implications for Future Research

The interventions discussed in this chapter offer some useful foundations on which to build as we begin to identify and meet the needs and priorities of AI/AN communities. Some themes found throughout the literature were the incorporation of assets such as community identity, respected elders, indigenous knowledge, and norms about sexual behavior and risks. The focus on holistic health or working with the whole person was also evident in the interventions and programs described and was key to intervention development, adaptation, and, theoretically, success [37, 72, 75, 76, 87, 102]. Often, the holistic health approach led to interventions and programs that targeted multiple issues at once. For example, Klein et al. addressed all of the following within their intervention: HIV prevention, reproductive health, parenting, fitness, nutrition, violence and trauma, substance abuse, community support, self-esteem, and welfare reform. Although unstated, the decision to offer HIV testing and prevention in a residential substance abuse center is a reflection of this holistic approach. Such approaches align with a broader focus to target social determinates of community health [76].

In addition, most of the prevention efforts explored included community partners, although the degree of power sharing differed by intervention. Some interventions were developed through consultations with tribal communities, using focus groups and interviews [76], in order to better understand indigenous knowledge and customs, whereas other interventions were developed, implemented, and tested by tribal members [2]. In their study, Klein and colleagues discussed the process of partnership and lessons learned to provide community partners and academic researchers insights into the complex dynamics that occur in a community–academic partnership [76].

In addition to assessing studies for the traditional marks of scientific rigor, we contend that the equity of the partnership between the community and academic researchers should also be critiqued. This point seems particularly important as we move toward addressing the social determinants of health and reducing health inequities, including HIV-related health inequities.

Although virtually all prevention interventions reviewed made reference to traditional or tribal values informing programming, only a small number made attempts to test the hypothesized relationship [2]. Explication and testing of such cultural assumptions should occur more often and—despite the obvious irony—more formally. Doing so, brings all involved closer to the underlying tension between world views and raises the question: Who's way of knowing is superior? By creating community partnerships that are respectful and open, HIV interventions and programs can be built on the best of both worlds: placing prevention in the context of holistic health and rigorously testing the interventions and programs to assess their effectiveness to address this growing social problem.

Discussion and Conclusion

To a large extent, we conclude where we began. The literature on HIV prevention for AI/AN communities highlights the historical and modern faces of colonialism. Although a desire to move beyond colonialism is understandable, it is sadly naive. Forces of oppression and privilege continue and increase HIV risk and related conditions in AI/AN communities. Some argue that the disparity in rates of HIV within AI/AN communities is not at the extreme levels of inequalities of other health issues facing this community (e.g., poverty, injuries, tuberculosis, and infant mortality); however, the presence of risk factors (including high rates of STIs), high levels of substance use, and sexual risk warrant concern. The disproportionate burden of HIV borne by AI/AN communities necessitates action, but we contend that this action must be done through engagement and partnership. We cannot confront HIV using approaches that align with colonialism; instead, we must work together to blend the perspectives and resources of diverse partners.

Despite the recognized need for evidence-based HIV prevention interventions and programs, the same colonial forces that created risk for HIV exposure and transmission within AI/AN communities complicate the honest attempts by indigenous, medical, and research communities to mount successful prevention efforts. In order to overcome these barriers and implement effective HIV prevention interventions and programs in AI/AN communities, efforts must come from within this community; respectful and trusting partnerships must be built and nurtured, and the capacity for research among tribal members must be developed. Although ideal research conditions have rarely been achieved in prevention science with this population, a number of community-driven HIV prevention interventions and programs have been developed grounded in the unique contexts of AI/AN communities. Those programs that have been most promising treat the whole person and provide templates for next steps in both research and practice.

Summary and Recommendations

- AI/AN communities may benefit from a raised consciousness about the impact of HIV and require a level of community "readiness" to both address HIV and engage and partner with others.
- In order to move forward with HIV prevention efforts, the understanding of HIV among AI/ANs must be developed and contextualized within the frame of indigenous knowledge and ways of knowing and "doing things."
- Academic researchers must be available to tribal communities to partner on program and intervention development, implementation, and evaluation when tribal communities are ready. This may require mutual trust and long-standing relationships.
- Capacity must be enhanced for academic researchers and providers to authentically partner with tribal communities and tribal communities to implement rigorous scientific methodologies.
- New research paradigms must be developed that include engagement, partnership, and self-determination.
- Community–academic partnerships must be authentic; power must be shared, and differences among partners should not be understood as differences in status.
- Existing barriers between Indian Health Service and local tribal government should be reduced so that information can be shared about the health needs of the tribal communities.

- Work should continue to be done to reduce the stigma attached to getting tested for or living with HIV.
- HIV prevention interventions and programs must be informed by the issues and dynamics of historical trauma.
- Tribal, cultural, and linguistic diversity must be recognized; stereotyping of any partner must be avoided.
- Individuals within tribal communities may be trained to successfully disseminate information, distribute risk reduction resources, build skills, combat stigma, and facilitate HIV testing.

The intersecting journeys of community engagement and participation and HIV prevention are not linear just as life is not linear. There will be ups and downs along the way. There is much hope because of the good work being conducted in partnership with communities on tribal lands and in cities around the country. It is vital that we continue to make progress. AI/AN communities must be a priority for the development, implementation, and evaluation of HIV prevention interventions and programs, and these efforts must be conducted through engagement and partnership. Authentic engagement and partnership is not easy, but the results, if done well, can be profound. We continue to face an epidemic and even after 30 years, our toolkit is limited. Community engagement and partnership not only have the potential to affect HIV among AI/AN communities but provide guidance to address other health disparities facing these and other communities and populations.

References

1. Said EW. Culture and imperialism. Vintage Books, New York, NY. 1993.
2. Duran B, Walters KL. HIV/AIDS prevention in „Indian country": current practice, indigenist etiology models, and postcolonial approaches to change. AIDS Educ Prev. 2004;16(3):187–201.
3. Jones DS. The persistence of American Indian health disparities. Am J Public Health. 2006;96(12):2122–34.
4. Vernon I, Jumper-Thurman P. The changing face of HIV/AIDS among Native populations. J Psychoactive Drugs. 2005;37(3):247–55.
5. Centers for Disease Control and Prevention. HIV Surveillance Report, 2011; 2013.
6. Prejean J, Song R, Hernandez A, Ziebell R, Green T, Walker F, et al. Estimated HIV incidence in the United States, 2006–2009. PloS ONE. 2011;6(8):e17502.
7. Alaska Department of Health and Human Services. 2010–2012 Alaska HIV Prevention Plan. Anchorage. Alaska: Alaska Department of Health and Human Services; 2010.
8. South Dakota Department of Health. South Dakota Epidemiologic Profile of HIV/AIDS 2011. Pierre, South Dakota: South Dakota Department of Health; 2011.
9. Minnesota Department of Health. HIV Surveillance Report. St. Paul, Minnesota: Minnesota Department of Health; 2011.
10. Bertolli J, Lee LM, Sullivan PS. Racial misidentification of American Indians/Alaska Natives in the HIV/AIDS Reporting Systems of five states and one urban health jurisdiction, U.S., 1984–2002. Public Health Rep. 2007;122(3):382–92.

11. Reilley B, Redd JT, Cheek J, Giberson S. A review of missed opportunities for prenatal HIV screening in a nationwide sample of health facilities in the Indian Health Service. J Community Health. 2011;36(4):631–4.

12. Vernon IS, Jumper-Thurman P. Prevention of HIV/AIDS in Native American communities: promising interventions. Public Health Rep. 2002;117(Suppl 1):S96–103.

13. Duran B, Bulterys M, Iralu J, Graham Ahmed Edwards CM, Edwards A, Harrison M. American Indians with HIV/AIDS: health and social service needs, barriers to care, and satisfaction with services among a Western tribe. Am Indian Alaska Native Ment Health Res. 2000;9(2):22–35 (Online).

14. Centers for Disease Control and Prevention. HIV/AIDS among American Indian and Alaska Natives; 2008.

15. Vernon IS. Killing us quietly: Native Americans and HIV/AIDS. Lincoln: University of Nebraska Press; 2001.

16. Walters KL, Simoni JM, Harris C. Patterns and predictors of HIV risk among urban American Indians. Am Indian Alaska Native Ment Health Res. (Online). 2000;9(2):1–21. [Epub 2001/03/30].

17. Gone JP. Reconsidering American Indian historical trauma: lessons from an early Gros Ventre war narrative. Transcult Psychiatry. 2013;0(0):1–20. doi:10.1177/1363461513489722.

18. Compton WM, Thomas YF, Stinson FS, Grant BF. Prevalence, correlates, disability, and comorbidity of DSM-IV drug abuse and dependence in the United States: results from the national epidemiologic survey on alcohol and related conditions. Arch Gen Psychiatry. 2007;64(5):566–76.

19. Grant BF, Dawson DA, Stinson FS, Chou SP, Dufour MC, Pickering RP. The 12-month prevalence and trends in DSM-IV alcohol abuse and dependence: United States, 1991–1992 and 2001–2002. Drug Alcohol Depend. 2004;74(3):223–34.

20. Center for Behavioral Health Statistics and Quality SAaMHSA. Injecting drug abuse adminssions to substance abuse treatment: 1992 and 2009. The TEDS Report. 2011.

21. Strathdee SA, Stockman JK. Epidemiology of HIV among injecting and non-injecting drug users: current trends and implications for interventions. Curr HIV/AIDS Rep. 2010;7(2):99–106.

22. Baldwin JA, Maxwell CJ, Fenaughty AM, Trotter RT, Stevens SJ. Alcohol as a risk factor for HIV transmission among American Indian and Alaska Native drug users. Am Indian Alaska Native Ment Health Res. 2000;9(1):1–16 (Online).

23. Frosch D, Shoptaw S, Huber A, Rawson RA, Ling W. Sexual HIV risk among gay and bisexual male methamphetamine abusers. J Subst Abuse Treat. 1996;13(6):483–6.

24. Substance Abuse and Mental Health Services Administration. Results from the 2011 National survey on drug use and health: summary of national findings. Rockville, MD: Substance Abuse and Mental Health Services Administration, 2012 Contract No.: NSDUH Series H-44, HHS Publication No (SMA) 12–4713.

25. Leigh BC. Peril, chance, adventure: concepts of risk, alcohol use and risky behavior in young adults. Addiction. 1999;94(3):371–83.

26. Fleming DT, Wasserheit JN. From epidemiological synergy to public health policy and practice: the contribution of other sexually transmitted diseases to sexual transmission of HIV infection. Sex Transm Infect. 1999;75(1):3–17.

27. Nelson KM, Simoni JM, Pearson CR, Walters KL. 'I've had unsafe sex so many times why bother being safe now?': the role of cognitions in sexual risk among American Indian/Alaska Native men who have sex with men. Ann Behav Med. 2011;42(3):370–80.

28. US Census Bureau. Profile America: facts for features: American Indian and Alaska Native Heritage Month: November 2012. Washington, DC: US Census Bureau; 2012.

29. Garrett MT, Pichette EF. Red as an apple: Native American acculturation and counseling with or without reservation. J Couns Dev. 2000;78(1):3–13.

30. Wolfley JE. Ecological risk assessment and management: their failure to value indigenous traditional ecological knowledge and protect tribal homelands. Am Indian Cult Res J. 1998;22:151–69.

31. Whitbeck LB, Walls ML, Johnson KD, Morrisseau AD, McDougall CM. Depressed affect and historical loss among North American Indigenous adolescents. Am Indian Alaska Native Ment Health Res. 2009;16(3):16–41 (Online).
32. Stevens SJ, Estrada AL. HIV and AIDS among American Indians and Alaska Natives. Am Indian Alaska Native Ment Health Res. 2000;9(1):v–ix (Online).
33. Lowe J. A cultural approach to conducting HIV/AIDS and hepatitis C virus education among native American adolescents. J Sch Nurs. 2008;24(4):229–38.
34. Stevens S, Estrada A. Editorial: HIV and AIDS among American Indians and Alaska Natives. Am Indian Alaska Native Ment Health Res. 2000;9(1):v–ix.
35. Dennis MK. Risk and protective factors for HIV/AIDS in Native Americans: implications for preventive intervention. Soc Work. 2009;54(2):145–54.
36. Duran B, Harrison M, Shurley M, Foley K, Morris P, Davidson-Stroh L, et al. Tribally-driven HIV/AIDS health services partnerships: evidence-based meets culture centered interventions. J HIV AIDS Soc Serv. 2010;9(1):110–29.
37. Lowe J. Research brief: the need for historically grounded HIV/AIDS prevention research among Native Americans. J Assoc Nurses AIDS Care. 2007;18(2):15–7.
38. Brave Heart MY, DeBruyn LM. The American Indian Holocaust: healing historical unresolved grief. Am Indian Alaska Native Ment Health Res. 1998;8(2):56–78 (Online).
39. Sotero M. A conceptual model of historical trauma: implications for public health practice and research. J Health Disparities Res Pract. 2006;1(1):93–108.
40. Wilson HW, Widom CS. Sexually transmitted diseases among adults who had been abused and neglected as children: a 30-year prospective study. Am J Public Health. 2009;99(Suppl 1):S197–203.
41. Evans-Campbell T. Historical trauma in American Indian/Native Alaskan communities. J Interpers Violence. 2008;23(3):316–38.
42. Oetzel J, Duran B. Intimate partner violence in American Indian and/or Alaska Native communities: a social ecological framework of determinants and interventions. Am Indian Alaska Native Ment Health Res. 2004;11(3):49–68.
43. Simoni JM, Sehgal S, Walters KL. Triangle of risk: urban American Indian women's sexual trauma, injection drug use, and HIV sexual risk behaviors. AIDS Behav. 2004;8(1):33–45.
44. Wu E, El-Bassel N, Witte SS, Gilbert L, Chang M. Intimate partner violence and HIV risk among urban minority women in primary health care settings. AIDS Behav. 2003;7(3):291–301.
45. Pharris MD, Resnick MD, Blum RW. Protecting against hopelessness and suicidality in sexually abused American Indian adolescents. J Adolesc Health. 1997;21(6):400–6.
46. Medrano MA, Zule WA, Hatch J, Desmond DP. Prevalence of childhood trauma in a community sample of substance-abusing women. Am J Drug Alcohol Abuse. 1999;25(3):449–62.
47. Fullilove MT, Lown EA, Fullilove RE. Crack 'hos and skeezers: traumatic experiences of women crack users. J Sex Res. 1992;29(2):275–87.
48. Thornton R. American Indian holocaust and survival: a population history since 1492. Norman: University of Oklahoma Press; 1987.
49. Benson T. Blinded with science: American Indians, the Office on Indian Affairs, and the federal campaign against trachoma, 1924–1927. Am Indian Cult Res J. 1999;23(3):119–42.
50. Jarrell RH. Native American women and forced sterilization, 1973–1976. Caduceus (Springfield, Ill). 1992;8(3):45–58.
51. Cross T. Spirituality and mental health: a Native American perspective. Focal Point. 2001;15(2):37–8.
52. Gilgun JF. Completing the circle: American Indian medicine wheels and the promotion of resilence of children and youth in care. J Human Behav Soc Environ. 2002;6(2):65–84.
53. Kulis S, Hodge DR, Ayers SL, Brown EF, Marsiglia FF. Spirituality and religion: intertwined protective factors for substance use among urban American Indian youth. Am J Drug Alcohol Abuse. 2012;38(5):444–9.
54. Institute of Medicine. Promoting health: intervention strategies from social and behavioral research. Washington, DC: National Academy Press; 2000.

55. Institute of Medicine. No time to lose: Getting more from HIV prevention. Washington, DC: National Academy Press; 2001.

56. Institute of Medicine. Unequal treatment: confronting racial and ethnic disparities in health care. Washington, DC: National Academy Press; 2003.

57. Institute of Medicine, Committee on Prevention and Control of Sexually Transmitted Diseases. The hidden epidemic: Confronting sexually transmitted diseases. Eng TR, Butlet WT, editors. Washington, DC: National Academy Press; 1997.

58. Rhodes SD, Malow RM, Jolly C. Community-based participatory research: a new and not-so-new approach to HIV/AIDS prevention, care, and treatment. AIDS Educ Prev. 2010;22(3):173–83.

59. Rhodes SD. Demonstrated effectiveness and potential of CBPR for preventing HIV in Latino populations. In: Organista KC, Editor. HIV Prevention with Latinos: theory, research, and practice. New York: Oxford University Press; 2012. p. 83–102.

60. Blankenship KM, Bray SJ, Merson MH. Structural interventions in public health. AIDS. 2000;14(Suppl 1):S11–21.

61. Rhodes SD, Hergenrather KC, Vissman AT, Stowers J, Davis AB, Hannah A, et al. Boys must be men, and men must have sex with women: a qualitative CBPR study to explore sexual risk among African American, Latino, and white gay men and MSM. Am J Men's Health. 2011;5(2):140–51.

62. Stone RA, Whitbeck LB, Chen X, Johnson K, Olson DM. Traditional practices, traditional spirituality, and alcohol cessation among American Indians. J Stud Alcohol. 2006;67(2): 236–44.

63. Farmer P. Infections and inequalities: the modern plagues. Berkeley: University of California Press; 1999.

64. Hertzberg HW. The search for an American Indian identity: modern Pan-Indian movements. Syracuse: Syracuse University Press; 1982.

65. Graham TLC. Using reasons for living to connect to American Indian healing traditions. J Sociol Soc Welf. 2002;29(1):55–75.

66. Hodge DR, Limb GE, Cross TL. Moving from colonization toward balance and harmony: a Native American perspective on wellness. Soc Work. 2009;54(3):211–9.

67. Marsiglia FF, Cross S, Mitchell-Enos V. Culturally grounded group work with adolescent American Indian students. Soc Work Gr. 1998;21(1/2):89–102.

68. Marsiglia FF, Nieri T, Stiffman AR. HIV/AIDS protective factors among urban American Indian youths. J Health Care Poor Underserved. 2006;17(4):745–58.

69. Davis SM, Reid R. Practicing participatory research in American Indian communities. Am J Clin Nutr. 1999;69(4 Suppl):755S–9S.

70. Caldwell JY, Davis JD, Du Bois B, Echo-Hawk H, Erickson JS, Goins RT, et al. Culturally competent research with American Indians and Alaska Natives: findings and recommendations of the first symposium of the work group on American Indian Research and Program Evaluation Methodology. Am Indian Alaska Native Ment Health Res. 2005;12(1):1–21 (Online).

71. Mitchell CM, Kaufman CE. Structure of HIV knowledge, attitudes, and behaviors among American Indian young adults. AIDS Educ Prev. 2002;14(5):401–18.

72. Baldwin JA, Rolf JE, Johnson J, Bowers J, Benally C, Trotter RT. Developing culturally sensitive HIV/AIDS and substance abuse prevention curricula for Native American youth. J Sch Health. 1996;66(9):322–7.

73. Gilley BJ, Co-Cke JH. Cultural investment: providing opportunities to reduce risky behavior among gay American Indian males. J Psychoactive Drugs. 2005;37(3):293–8.

74. Naughton MJ, Rhodes SD. Adoption and maintenance of safer sex practices. In: Shumaker SA, Ockene JK, Riekert K, editors. The handbook of health behavior change. 3 ed. New York: Springer; 2009. p. 253–69.

75. Kaufman CE, Litchfield A, Schupman E, Mitchell CM. Circle of Life HIV/AIDS-prevention intervention for American Indian and Alaska Native youth. Am Indian Alaska Native Ment Health Res. 2012;19(1):140–53 (Online).

76. Klein D, Williams D, Witbrodt J. The collaboration process in HIV prevention and evaluation in an urban American Indian clinic for women. Health Educ Behav. 1999;26(2):239–49. [Epub 1999/03/31].
77. Weaver HN. Through indigenous eyes: native Americans and the HIV epidemic. Health Soc Work. 1999;24(1):27–34.
78. Laveaux D, Christopher S. Contextualizing CBPR: key principles of CBPR meet the indigenous research context. Pimatisiwin. 2009;7(1):1.
79. Rhodes SD, Duck S, Alonzo J, Downs M, Aronson RE. Intervention trials in community-based participatory research. In: Blumenthal D, DiClemente RJ, Braithwaite RL, Smith S, editors. Community-based participatory research: issues, methods, and translation to practice. New York: Springer 2013. p. 157–80.
80. Foley K, Duran B, Morris P, Lucero J, Jiang Y, Baxter B, et al. Using motivational interviewing to promote HIV testing at an American Indian substance abuse treatment facility. J Psychoactive Drugs. 2005;37(3):321–9.
81. Jackson KF, Hodge DR. Native American youth and culturally sensitive interventions: a systematic review. Res Soc Work Pract. 2011;21(2):212–21.
82. Rhodes SD, Daniel J, Alonzo J, Vissman AT, Duck S, Downs M, et al. A snapshot of how Latino heterosexual men promote sexual health within their social networks: process evaluation findings from an efficacious community-level intervention. AIDS Educ Prev. 2012;24(6):514–26.
83. Rhodes SD, Duck S, Alonzo J, Daniel J, Aronson RE. Using community-based participatory research to prevent HIV disparities: assumptions and opportunities identified by the Latino partnership. J Acquir Immune Defic Syndr. 2013;63(Suppl 1):S32–S5.
84. Rolf JE, Nansel TR, Baldwin JA, Johnson K, Benally C. HIV/AIDS and substance abuse prevention in Native American communities: behavioral and community effects. In: Mail PD, Heurtin-Roberts S, Martin SE, Howard J, editors. Alcohol use among American Indians: multiple perspectives on a complex problem. Bethesda: National Institute on Alcohol Abuse and Alcoholism; 2002.
85. Baldwin JA, Trotter RT, 2nd, Martinez D, Stevens SJ, John D, Brems C. HIV/AIDS risks among Native American drug users: key findings from focus group interviews and implications for intervention strategies. AIDS Educ Prev. 1999;11(4):279–92.
86. Wiechelt SA, Gryczynski J, Johnson JL. Designing HIV prevention interventions for urban American Indians: evolution of the don't forget us program. Health Soc Work. 2009;34(4):301–4.
87. Kaufman CE, Mitchell CM, Beals J, Desserich JA, Wheeler C, Keane EM, et al. Circle of life: rationale, design, and baseline results of an HIV prevention intervention among young American Indian adolescents of the Northern plains. Prev Sci. 2010;11(1):101–12.
88. Rhodes SD, McCoy TP, Vissman AT, DiClemente RJ, Duck S, Hergenrather KC, et al. A randomized controlled trial of a culturally congruent intervention to increase condom use and HIV testing among heterosexually active immigrant Latino men. AIDS and Behav. 2011;15(8):1764–75.
89. Nelson K, Tom N. Evaluation of a substance abuse, HIV and hepatitis prevention initiative for urban Native Americans: the Native voices program. J Psychoactive Drugs. 2011;43(4):349–54.
90. Chino M, Debruyn L. Building true capacity: indigenous models for indigenous communities. Am J Public Health. 2006;96(4):596–9.
91. Aguilera S, Plasencia AV. Culturally appropriate HIV/AIDS and substance abuse prevention programs for urban Native youth. J Psychoactive Drugs. 2005;37(3):299–304.
92. Miller WR, Rollnick S. Motivational Interviewing: Helping people change. 3 ed. New York: Guilford; 2012.
93. Prochaska JO, Redding CA, Evers KE. The transtheoretical model and stages of change. In: Glanz K, Rimer BK, Lewis FM, editors. Health behavior and health education: theory, research and practice. San Francisco: Jossey-Bass; 2002. p. 99–120.

94. DePoy E, Bolduc C. AIDS prevention in a rural Native American population: an empirical approach to program development. J Multicult Soc Work. 1992;2(3):51–70.
95. Jumper Thurman P, Vernon IS, Plested B. Advancing HIV/AIDS Prevention among American Indians through capacity building and the community readiness model. J Public Health Manag Pract. 2007:S49–54.
96. Baldwin JA, Johnson JL, Benally CC. Building partnerships between indigenous communities and universities: lessons learned in HIV/AIDS and substance abuse prevention research. Am J Public Health. 2009;99(Suppl 1):S77–82.
97. Castro FG, Barrera M, Jr., Martinez CR, Jr. The cultural adaptation of prevention interventions: resolving tensions between fidelity and fit. Prev Sci. 2004;5(1):41–5.
98. Green LW, Glasgow RE. Evaluating the relevance, generalization, and applicability of research: issues in external validation and translation methodology. Eval Health Prof. 2006;29(1):126–53.
99. Wingood GM, DiClemente RJ. The ADAPT-ITT model: a novel method of adapting evidence-based HIV Interventions. J Acquir Immune Defic Syndr. 2008;47(Suppl 1):S40–6.
100. Falicov CJ. Commentary: on the wisdom and challenges of culturally attuned treatments for Latinos. Fam Process. 2009;48(2):292–309.
101. McKleroy VS, Galbraith JS, Cummings B, Jones P, Harshbarger C, Collins C, et al. Adapting evidence-based behavioral interventions for new settings and target populations. AIDS Educ Prev. 2006;18(4 Suppl A):59–73.
102. Solomon J, Card JJ, Malow RM. Adapting efficacious interventions: advancing translational research in HIV prevention. Eval Health Prof. 2006;29(2):162–94.
103. DiClemente RJ, Wingood GM. A randomized controlled trial of an HIV sexual risk-reduction intervention for young African-American women. JAMA. 1995;274(16):1271–6.
104. Inter Tribal Council of Arizona I. Connecting the past, present and future. 2010 Annual Report. 2010 http://itcaonline.com/wp-content/uploads/2012/01/2010-Annual-Report.pdf.

Chapter 7
CBPR to Prevent HIV within Racial/Ethnic, Sexual, and Gender Minority Communities: Successes with Long-Term Sustainability

Scott D. Rhodes, Lilli Mann, Jorge Alonzo, Mario Downs, Claire Abraham, Cindy Miller, Jason Stowers, Barry Ramsey, Florence M. Simán, Eunyoung Song, Aaron T. Vissman, Eugenia Eng and Beth A. Reboussin

Now in its fourth decade, HIV remains an epidemic that has a profound impact on all communities, particularly vulnerable ones, such as minority (e.g., racial/ethnic, sexual, and gender) and economically disadvantaged communities. Innovative approaches have emerged that are designed to improve the success of intervention research and practice to reduce and eliminate health disparities generally and HIV-related dis-

S. D. Rhodes (✉) · L. Mann · J. Alonzo · M. Downs · C. Abraham · C. Miller · E. Song
Department of Social Sciences and Health Policy, Division of Public Health Sciences, Wake Forest University School of Medicine, Medical Center Blvd., Winston-Salem, NC 27157, USA
e-mail: srhodes@wakehealth.edu

L. Mann
e-mail: lmann@wakehealth.edu

J. Alonzo
e-mail: jalonzo@wakehealth.edu

M. Downs
e-mail: mdowns@wakehealth.edu

C. Abraham
e-mail: cabraham@wakehealth.edu

C. Miller
e-mail: cytmill@wakehealth.edu

J. Stowers
Triad Health Project, 801 Summitt Avenue, Greensboro, NC 27405, USA
e-mail: jstowers@triadhealthproject.com

B. Ramsey
Center for Health Promotion and Disease Prevention, University of North Carolina at Chapel Hill, 1700 Martin Luther King Blvd., CB#7426, Chapel Hill, NC 27599-7426, USA
e-mail: barry_ramsey@unc.edu

F. M. Simán
El Pueblo, Inc., 2321 Crabtree Boulevard, Suite 105, Raleigh, NC 27604, USA
e-mail: florence@elpueblo.org

E. Song
e-mail: esong@wakehealth.edu

S. D. Rhodes (ed.), *Innovations in HIV Prevention Research and Practice through Community Engagement,* DOI 10.1007/978-1-4939-0900-1_7,
© Springer Science+Business Media New York 2014

parities specifically. One such approach is community-based participatory research (CBPR). CBPR is based on the premise that so-called outside-experts (e.g., scientists from academic, government, and some nongovernment institutions) can promote health and prevent disease more effectively and efficiently in authentic equitable partnership with community members who themselves are experts [1].

Traditional outside-experts may have limited understanding and appreciation of how social, cultural, political, and economic contexts and individuals interact within a specific community [2, 3]. Thus, understanding and intervening on the complex behavioral, contextual, and environmental factors that influence HIV exposure and transmission in a community benefit from multiple perspectives, insights, and experiences.

Our partnership, comprised of scientists and lay-experts from academic, government, and nongovernment institutions, including community-based organizations and businesses and the community at large, has more than a decade-long history of successful and sustained CBPR to reduce HIV risk among vulnerable communities. Thus, given our long-standing history with CBPR, members of our partnership sought to identify and describe our partnership's underlying values; predisposing, enabling, and reinforcing factors that influence and sustain our approach to CBPR; and our own real-world challenges to engagement, partnership, and CBPR.

CBPR Defined

CBPR is a collaborative research approach designed to improve health and well-being through participatory and better-informed inquiry, always with an eye on how the knowledge generated can be translated and applied. A hallmark of CBPR is that research is conducted to improve health through action, including change at the individual, group, community, policy, and social levels. CBPR emphasizes co-learning; reciprocal transfer of expertise; sharing of decision-making power; and mutual ownership of the processes and products of research [1, 3–5]. Rather than scientists from universities, government, or other types of nongovernmental research organizations "approaching" and "entering" a community with a preconceived notion of

A. T. Vissman
Department of Behavioral Sciences and Health Education, Rollins School of Public Health, Emory University, 1518 Clifton Road NE, Atlanta, GA 30322, USA
e-mail: aaron.vissman@emory.edu

E. Eng
Department of Health Behavior, Gillings School of Global Public Health, University of North Carolina at Chapel Hill, 360 Rosenau Hall, Campus Box 7440, Chapel Hill, NC 27599, USA
e-mail: eugenia_eng@unc.edu

B. A. Reboussin
Department of Biostatistical Sciences, Division of Public Health Sciences Wake Forest University School of Medicine, Medical Center Blvd., Winston-Salem, NC 27157, USA
e-mail: brebouss@wakehealth.edu

what is best for a community, CBPR involves lay community members and representatives from community-based organizations sharing research roles with these scientists. CBPR moves from treating individuals within a community as targets of research to engaging them fully as nontoken research partners.

CBPR has the potential to improve health and well-being, aid in disease prevention, and reduce health disparities because, among its strengths, it builds bridges between communities and scientists. Blending the experiences of community members and of organization representatives in public health practice and service provision with sound science can help develop deeper and more informed understanding of health-related phenomena and produce interventions and programs that are more relevant, culturally congruent, and more likely to be effective and to be adopted and sustained if effective and warranted [1, 3, 6–8]. Similarly, study designs, including those used to evaluate actions (including interventions, programs, and other types of actions), that are informed by multiple perspectives may be more authentic to the community and to ways that community members engage, convene, interact, and take action. Thus, interventions may be more innovative; recruitment benchmarks, including participation and retention rates, may be higher; measurements may be more precise; data collection may be more acceptable, complete, and meaningful; analysis and interpretation of findings may be more accurate; and sustainability and meaningful dissemination may be more likely [8].

Furthermore, a distinguishing feature of CBPR is the recognition of community as a social entity with a sense of identity and a shared fate. Working with rather than merely in communities, partners applying CBPR approaches may strengthen a community's overall capacity to problem-solve and reduce health disparities through engagement and ongoing participation in the research process.

Our CBPR Partnership

Members of our partnership focus on the health of ethnic/racial, sexual, and gender minorities and economically disadvantaged comunities. Over the past 13 years, our partnership has evolved to reflect demographic trends and the evolving impact of the HIV epidemic. Current partners include representatives from North Carolina public health departments (local and state level); six AIDS service organizations; community-based organizations, including Latino soccer leagues and teams, the North Carolina lesbian, gay, bisexual, and transgender (LGBT) pride organization, and Latino-serving organizations; a local LGBT foundation; local businesses, including media organizations, Internet companies, bars and clubs, a video production company, and *tiendas* (Latino grocers); the Centers for Disease Control and Prevention (CDC); and five universities. Our partnership consists of a variety of members working on multiple projects; members may be involved with and committed to different projects; however, our partnership is not study-specific. Members may join and leave, and be more or less involved, but despite transitions, the partnership remains.

Currently, members of our CBPR partnership are involved with the following:

- Exploring sexual risk behavior and testing potential intervention strategies among Latino gay and bisexual men, men who have sex with men (MSM), and transgender persons
- Developing a new partnership with, and documenting the needs and priorities of, Latina transgender women
- Evaluating the sustainability of effects of a male-focused lay health advisor intervention designed to increase sexual health among predominately heterosexual, Latino soccer team members
- Testing the processes of dissemination of an evidence-based intervention to increase condom use among male, predominately heterosexual, Latino soccer team members
- Designing a lay health advisor intervention to promote reproductive and sexual health among Latina women
- Studying risk among Guatemalan gay and bisexual men, MSM, and transgender persons
- Implementing and evaluating an intervention designed to promote HIV testing among MSM who use social media and online settings (e.g., chat rooms, craigslist, and mobile application software or "apps") for social and sexual networking
- Documenting the impact of immigration policies on accessing and utilizing public health and other medical services among Latinos
- Studying the process of community engagement within a national sample of programs for the prevention of HIV and sexually transmitted infection (STI)

The key is that CBPR requires an ongoing partnership that is not tied to a single study or funding source; in fact, partnership members are committed to, and involved in, the partnership, with or without funding.

Evaluating our Partnership's Approach to CBPR

As part of our ongoing efforts to conduct authentic, equitable, and sustained community engagement and partnership and take experiences and lessons learned to improve our processes, members of our CBPR partnership have worked with an external researcher to evaluate our approach to CBPR since 2008. Our partnership chose an outside evaluator with whom we had an established relationship. This evaluator has postdoctoral training in CBPR, experience as a director within an AIDS service organization, and more than a decade of work as an academic scientist using community engagement and partnership approaches along a continuum. He was well known, trusted, and well liked by many members of our partnership. The research he is involved with parallels the types of research that members of our partnership engage in. He does not work within our region of the country, which appealed to us because we thought he would be less likely to have preconceived notions; his only allegiance was authentic CBPR.

Members of our partnership wanted to ensure that our approach to CBPR was not CBPR merely because we said it was; rather, we wanted to constantly strive for values, principles, and processes typically associated with CBPR, including

Table 7.1 Common values underlying our approach to community-based participatory research

Participation of scientists and lay-experts from academic, government, and nongovernment institutions, including community-based organizations and businesses, and the community at large throughout all phases of the research process
Agreement among partners on the goals and aims of the research
Ongoing commitment, cooperation, and negotiation among partners to work toward and meet agreed-upon goals
Transparent processes with and open communication within the partnership
Multidirectional exchange of information and learning among partners
Capacity development among partners
Focus on community empowerment and an assets orientation to health promotion and disease prevention
Ongoing reflection among partners to ensure inclusion and adherence to values, partnership principles, and goals and aims
Conflict among partners as a catalyst to improve research processes and outcomes
Shared power and resources among partners
Movement of research to community change and improved health

openness, inclusion, transparent communication, a focus on community priorities and action, etc. [3, 5, 9–14]. Because reflexivity and reflection tend to be key strategies to ensure that one's intentions remain centered on good processes associated with CBPR to identify and meet community priorities (see Chap. 10 for a summary of reflexivity), including an evaluator to gain insights into our approach to CBPR made sense for our partnership. Basically, members of our partnership believed that we must explore our CBPR-related processes if we wanted to understand outcomes and what contributes to the sustainability of our CBPR.

To assess our CBPR approach, the outside evaluator conducted iterative individual in-depth interviews and facilitated group discussions with members of our CBPR partnership; directly observed partnership meetings, intervention implementation, and informal interactions; and reviewed documents (e.g., meeting notes). The evaluator and an ad hoc subcommittee from the CBPR partnership conducted preliminary data analysis. Members of our partnership used a nominal group process to refine and finalize findings.

Values

Eleven values emerged from this data collection, analysis, and interpretation (Table 7.1).

Broad Partnerships

The first value is a commitment to partnership that spans the types of individuals living and working within communities throughout all phases of the research process. Our partnership includes those primarily at risk for HIV exposure and transmission as well as community members who are involved in HIV prevention, care, and treatment, and Latino and LGBT health. We are dedicated to bringing various perspectives, insights, and experiences together to ensure the most informed understanding of health-related phenomena possible, which helps lead to improved interventions and programs. Furthermore, this commitment to a broad inclusion of partners and perspectives reflects our dedication to improved decision-making regarding studies and research questions; study designs; methods; instrumentation; data collection, analysis, and interpretation; and the dissemination of findings. The inclusion of diverse partners helps to ensure that all decisions are carefully considered by blending insider (emic) and outsider (etic) perspectives. Without such inclusion and active and meaningful participation, it can be easy to cut corners, fall back on assumptions, and be less innovative.

Consensus on the Goals of Our Research

Throughout the research process (including initial conceptualization of the study and the research question), we agree on what we are working toward. For example, within our intervention research, partners agree that we are testing interventions to determine their efficacy. This focus is particularly important, given that staff from community-based organizations often deliver interventions and programs, as opposed to testing them. Testing an intervention adds complexity beyond the challenges typically associated with delivery and includes issues related to sample size and power, randomization, measurement, data collection methods, fidelity, and validity.

We have made changes to studies over time through involvement of all partners, including study statisticians, but there may be less flexibility after an intervention study has been funded and is in implementation. Thus, broad partnership ensures that study designs, methods, and analysis plans are as realistic from the beginning, challenges are minimized, and creative and meaningful solutions to unforeseen challenges are developed as needed.

Commitment, Cooperation, and Negotiation

Our work together is a marathon rather than a sprint. To reach agreed-upon goals and aims, members of our partnership recognize that we must be committed to working together and sustaining our work. This commitment includes a thoughtful and stepwise approach to capacity building. For example, an organizational partner may not be ready to handle all aspects of a project. We may decide that developing fiscal management infrastructure is an initial priority, so that hiring and supervising project staff over time may be more realistic. Furthermore, this commitment includes ongoing revisiting of roles, responsibilities, and partnership structures as community and partner priorities and needs change and recognizing when and how to bring closure to a CBPR partnership that is not working.

Transparency and Open Communication

It is important that each partner's voice is heard, but this can be difficult when power differentials exist or when those who have felt unheard for so long are "suddenly" heard but still must hear others. For example, partners who are gay men may find it challenging to listen to the perspectives of others whom they think do not understand gay men. However, within this space of open and clear communication assumed knowledge can benefit from critical analysis through clarification, refinement, and revision. Assumed knowledge may be based on one partner's experiences and not based on broader perspectives. We have seen when assumed knowledge is limited knowledge.

We contend that there must be space for each perspective to be heard and assertions to be questioned, as well as ongoing discussion, negotiation, and compromise. For example, because of our commitment to interventions and programs that build communities, we moved from the term "MSM" to language that includes identities. After all, a tenet of CBPR is the harnessing of identities of community members and not removing them from their contexts and supports [5, 8, 9, 15–17]. Although there is discussion in Chap. 4 of the term "MSM" becoming an identity, we have not found that to the case within the communities we work; rather, we have found that those who do not self-identify as gay or bisexual tend self-identify as heterosexual or straight. Thus, we designed our interventions to be inclusive of gay and bisexual men, MSM, and transgender persons. We knew that we had substantial percentages of transgender persons in our previous studies [18, 19]; however, we realized that our partnership-developed interventions did not acknowledge and address the concerns and contexts of transgender persons. For instance, the "H" in our HOLA and HOLA en Grupos interventions stood for "hombres" (men) [20, 21], and yet, some participants who met inclusion criteria may not self-identify as men. When an academic scientist brought this concern to members of the partnership, a Latino gay man noted that the partnership should not worry about the lack of inclusive language and intervention activities, because transgender persons were "accustomed" to being excluded. Upon hearing this verbalized, others in the partnership realized that such a response was not in line with the values and principles of our partnership, and an open and honest discussion ensued that prompted members of our partnership to choose more inclusion language. We quickly revised the curricula for both interventions. We no longer defined and gave meaning to the letters within the acronym HOLA in the intervention titles; for example, we removed the meaning of the acronym HOLA from logos, t-shirts, caps, and all printed materials. We also revised all facilitator language to include "transgender persons," in addition to "gay and bisexual men and other MSM" in Spanish. We updated information to include rates of HIV and STI among transgender persons, revised role plays to include realistic transgender scenarios, and ensured that all visuals included images of transgender persons. We also successfully developed and implemented a transgender photovoice project to build trust with transgender persons and better understand their needs and priorities [22].

Multidirectional Exchange of Information and Learning

Discovery in our CBPR occurs both as the research process unfolds through process evaluation and as research goals are met in the form of study outcomes. We are committed to learning throughout the process: how to work together more effectively, how to problem-solve, and how to accomplish study-related tasks. This learning also includes the discovery associated with primary study outcomes. Thus, partners representing community members or community-based organizations contribute and learn throughout the process; they are involved not only in overcoming hurdles related to recruitment, for example, but are involved throughout the entire study, including conceptualization, study design and conduct, data analysis and interpretation, and the dissemination of findings.

Capacity Development

The capacity built among scientists is commonly acknowledged (e.g., improved understanding of health and health phenomena, study methods, writing skills, and professional reputation); in fact, scientists gain subsequent opportunities through their involvement in research. It is important to members of our partnership that all partners grow and develop. For our partners, developed capacities have included improved problem-solving, community mobilization, public speaking, organizational and grant writing skills; greater awareness of health and well-being, health disparities, and social determinants of health; and enhanced reach through newly formed networks and access to new resources. Partners have presented at local, regional, national, and international conferences, and led training workshops in person and through webinars. We hope that the development of expertise leads to next steps that promote growth for each partner, not merely for the academic partners.

Community Empowerment

Members of our partnership are committed to community empowerment and an assets orientation to health promotion and disease prevention. We do not want to perpetuate a paternalistic approach to public health and medicine in which scientists have the answers and communities have the problems. For example, our Cyber-Based Education and Referral/testing (CyBER/testing) intervention focuses on supporting technology-using gay and bisexual men, MSM, and transgender persons to get tested for HIV. We do not view social media, including online sites and mobile apps, that promote social and sexual networking as health compromising; rather, we see these settings as community assets. We harness these assets and contribute to them as community members and participants by supporting users in multiple ways, including by building trust, offering social support, and providing information and referrals that users want. We have only recently expanded to apps, but examples of our CBPR with gay and bisexual men, MSM, and transgender persons using social media and online settings have been published [23–27].

Ongoing Reflection

We are committed to continually evaluating what we think, say, and do. This self and group reflection is particularly important to keep members of our partnership as grounded as possible, to remain focused, and to stay as close to possible on authentic community engagement and partnership to promote community health in the ways we agree upon and value. This continual reflection, along with our lessons learned, contribute to the quality, improvement, and sustainability of engagement, partnership, and CBPR.

Embracing Conflict

True partnerships are not without conflict, and we attempt to embrace conflict as a method to improve our research processes and outcomes. Conflict can be intense as partners come together for a common cause. Partners always have different levels of perceived trust, various communication styles and skills, and their own histories and perceptions of power, but we prefer to learn from the perspectives, insights, and experiences of diverse partners for the greater good of our research than to have a smooth process. Conflict requires clarification, explanation, and rethinking, all of which have the potential to benefit all phases of the research process. As Saul Alinsky, a strong proponent of the need for conflict and controversy to achieve meaningful change, wrote, "Change means movement. Movement means friction. Only in the frictionless vacuum of a nonexistent world can movement or change occur without that abrasive friction of conflict" (p. 21; [28]).

Sharing Power and Resources

In all of our CBPR studies, community members and/or organization representatives serve as co-investigators, project managers and coordinators, data collectors, health educators, and interventionists. However, it remains difficult to ensure that all partners feel that they hold power, particularly when research is federally funded. For federally funded CBPR, an academic partner often serves as the principal investigator; community partners often have not had opportunities to develop their research expertise and reputation sufficiently to convince members of federal study sections or grant review panels that they may be appropriate principal investigators. However, some large community-based organizations with missions that include research and departments focusing on research and evaluation may be successful in obtaining principal investigator status. In contrast, some community partners do not want the responsibilities associated with serving as principal investigators.

Members of our partnership use many techniques to ensure that members have the opportunity to share power and resources. For example, we view financial resources as a proxy of power sharing; in our CBPR, 40–50 % of direct costs are in the budgets of community-based organizations through subcontracts. However, some partners may still feel they have little or no power because their funding is funneled through a university. Other ways of power sharing include shared authorship in manuscripts and publications and participation in conferences, meetings, webinars, webcasts, workshops, and other forms of dissemination. Basically, we are careful to ensure that partners do not represent the research of the partnership without fully acknowledging and crediting the partnership's collective efforts and vital contributions.

Focusing on Community Change and Improved Health

A distinct hallmark of CBPR is the purposeful and strategic movement of formative research to community change and improved health. Thus, CBPR is inherently translational; it ensures that basic, more formative research is conducted with a goal of practical use to improve community health. Research may begin with an assessment of needs, and to understand phenomena through community perceptions and epidemiologic data, but research findings must be translated into some type of action for positive community change [1, 4, 8, 12, 20, 29–31]. Members of our partnership know that there is a long history of research to answer interesting and potentially important questions but that those answers have not been consistently applied to effect community change and promote health. We do not want to solely add to the body of knowledge; instead, we are committed to movement to action, including individual, group, and community action, as well as policy and social change. Unfortunately, the use of findings can be slow. Our initial formative research with a soccer league did not yield implementation of the HoMBReS intervention for that soccer league until 4 years after formative data were collected [16, 20, 32–34], but the partners were committed to and explicitly working together toward action. Furthermore, by engaging and partnering, change may be occurring; that change, however, can be difficult to quantify.

Some formative methods associated with CBPR promote action more rapidly. These methods include photovoice [35–39], systematic and well-facilitated community forum [6] environmental mapping and audits [40], rapid ethnographic assessment [19, 41–43], community or venue-based HIV counseling and rapid testing [44], and action-oriented community diagnosis [31, 45]. These types of formative data collection methods that are designed to inform next research steps are unique because they produce immediate, meaningful, positive, and measureable changes about the issue being explored among the participants themselves. Simply, the beneficiaries are those directly involved in the formative research as well as those who participate in subsequent research.

Table 7.2 Factors affecting our approach to community-based participatory research

Predisposing factors
Existing partnership
Alignment among partner priorities, organizational missions, and research questions
Commitment to social inclusion
"Can-do" attitude
Enabling factors
Agreement on priorities
Capacity to move beyond service and individual or case management
Financial stability of involved organizations
Flexibility
Commitment to positive and ecologic perspectives
Reinforcing factors
Operationalized principles of partnership
Friendships among partners
Immediate use of findings by partners
Stepwise building on successful history of CBPR
Comprehensive engagement of research team in core functions of agency

In summary, the 11 values underlying our CBPR partnership serve as principles that guide our decisions and actions; however, we acknowledge that we may stray from following these principles in practice. As individuals working within our own contexts and with our own challenges, expectations, perspectives, motivations, and assumptions about the decisions and behaviors of others, a set of principles for engagement and partnership provides a touchstone for sustaining the partnership. Fortunately, even in situations when we are not able to fulfill all of our principles, we learn about ways to refine and enhance our CBPR approach.

Factors Facilitating CBPR Success

We have identified four predisposing, five enabling, and five reinforcing factors [46] that contribute to the success and sustainability of our approach to CBPR. These factors are outlined in Table 7.2.

Predisposing Factors

In the context of CBPR, we define predisposing factors as preexisting factors that facilitate community engagement and partnership among individuals, groups, and organizations.

Existing Partnership Our CBPR partnership is based on a firm foundation laid by a North Carolina Community-Based Public Health Initiative (CBPHI)-organized CBPR partnership that had a history of successfully implementing community-based diabetes interventions within African-American/black faith communities in rural North Carolina [20, 33, 47, 48]. This CBPHI partnership wanted to explore the health priorities and needs of the growing immigrant Latino community because they were concerned that these priorities and needs were being neglected [20, 33, 49]. This concern was related to a well-publicized anti-Latino immigration rally on the steps of the community's town hall, led by David Duke, a former Grand Wizard of the Ku Klux Klan. Our CBPR partnership has evolved substantially and now includes a broader and larger membership [20, 50].

Aided by an outside consultant, partners went through a facilitated 2-day visioning process to refine their focus. The focus that emerged and was mutually agreed upon was the following:

> A collaboration of community members, organization and business representatives, and academic partners founded on the principles of mutual respect and open communication working together to synergistically, creatively, and revolutionarily address community needs to promote sexual and reproductive health for the mutual benefit of the community, university, and ultimately the world.

This vision has guided our CBPR projects and process ever since. During our data collection, analysis, and interpretation, this vision emerged as essential to our success and sustainability.

Alignment of Partner Priorities Clearly linked to the first predisposing factor is the alignment of partner priorities, organizational missions, and research questions. Overall, partners are committed to HIV prevention for racial/ethnic, sexual, and gender minority and economically disadvantaged communities through increased understanding of health and the development, careful implementation, and comprehensive evaluation of interventions. In fact, this commitment was identified early on and subsequently documented during formative research [17, 19, 20, 23, 24, 33, 34, 39, 50, 51]. This alignment was strengthened by a request for proposals from the North Carolina Department of Health and Human Services, Division of Public Health, Communicable Disease Branch, to fund behavioral HIV prevention interventions for communities at increased risk, including racial/ethnic, sexual, and gender minority communities. The request for proposals required the use of evidence-based interventions included with the *Compendium of Evidence-Based HIV Prevention Interventions*; however, at this time, there were no efficacious Spanish-language or Internet-based interventions within the *Compendium* (see Chap. 11 for a description and summary of the *Compendium*). Thus, members of the partnership mobilized around their first CBPR project—to develop, implement, and evaluate a Spanish-language intervention for immigrant Latino populations in the Southeast. As a Latino partner noted at that time, "*Latinos want and need information and help to be safe, but nothing exists that we can point to that shows promise to save the lives of Latinos living here in our community.*"

Thus, there is overlap in the priorities of communities, the primary focuses of government and nongovernment organizations, and the research strengths of academic partners. Although each partner may not set HIV as a priority in its mission (e.g., some may have as a priority Latino health more broadly or social justice), each partner is committed to the health and well-being of racial/ethnic, sexual, and

Fig. 7.1 Arnstein's ladder of citizen participation [52]

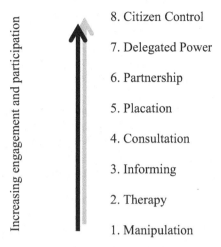

Increasing engagement and participation

8. Citizen Control

7. Delegated Power

6. Partnership

5. Placation

4. Consultation

3. Informing

2. Therapy

1. Manipulation

gender minorities, and HIV prevention is an area of common interest and skills, even if from different vantage points. Furthermore, partners recognize a broad and holistic definition of sexual and reproductive health while maintaining a focus on HIV prevention.

Social Inclusion As we operationalize it, social inclusion involves the authentic inclusion of perspectives, insights, and experiences of those in the community, those who provide services within communities, and scientists. The idea is that all members of communities have both the rights and the responsibilities to play an active role throughout the research, and differences in race/ethnicity, gender, sexual orientation, age, educational attainment, and social and economic status should not lead to exclusion [27]. In fact, our partnership thrives on the inclusion of diversity based on these types of variables; we contend that our success is based on the heterogeneity of backgrounds, characteristics, and, thus, voices within our partnership. Social inclusion also occurs when engagement and partnership are demonstrated to be authentic rather than tokenistic or manipulative. Thus, engagement and partnership only occur when they reach the top three tiers of Arnstein's ladder of citizen participation: partnership, delegated power, and citizen control (Fig. 7.1; [52]).

"Can-do" Attitude Members of our partnership are usually quite confident that we can realize our goals and aims and work diligently to realize our research potentials. For example, across all of our studies, we have high recruitment and retention rates; this is particularly noteworthy, given that immigrant Latino populations are assumed by outsiders to be transient, "hidden," or "hard to reach" over time. Being considered hidden or hard to reach is purely subjective and most often describes being difficult to reach by community outsiders, such as scientists.

In one of our partnership's recent CBPR study designed to test the HoMBReS Por un Cambio (Men For Change) intervention (an HIV-prevention intervention for predominately heterosexual adult Latino men who are part of soccer teams), we had an 85.5% retention rate at 12-month follow-up. This retention rate was lower than that in other studies that members of our partnership have conducted [20, 34, 53, 54], but we achieved this rate despite the resignation and departure of a key project coordinator who was the study contact person and had established trust with the 258 participants. Without this project coordinator, members of our partnership found initial participants and rebuilt trust in order to locate other participants and obtain their follow-up data.

Furthermore, when members of our partnership decided to test the feasibility of recruiting and assessing sex workers and clients of sex workers to design a larger study, representatives from an AIDS service organization thought that they would have no difficulty in conducting the study. They led the charge by designing a protocol and successfully completing the agreed-upon number of in-depth interviews [55].

Enabling Factors

Enabling factors are characteristics that facilitate engagement and partnership.

Agreement on Priorities Members of our partnership identified agreement on priorities as essential to engagement and partnership. Together, we come to consensus on where and how to focus resources and skills through ongoing dialogue that combines local perspectives and theory about what is going on in communities and epidemiologic data. We also include frank discussions about what is do-able. Although there is much to be done that aligns with community priorities, we are careful to discuss what resources, talents, and interests members of our partnership have and their fit with identified priorities. We recognize that if we need funding to do meaningful CBPR, our proposals must have some viability to be fundable. It is impossible to predict what will be funded, but we try to move ideas forward that fit with our own resources, talents, and interests.

Capacity to Move Beyond Service Members of our partnership and the organizations some of them represent must have the capacity to move beyond service. Provision of services and individual patient or case management differs from CBPR. Different partners have different levels of experience with research and different types of research skills to offer, but there must be a willingness, interest, and capacity to learn more about and contribute to research. An academic partner in our partnership has learned the need to continue to remind organizational partners that what we are doing is innovative, has not been done before (otherwise we would not have received research funding), and can influence prevention locally, nationally, and internationally. At the same time, however, to reach potentials, partners must stretch and move beyond what has been done in the past.

Financial Stability We found that partner organizations must be financially stable to adhere to our CBPR values, vision, established priorities, and research questions. Given the current funding environment for health promotion and disease prevention generally and HIV specifically, staff within community-based organizations and AIDS service organizations are struggling to keep their doors open and provide the services that so many people rely on, especially some within racial/ethnic, sexual, and gender minority and economically disadvantaged communities and others disproportionately affected by HIV. Academic scientists may feel that research funding for HIV is difficult to obtain; however, for staff at community-based organizations and AIDS services organizations the landscape has changed even more dramatically, and change will continue into the foreseeable future. These organizations have been required to change focus if they want to obtain federal and state funding. For example, funding priorities for prevention programming have shifted from implementation of interventions (including those outlined in Chap. 11), to HIV testing of high-risk populations labeled by outsiders as hidden or hard to reach and case management of those with HIV.

Furthermore, HIV has lost its urgency as it has become to be known as a chronic and thus manageable disease. As such, it competes with other diseases for support from foundations and private donors. Community support for HIV prevention is much more difficult to garner than in the past, and this lack of support has led to some community-based organizations and AIDS services organizations closing their doors as well [56, 57].

In our CBPR partnership, one partner organization, which was home to a co-investigator and intervention implementation team and held a subcontract from the institution of an academic partner, had such intense financial challenges that it did not spend grant funds on the supports necessary to fulfill research aims. Instead, it initiated such extreme cost transfers that the research aims would have been impossible to meet. The organization was not adhering to the research protocol, dramatically exceeded line items (e.g., rent and co-investigator administrative effort, two line items that are difficult to get funded on service delivery grants), and was on a trajectory that would lead to its subcontracted annual budget being exhausted within the first 6 months of a fiscal year. Representatives from this partner organization began to avoid communicating with other partners and did not attend partnership meetings, and engagement and partnership become strained. These strains lead to partner suspicion and mistrust. Ultimately, after it was clear that representatives from the subcontracted organization would not or could not get the project back on focus, its subcontract was terminated and it left the overall CBPR partnership. The organization was able to refocus on its immediate priority—the needs of those with HIV as opposed to primary prevention—and survived. However, it has not re-emerged as a partnership member.

Flexibility Both partners and funders are flexible to protocol revisions and changes during study implementation. Although we work closely as a partnership during study conceptualization and the grant application process, what was planned and seemed possible at the time of grant submission and what becomes realistic for partners as implementation begins may differ. Through careful negotiation and consultation with federal funders, members of our partnership have been able to revise the study design. Moreover, because the time between conceptualizing a study and getting it funded can be protracted, we usually include within the research strategy and time line an opportunity for revisions of the study and study design to allow for modest adjustments if needed and agreed upon.

Commitment to Positive and Ecologic Perspectives Members of our partnership are committed to positive and ecologic approaches to health promotion and disease prevention that also may question the directionality and intersectionality of causal reasoning. For example, our HIV-prevention interventions do not focus only on condom use, but rather they also focus on community change. Our research explores and reframes community norms about masculinity, identity as an immigrant, being raised as a man, and being a sexual and/or gender minority. We also focus on communication about sexual health with partners, peers, and providers, etc.

Moreover, we do not provide HIV testing; we want intervention participants to pursue and experience the process of testing at health departments. We believe that facing and successfully overcoming obstacles related to HIV testing (e.g., a security guard at the entrance of a health department and limited interpretation services) may ensure that some participants will access services in the future after the intervention is over, which is a form of sustainability of intervention effects. Thus, our HIV-prevention interventions are designed to prepare participants for the obstacles they will face and to provide vicarious learning about overcoming these obstacles. We know that we cannot foresee all challenges, but we can build self-efficacy among participants to handle what they encounter. We also contend that when they access services, participants may learn about additional services available, and they may share this information with others; for example, they may learn about women's health services, share information about their own experiences facing and successfully overcoming obstacles to access services, and thus, reduce delay in prenatal care by a partner, sister, or aunt.

Reinforcing Factors

In the context of CBPR, we define reinforcing factors as rewards that are associated with and further bolster engagement and partnership.

Operationalized Principles of Partnership We established operationalized principles of partnership through which we build and maintain trust among each of us— community members; representatives of organizations, agencies, and businesses; researchers; and clinicians—with the ultimate goal of improving community health (Table 7.3). These principles reflect and expand on our values, but are more concrete. For example, although we rely on the perspectives, insights, and experiences of diverse partners, we also recognize that we may not always have the expertise needed. Thus, one partnership principle is that we develop and use relationships and networks outside of the partnership. In all of our CBPR studies, we have had to connect with networks and develop relationships with representatives from community-based organizations and scientists who may not be part of our partnership and/or may not be geographically local but have skill sets and expertise that can be applied to meeting the priorities of the local community.

Friendship We contend that friendship among partners is invaluable to reinforcing our research together. We care about one another as individuals within communities, within communities of identity and shared geography, as two examples, and we

Table 7.3 Operationalized principles of community-based participatory research partnership

Show mutual respect and genuineness
Establish, develop, and use formal and informal networks and structures inside and outside of the partnership
Commit to transparent processes and clear and open communication
Allow roles, norms, and processes to evolve from the input and agreement of all partners
Agree on the values, goals, and objectives of research and practice
Build on each partner's strengths and assets
Offer continual feedback among members
Ensure balance of power and sharing of resources
Share credit for the accomplishments of the partnership
Face challenges together
Question the directionality and intersectionality of causal reasoning
Incorporate existing environmental structures to address partnership focuses
Take responsibility for the partnership and its actions
Disseminate conclusions and findings to research and clinical audiences, community members, and policy makers

care about one another as individuals within the community of our partnership. The provision of social support is vital to our partnership.

Immediate Use of Findings The immediate use of findings by all partners is a priority. Often, the extended time between data collection to analysis and interpretation can be frustrating for partners who want to apply what they have learned as quickly as possible. We recognize that, together, partners own and have right to the data and their use. Thus, we often will work together to develop preliminary findings, which can be used in service grant proposals by community members and organizational partners, for example.

Stepwise Approach Our success in using and sustaining CBPR has been characterized by partners as slow and steady. We began our research process modestly, incrementally building a history of success. We chose a stepwise approach that moved in a linear manner from formative data collection to intervention design, implementation, and evaluation. This was a carefully calibrated and orchestrated process because reasonable scopes of work help to ensure early successes, which, in turn, develop capacities and help maintain enthusiasm and involvement among partners.

Engagement in Core Functions The last reinforcing factor is the comprehensive engagement of research staff in the core functions of community-based organizational partners. Much has been written in the CBPR literature about academic partners getting out of the office and into the community. In many cases, this is about being seen in the community to build trust through attending celebrations, sporting events, etc; however, there are other ways to build trust. For example, to better understand and build trust with both the Latino community and the leadership at a Latino community-serving organization, an academic partner (the first author) volunteered to staff the reception desk and provide general office support at a Latino-serving community-based organization a half-day each week. He offered

Table 7.4 Challenges faced by our community-based participatory research partnership

Determining who represents the community and how community is defined

Becoming dependent on the research agenda as a motivating factor for organization direction and planning

Having passion for a cause is not sufficient

Dealing with conflicts over funding

Having different emphases on processes and outcomes

Accepting that the CBPR process can be time-consuming

Maintaining relationships during transition to achieve continuity of work and goals when leaders change

a service that was needed and appreciated by the organization; he was not asking for something from an understaffed and not well-resourced organization but rather was investing in the organization. More currently, an academic partner who handles budgets (both for proposals and post-award) at our university, has applied her skill set to help staff at community-based organizations develop budgets, documentation procedures, and internal financial policies. This support may not directly link to the research being conducted within the partnership but it may link to the broad needs and functions of an organization and develop staff capacities.

Challenges

Seven challenges to our CBPR emerged (Table 7.4).

Representing and Defining Community

A common challenge identified by members of our partnership is determining who represents the community and how community is defined. Communities do not speak in one voice, and in fact, scientists and lay-experts, and the community at large may have very different backgrounds, experiences, and perspectives. No one voice will represent the community; rather, there are many voices and some will contradict each other. Thus, it is important to have a broad spectrum of partners in order to ensure that one voice is not guiding the process.

Dependence on a Research Agenda

We have seen how an organizational partner can become dependent on a research agenda as the motivating factor for organizational direction and programming. Representatives of a community-based organization can deviate from their organization's mission and instead change how they participate in a partnership because they want to maintain a funding stream that is linked to research. This is a challenge particularly for representatives from organizations that are less financially sound. Representatives from financially stronger organizations tend to feel more confident about asserting their perspectives. All members of our partnership are responsible for ensuring mechanisms are in place for engagement and authentic participation.

Passion is Not Enough

Although passion can help bring partners together, engagement, partnership, participation, and research are difficult. We have discussed much of the process of engagement and partnership within this chapter, but it is important to note that CBPR is indeed research. Our experiences suggest that CBPR does not make research easier; in fact, it makes the research process more difficult. However, that research is both more informed, and as such, its contribution is greater because CBPR brings together various perspectives, insights, and experiences during the conduct of discovery, the generation of knowledge, and the implementation of action. Traditional research tends to provide a framework through the consideration of internal and external validity, the reduction of bias, and the control of the experimental process. CBPR adds to the strength of research, but in our case, it clearly adds new, and at times unpredictable, perspectives to this framework. Blending and balancing various perspectives, insights, and experiences to improve research is important but is not easy. Thus, passion for HIV prevention is not sufficient; within CBPR, partners must be committed to working together to conduct sound science.

Conflicts About Funding

We also found that conflicts over funding can lead to problems within a partnership. Within the section on enabling factors, we described an example of an organizational partner not spending allocated funds in a manner consistent with the research aims and the risks that placed on the science-related outcomes, health promotion and disease prevention, and the sustainability of our partnership's CBPR. Moreover, intra-partnership conflict also may occur. For example, our partnership had a project that included multiple organizations implementing an intervention at their own sites. Several times during the implementation of the project, representatives of the organizations proposed taking on the project from the other partners. This idea was presented as a cost-saving step but may have been founded on the financial instability of the organization proposing the expansion. There is much competition for resources among community-based organizations and AIDS service organizations providing HIV prevention and care, and this competition can jeopardize partnerships and CBPR study outcomes.

Different Emphases on Processes and Outcomes

Representatives from community-based organizations tend to have a task and process orientation whereas traditional research partners tend to have an outcome orientation. This tension can be profound if there is not mutual respect by partners regarding the value of each perspective and the ability to integrate them to better CBPR. Much of the CBPR literature is replete with examples of the development and maintenance of partnerships; there is much less attention given to whether an intervention or program, for example, effects community health outcomes [8, 11, 17]. Members of our partnership are committed to moving toward measurable health outcomes, and although this may be difficult, we attempt to balance tasks and processes and outcomes. After all, as one partner noted, *"If we weren't trying to make a real difference in the community, we wouldn't be working together."*

Similarly, there is much discussion within CBPR that the process builds capacity of partners that are transferable to other health disparities; partners gain skills to lead, mobilize, and problem-solve. The idea is that building capacity and skills have an impact on health upstream. Thus, these types of outcomes may not be identifiable in the short-term, but overall community capacity and community health may be changing. However, members of our partnership acknowledged that we have not designed studies sufficiently to explore the development of these capacities.

Time-Consuming Process

It has been widely acknowledged that CBPR can be a time-consuming process, and members of our partnership agreed. However, members also concluded that the products are stronger. For example, as we develop interventions, many perspectives are integrated to ensure that the intervention strategy is innovative and makes sense for the community and that the messages and components (e.g., activities) are as sound and as meaningful as possible. Because we know that partnership members quickly become different from their peers by the fact that they come to meetings, engage with one another, and hear different perspectives, members of our partnership go back to uninvolved community members to hear from them throughout the data analysis and interpretation and intervention development processes. Thus, we do not merely collect formative data and blend with health behavior theory to develop an intervention. Rather, we continually engage different community members who are not part of our partnership to get feedback, resolve differences of opinion, and refine our understanding.

We also tend to refine an intervention as we progress through implementation. These refinements may not be profound; however, because the time for an intervention to be available for broad dissemination and adaption may be protracted, we are committed to having the most current products possible. Our approach may conflict somewhat with the gold standard of controlled clinical trials. However, behavior is not the same as a physiologic reaction (e.g., as one might expect to see in a clinical trial comparing two drugs); it is a complex interplay that heavily includes context. Context changes in different ways at different rates for different reasons, but it always changes. Furthermore, we tend to know that our revisions strengthen the intervention. They are not haphazard and are based in what we are learning throughout the process. In addition, our approach is in line with community priorities: to have the most innovative and effective interventions and programs possible to meet real needs built on continually more informed understanding.

Maintaining Relationships Through Transitions

It is difficult to maintain relationships during transition to achieve continuity of CBPR and achieve goals. For example, when leadership at an organizational partner changes, members of our partnership have seen profound changes in skills and capacities; in some cases, capacity has been reduced so severely that the research aims were in jeopardy. This challenges all partners as well as the productivity of the CBPR. Leadership changes have also occurred when partners moved on to larger agencies and to jobs with greater responsibilities based on the capacities they had developed as a direct result of their involvement in CBPR. This is indeed a good outcome, but these types of partner changes have negatively affected the CBPR we have been engaged in.

Discussion and Conclusion

Our partnership is strong and well established. Members are committed and dedicated to addressing the health-care disparities within vulnerable communities and populations, including racial/ethnic, sexual, and gender minorities and low-income, rural, and inner-city communities. Because CBPR is well recognized as a promising approach to effecting the health and well-being of these vulnerable communities and populations, [1, 5, 9, 11, 16, 31], we are committed to moving both community health and the science of CBPR forward.

To facilitate our CBPR, we have established partnership principles to which partners try to adhere. We work together, recognizing that no one person or type of person (e.g., community member, organization representative, or scientist) has the answer to important research questions to promote community health and well-being. No one can identify and meet the priorities and needs of communities alone. Because we want to make a difference in the HIV epidemic, members of our partnership are committed to working together to blend perspectives, insights, and experiences. We have found CBPR to be an effective approach to meaningful research, to identifying community needs and priorities, and to effecting positive community change. CBPR requires a firm foundation and ongoing partner commitment and dedication.

Our work as a partnership has not been done without challenges. Community members and organization representatives face the realities of HIV infection every day and know that something must be done for the communities they belong to. The slow pace of securing research funding and conducting sound research is an ongoing frustration.

Furthermore, communities themselves are not infallible; community members and members of CBPR partnerships may have strongly held prejudices about one another. For example, some members who were part of the original CBPR partnership advocated against prioritizing Latino health. They had negative feelings about Latinos, whom they perceived as undocumented and unwelcome. In addition, when Latino gay men stepped forward to advocate for HIV-prevention programming, some Latino partners had initial misconceptions about Latino gay men. Facilitating a partnership around sensitive issues that include race and sexuality has required, and we predict will continue to require, ongoing attention and work.

Members of our partnership have multiple projects that have grown and developed synergistically. Although this growth has seemed slow, the products of our research have been profound. We now have three HIV-prevention interventions designed for heterosexually active Latino men that have evidence of effectiveness: HoMBReS, HoMBReS 2, and HoMBReS Por un Cambio [20, 34, 53, 54]. We also have an intervention (CyBER/testing) with evidence of increasing HIV testing among gay and bisexual, MSM, and transgender persons who use online settings, such as chat rooms for social and sexual networking [25]. These interventions have a high level of cultural congruence, given the iterative process of community engagement and participation in their development and implementation. Further studies have been built on these initial projects. We start slow, build capacity, and expand on our successes over time.

Our partnership has since developed three other interventions: two for Latino gay and bisexual men, MSM, and transgender persons, and one for Latina women; some of which are currently being tested. During the development of interventions, partners continued to use an approach that ensured that the interventions were built on the expertise of scientists and lay-experts, including community-based organizations and businesses, and the community at large.

We have had great success using systematic CBPR processes to meet the priorities and needs of racial/ethnic, sexual, and gender minorities this part of the country. We are committed to CBPR as an innovative approach to HIV-prevention research because it maximizes the probability that what we do together is based on what the community itself sets as a priority; is more informed because of the sharing of broad perspectives, insights, and experiences; builds capacity of all partners to solve community problems, use community assets, and conduct meaningful research; and promotes sustainability.

References

1. Rhodes SD, Malow RM, Jolly C. Community-based participatory research: a new and not-so-new approach to HIV/AIDS prevention, care, and treatment. AIDS Educ Prev. 2010;22(3):173–83.
2. Minkler M, Wallerstein N. Introduction to community based participatory research. In: Minkler M, Wallerstein N, editors. Community-based participatory research for health. San Francisco: Jossey-Bass; 2003. p. 3–26.
3. Cashman SB, Adeky S, Allen AJ, Corburn J, Israel BA, Montaño J, et al. The power and the promise: working with communities to analyze data, interpret findings, and get to outcomes. Am J Public Health. 2008;98(8):1407–17.
4. Israel BA, Eng E, Schulz AJ, Parker EA. Introduction to methods in community-based participatory research for health. In: Israel BA, Eng E, Schulz AJ, Parker EA, editors. Methods in community-based participatory research. San Francisco: Jossey-Bass; 2005.
5. Israel BA, Krieger J, Vlahov D, Ciske S, Foley M, Fortin P, et al. Challenges and facilitating factors in sustaining community-based participatory research partnerships: lessons learned from the Detroit, New York City and Seattle Urban Research Centers. J Urban Health. 2006;83(6):1022–40.
6. Rhodes SD, Hergenrather KC, Vissman AT, Stowers J, Davis AB, Hannah A, et al. Boys must be men, and men must have sex with women: a qualitative CBPR study to explore sexual risk among African American, Latino, and white gay men and MSM. Am J Mens Health. 2011;5(2):140–51.
7. Wallerstein N, Oetzel J, Duran B, Tafoya G, Belone L, Rae R. What predicts outcomes in CBPR? In: Minkler M, Wallerstein N, editors. Community-based participatory research: from process to outcomes. San Francisco: Wiley; 2008. p. 371–92.
8. Rhodes SD, Duck S, Alonzo J, Downs M, Aronson RE. Intervention trials in community-based participatory research. In: Blumenthal D, DiClemente RJ, Braithwaite RL, Smith S, editors. Community-based participatory research: issues, methods, and translation to practice. New York: Springer; 2013. p. 157–80.
9. Israel BA, Schulz AJ, Parker EA, Becker AB. Review of community-based research: assessing partnership approaches to improve public health. Annu Rev Public Health. 1998;19:173–202.
10. Seifer SD. Building and sustaining community-institutional partnerships for prevention research: findings from a national collaborative. J Urban Health. 2006;83(6):989–1003.
11. Viswanathan M, Eng E, Ammerman A, Gartlehner G, Lohr KN, Griffith D, et al. Community-based participatory research: assessing the evidence. Evidence Report/Technology Assessment. Rockville, MD: Agency for Healthcare Research and Quality, 2004 July. Report No.: 99.
12. Reece M, Dodge B. A study in sexual health applying the principles of community-based participatory research. Arch Sex Behav. 2004;33(3):235–47.
13. Reece M, Herbenick D, Sherwood-Puzzello C. Sexual health promotion and adult retail stores. J Sex Res. 2004;41(2):173–80.
14. Seifer SD, Maurana CA. Developing and sustaining community-campus partnerships: putting principles into practice. Partnersh Perspect. 2000;1(2):7–11.
15. Rhodes SD, Yee LJ. Public health and gay and bisexual men: A primer for practitioners, clinicians, and researchers. In: Shankle M, editor. The handbook of lesbian, gay, bisexual, and transgender public health: a practitioner's guide to service. Binghamton: Haworth; 2006. p. 119–43.
16. Rhodes SD. Community-based participatory research. In Blessing JD, Forister JG, editors. Introduction to research and medical literature for health professionals. 3rd ed. Burlington: Jones & Bartlett; 2013. p. 167–87.

17. Rhodes SD, Duck S, Alonzo J, Daniel J, Aronson RE. Using community-based participatory research to prevent HIV disparities: assumptions and opportunities identified by the Latino partnership. J Acquir Immune Defic Syndr. 2013;63(Suppl 1):S32–5.

18. Rhodes SD, McCoy TP, Hergenrather KC, Vissman AT, Wolfson M, Alonzo J, et al. Prevalence estimates of health risk behaviors of immigrant Latino men who have sex with men. J Rural Health. 2012;28(1):73–83.

19. Rhodes SD, Hergenrather KC, Aronson RE, Bloom FR, Felizzola J, Wolfson M, et al. Latino men who have sex with men and HIV in the rural south-eastern USA: findings from ethnographic in-depth interviews. Cult Health Sex. 2010;12(7):797–812.

20. Rhodes SD. Demonstrated effectiveness and potential of CBPR for preventing HIV in Latino populations. In: Organista KC, editor. HIV Prevention with Latinos: theory, research, and practice. New York: Oxford University Press; 2012. p. 83–102.

21. Rhodes SD, Daniel J, Alonzo J, Duck S, Garcia M, Downs M, et al. A systematic community-based participatory approach to refining an evidence-based community-level intervention: the HOLA intervention for Latino men who have sex with men. Health Promot Pract. 2013;14(4):607–16.

22. Rhodes SD, Mann L, Alonzo J, Simán M. F. Immigrant Latina transgender women: exploring health priorities through photovoice. In review.

23. Rhodes SD. Hookups or health promotion? An exploratory study of a chat room-based HIV prevention intervention for men who have sex with men. AIDS Educ Prev. 2004;16(4):315–27.

24. Rhodes SD, Hergenrather KC, Duncan J, Ramsey B, Yee LJ, Wilkin AM. Using community-based participatory research to develop a chat room-based HIV prevention intervention for gay men. Prog Community Health Partnersh. 2007;1(2):175–84.

25. Rhodes SD, Hergenrather KC, Duncan J, Vissman AT, Miller C, Wilkin AM, et al. A pilot intervention utilizing Internet chat rooms to prevent HIV risk behaviors among men who have sex with men. Pub Health Rep. 2010;125(Suppl 1):29–37.

26. Rhodes SD, Vissman AT, Stowers J, Miller C, McCoy TP, Hergenrather KC, et al. A CBPR partnership increases HIV testing among men who have sex with men (MSM): outcome findings from a pilot test of the CyBER/testing Internet intervention. Health Educ Behav. 2011;38(3):311–20.

27. Dolwick Grieb SM, Amutah N, J. S, Smith H, Hammonds K, Rhodes SD. Preventing HIV through social inclusion using community-based participatory research. In: Taket A, Crisp BR, Graham M, Hanna L, Goldingay S, Wilson L, editors. Practising social inclusion. Oxford: Routledge; 2014. p. 193–204.

28. Alinsky S. Rules for radicals. New York: Random House; 1971.

29. Minkler M. Community-based research partnerships: challenges and opportunities. J Urban Health. 2005;82(2 Suppl 2):ii3–i12.

30. Cornwall A, Jewkes R. What is participatory research? Soc Sci Med. 1995;41(12):1667–76.

31. Eng E, Moore KS, Rhodes SD, Griffith D, Allison L, Shirah K, et al. Insiders and outsiders assess who is "the community": participant observation, key informant interview, focus group interview, and community forum. In: Israel BA, Eng E, Schulz AJ, Parker E, editors. Methods for conducting community-based participatory research for health. 2nd ed. San Francisco: Jossey-Bass; 2013. p. 133–60.

32. Rhodes SD, Daniel J, Alonzo J, Vissman AT, Duck S, Downs M, et al. A snapshot of how latino heterosexual men promote sexual health within their social networks: process evaluation findings from an efficacious community-level intervention. AIDS Educ Prev. 2012;24(6):514–26.

33. Rhodes SD, Eng E, Hergenrather KC, Remnitz IM, Arceo R, Montano J, et al. Exploring latino men's HIV risk using community-based participatory research. Am J Health Behav. 2007;31(2):146–58.

34. Rhodes SD, Hergenrather KC, Bloom FR, Leichliter JS, Montaño J. Outcomes from a community-based, participatory lay health advisor HIV/STD prevention intervention for recently

arrived immigrant Latino men in rural North Carolina, USA. AIDS Educ Prev. 2009;21(Suppl 1):104–9.

35. Hergenrather KC, Rhodes SD, Cowan CA, Bardhoshi G, Pula S. Photovoice as community-based participatory research: a qualitative review. Am J Health Behav. 2009;33(6):686–98.

36. Streng JM, Rhodes SD, Ayala GX, Eng E, Arceo R, Phipps S. Realidad Latina: Latino adolescents, their school, and a university use photovoice to examine and address the influence of immigration. J Interprof Care. 2004;18(4):403–15.

37. Lopez EDS, Robinson N, Eng E. Photovoice as a CBPR method: a case study with African American breast cancer survivors in rural eastern North Carolina. In: Israel BA, Eng E, Schulz AJ, Parker EA, editors. Methods for community-based participatory research for health. 2nd ed. San Francisco: Jossey-Bass; 2013. p. 489–515.

38. Rhodes SD, Hergenrather KC, Griffith D, Yee LJ, Zometa CS, Montaño J, et al. Sexual and alcohol use behaviours of Latino men in the South-eastern USA. Cult Health Sex. 2009;11(1):17–34.

39. Rhodes SD, Hergenrather KC. Recently arrived immigrant Latino men identify community approaches to promote HIV prevention. Am J Public Health. 2007;97(6):984–5.

40. Berry NS, McQuiston C, Parrado EA, Olmos-Muniz JC. CBPR and ethnogrpahy: the perfect union. In: Israel BA, Eng E, Schulz A, Parker EA, editors. Methods for community-based participatory research for health. 2nd ed. San Francisco: Jossey-Bass; 2013. p. 305–34.

41. Beebe J. Rapid assessment process: an introduction. Walnut Creek: AltaMira Press; 2001.

42. Bloom F. Research report. Rapid assessment and syphilis. Anthropology News. 2001;42(2):56.

43. Trotter RT, Needle RH, Goosby E, Bates C, Singer M. A methodological model for rapid assessment, response, and evaluation: the RARE program in public health. Field Method. 2001;13(2):137–59.

44. Sena AC, Hammer JP, Wilson K, Zeveloff A, Gamble J. Feasibility and acceptability of door-to-door rapid HIV testing among latino immigrants and their HIV risk factors in North Carolina. AIDS Patient Care STDS. 2010;24(3):165–73.

45. Eng E, Blanchard L. Action-oriented community diagnosis: a health education tool. Int Q Community Health Educ. 1991;11(2):93–110.

46. Green LW, Krueter M, Krueter MW. Health promotion planning: an educational and environmental approach. 3rd ed. Mountain View: Mayfield Publications; 1999.

47. Margolis LH, Stevens R, Laraia B, Ammerman A, Harlan C, Dodds J, et al. Educating students for community-based partnerships. J Community Pract. 2000;7(4):21–34.

48. Parker EA, Eng E, Laraia B, Ammerman A, Dodds J, Margolis L, et al. Coalition building for prevention: lessons learned from the North Carolina community-based public health initiative. J Public Health Manag Pract. 1998;4(2):25–36.

49. Cuadros P. A home on the field: How one championship team inspires hope for the revival of small town America. New York: HarperCollins; 2006.

50. Rhodes SD, Hergenrather KC, Montano J, Remnitz IM, Arceo R, Bloom FR, et al. Using community-based participatory research to develop an intervention to reduce HIV and STD infections among Latino men. AIDS Educ Prev. 2006;18(5):375–89.

51. Rhodes SD, Hergenrather KC, Wilkin AM, Jolly C. Visions and voices: indigent persons living with HIV in the southern United States use photovoice to create knowledge, develop partnerships, and take action. Health Promot Pract. 2008;9(2):159–69.

52. Arnstein SR. A ladder of citizen participation. J Am Inst Plan. 1969;35:216–24.

53. Rhodes SD, McCoy TP, Vissman AT, DiClemente RJ, Duck S, Hergenrather KC, et al. A randomized controlled trial of a culturally congruent intervention to increase condom use and HIV testing among heterosexually active immigrant Latino men. AIDS Behav. 2011;15(8):1764–75.

54. Painter TM, Organista KC, Rhodes SD, Sañudo FM. Interventions to prevent HIV and other sexually transmitted diseases among Latino migrants. In: Organista KC, editor. HIV prevention with Latinos: theory, research, and practice. New York: Oxford University Press; 2012. p. 351–81.

55. Rhodes SD, Tanner A, Duck S, Aronson RE, Alonzo J, Wilkin AM, et al. Female sex work within the Latino community in central North Carolina: an exploratory qualitative community-based participatory research study. Prog Community Health Partnersh. 2012;6(4):417–27.
56. Catania DA. Damaging Whitman-Walker. The Washington Post. 2009 May 5, 2009.
57. Pollack H. In the US, the HIV prevention fight has stalled. The Washington Post. 2013.

Chapter 8
Community Involvement in HIV-related Policy Initiatives: History, Experiences, and Next Steps

Jason Daniel-Ulloa, Briana Woods-Jaeger, Melvin Jackson, Dominica Rehbein, Alexandra Lightfoot, Linda Riggins, Robert E. Aronson and Scott D. Rhodes

Community mobilization and organization have clearly made important impacts on HIV-related policies in the USA. Members from diverse communities across the country have advocated for, and changed policies directly related to, the prevention of HIV exposure and transmission and the care of persons with HIV. These efforts have resulted in the development and use of, and access to, evidence-based prevention and state-of-the-science treatment for HIV. Because of the tireless work of individuals involved in HIV-related policy initiatives, the process used by the US Food and Drug Administration (FDA) to develop, test, and approve potentially lifesaving HIV medications was revised and expedited; the involvement of persons with HIV on patient advisory boards ensuring consumer involvement in prevention and treatment is now expected and common; women and children must be included in community and clinical trials, and if not, a rationale must be offered and approved; needle-exchange programs have been established; access to substance

J. Daniel-Ulloa (✉)
Department of Community and Behavioral Health, University of Iowa College of Public Health, N438 CPHB, 145 Riverside Dr., Iowa City, IA 52242, USA
e-mail: Jason-daniel@uiowa.edu

B. Woods-Jaeger
Department of Community and Behavioral Health, University of Iowa College of Public Health, N426 CPHB, 145 Riverside Dr., Iowa City, IA 52242, USA
e-mail: briana-woods@uiowa.edu

M. Jackson
Strengthening The Black Family, Inc., 568 E Lenoir St Suite 001, Raleigh, NC 27601, USA
e-mail: Melvin.Jackson@wakegov.com

D. Rehbein
Department of Health Management and Policy, University of Iowa College of Public Health, 145 Riverside Dr., Box 312 CPHB, Iowa City, IA 52242, USA
e-mail: dominica-rehbein@uiowa.edu

A. Lightfoot
Community Based Participatory Research Core Center for Health Promotion and Disease Prevention, University of North Carolina at Chapel Hill, Campus Box #7426, 1700 Martin Luther King, Jr. Blvd, Chapel Hill, NC 27599, USA
e-mail: aflight@email.unc.edu

S. D. Rhodes (ed.), *Innovations in HIV Prevention Research and Practice through Community Engagement,* DOI 10.1007/978-1-4939-0900-1_8, © Springer Science+Business Media New York 2014

abuse treatment programs has increased; and condom use within the adult film industry is now mandated (although currently not enforced) within Los Angeles County. These examples are just a few ways communities have affected HIV-related policy. "Outside experts," including researchers and practitioners (e.g., scientists from academic, government, and some nongovernment institutions), can learn from these successful initiatives, and others like them, that have contributed to improved HIV prevention, treatment, and care in the USA, and build on them to move forward both the science and practice of community engagement within HIV-related policy initiatives.

Community engagement within the HIV epidemic began within the gay community. Gay men and their close allies acted when other organizations, including the US government, did not. In the early years of the epidemic, the prevention of HIV exposure and transmission among gay men and the care and treatment of those with HIV were decidedly not priorities for the "mainstream" in the USA (as well as globally). Thus, early prevention and treatment initiatives were led by gay men themselves, community insiders who responded to the HIV epidemic that was dramatically affecting their friends and neighbors, some of whom were living with HIV themselves; this history is introduced in Chap. 4.

A pivotal and early step in community mobilization and organization in response to the HIV epidemic occurred in 1983. A group of advocates met in Denver, Colorado, to develop goals and objectives related to HIV policies in the USA and established what are known as the Denver Principles. These principles asserted the dignity of all persons with HIV by calling for communities to organize to prevent workplace and housing discrimination based on HIV status (at the time discrimination was common); and to end scapegoating of people with, or assumed to be at risk for, HIV. These principles also recommended that persons with HIV and those closely aligned with them take several actions:

- Form caucuses to develop and plan strategies to meet their own priorities
- Participate at every level of decision-making and serve on the boards of prevention and provider organizations
- Share their own knowledge and lived experiences
- Substitute low-risk sexual behaviors for behaviors that could endanger their health and/or the health of their sexual partners.

L. Riggins
Focus on Youth Project, Strengthening the Black Family, Inc., 568 E, Lenoir St Suite 001, Raleigh, NC 27601, USA
e-mail: Linda.Riggins@wakegov.com

R. E. Aronson
Public Health Program, School of Natural and Applied Sciences, Taylor University, 236 West Reade Avenue, Upland, IN 46989, USA
e-mail: bob_aronson@taylor.edu

S. D. Rhodes
Department of Social Sciences and Health Policy, Division of Public Health Sciences, Wake Forest University School of Medicine, Winston-Salem, NC 27157, USA
e-mail: srhodes@wakehealth.edu

The principles also asserted the rights of persons with HIV, including the right to full and satisfying sexual and emotional lives; to high-quality medical treatment and social services without discrimination of any form based on sexual orientation, gender, diagnosis, economic status, or race; to full explanations of all medical procedures and risks, with the right to choose or refuse their treatment, to refuse to participate in research without jeopardizing their treatment, and to make informed decisions about their lives; to privacy, medical record confidentiality, and respect; and to dignity in life and death. The establishment of the Denver Principles illustrates how members of communities affected by a health problem convened and became involved in health-related policy initiatives rather than passively waiting for unwilling others to act [1]. These principles were used to guide priorities and strategies, laying a firm foundation for HIV-related policy initiatives.

We have come a long way since these early days of the HIV epidemic when a small group of community members laid this foundation. The *National HIV/AIDS Strategy* is a more recent HIV-related policy initiative that included a strong component of community engagement in its development. In fact, community input into the development of the *National HIV/AIDS Strategy* was systematic and came through multiple channels. Beginning in 2009, staff from the Office of National AIDS Policy convened 14 community forums across the country, which engaged more than 4,200 participants (http://www.whitehouse.gov/administration/eop/onap/nhas/activities). Input also was sought from representatives of the American–Indian/Alaska Native communities; people with HIV in rural communities in the South, a region of the country experiencing disproportionate HIV rates, and northeast; Asian and Pacific Islanders; African immigrants; business and philanthropic leaders; among others. The Office of National AIDS Policy further engaged community members and gathered perspectives, experiences, and insights through an online process that generated more than 800 submissions. The Office also held a series of expert meetings to explore more in-depth issues related to youth, women, and housing. Thus, through ongoing broad community engagement, the *National HIV/AIDS Strategy* was developed and designed to be a roadmap for next steps for the general public and policymakers based on the perspectives, experiences, and insights from a variety of stakeholders at all levels, such as community members, representatives from community-based organizations, academic researchers, government personnel, business persons, and philanthropic leaders. The *National HIV/AIDS Strategy* outlines four main goals: to reduce HIV incidence, increase access to care and improve health outcomes for persons with HIV, reduce HIV-related health disparities and inequities, and achieve a more coordinated national response to the HIV epidemic in the USA. The *Strategy* highlights areas that require the most immediate attention and change; action steps that must be taken, including policy changes; and targets for measuring progress toward the achievement of goals.

Despite these two examples of successful HIV-related policy initiatives (the development of the Denver Principles early on and of the *National HIV/AIDS Strategy* more recently), little research has evaluated HIV-related policy initiatives that involve partnerships among community members; representatives from community-based organizations, government agencies, and businesses; and academic researchers. In this chapter, we review five policy-change frameworks and the ways in which communities are engaged and partnerships are developed. We then build a rationale for the application of community-based particularity research (CBPR) in HIV-related policy initiatives, providing examples of policy initiatives and lessons learned from such efforts. Lastly, we propose a health-related and community-engaged framework that is informed by existing policy-change frameworks and experiences with policy initiatives that harnessed the strengths of partnerships that included community members; representatives from community-based organizations, government agencies, and businesses; and academic researchers.

Policy-change Frameworks and Community Engagement

Effective policies have been shown to improve community health and well-being. It has been suggested that some of the most important public health successes in the USA have resulted from policy changes; these successes include reduced rates of childhood lead poisoning, adolescent sexual activity, tobacco use, and workplace injuries; increased rates of vaccination; and improved motor vehicle safety [2–5]. Policy initiatives have at least three key advantages in promoting health and preventing morbidity and mortality. First, policy initiatives potentially can reach large numbers of community members as opposed to individual-change interventions, which, for the most part, affect the health and well-being of fewer individuals. Second, policy initiatives are not based on the idea that people make decisions rationally. Most individual-health-behavior theories are based somewhat on expectancy, assuming that an individual will choose to behave a certain way based on the desirability of an outcome. Policy initiatives, however, alter the context to one that supports health and well-being; there is less space for individuals to decide between healthier and less healthy options. Third, because of the context change, policies tend to have a lasting impact, as long as they are established as a priority and enforced by those charged with these responsibilities.

In Fig. 8.1, we present an adaptation of a health impact pyramid [6]. In this 5-tiered pyramid, the top tier, *HIV prevention education and risk reduction counseling*, includes individual- and group-level interventions, including the HIV and sexually transmitted infection (STI) interventions that are commonly disseminated by the Centers of Disease Control and Prevention (CDC) and implemented by health departments, community-based organizations, and medical settings that provide HIV-prevention services. These types of interventions are outlined in the CDC's *Compendium of Evidence-based HIV Behavioral Interventions* (www.cdc.gov/hiv/topics/research/prs/compendium-evidence-based-interventions.htm). This tier requires the most individual motivation and effort and has the lowest impact at the population level.

The next tier represents *clinical interventions*. These interventions include HIV preexposure prophylaxis; management of HIV in persons with HIV to maintain low viral loads and thus their infectivity; STI treatment, given the association of STIs

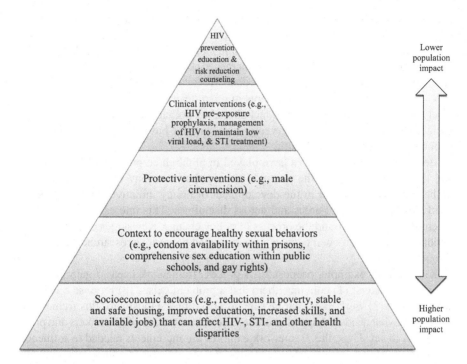

Fig. 8.1 An adaption of the public health pyramid [6]

and HIV infection; and treatment of factors associated with risk. Substance abuse treatment can be a clinical treatment related to HIV.

The third tier represents *protective interventions*. These are interventions, which generally include one-time or infrequent interventions and do not require ongoing clinical care. Male circumcision is an example of an HIV-related protective intervention that may have a profound impact on the HIV epidemic in at least some parts of the world. Male circumcision has been found to reduce female-to-male HIV transmission by 50–60 % [7]. Vaccination against human papillomavirus (HPV) is an example of a protective intervention designed to reduce the risk of health problems that HPV infection can cause, including genital warts, cancers of the anus, vagina, vulva, penis, and oropharynx [8].

The fourth tier is the *context to encourage healthy sexual behaviors include policies that promote health*. This level includes policies that make condoms readily available (a current challenge facing the reduction of HIV exposure and transmission within prisons), access to clean needles, and use of evidence-based HIV-prevention interventions. Even policies around gay rights and gay marriage affect HIV exposure and transmission, as supportive policies can reduce HIV risk [9, 10]. At the same time, the context to encourage healthy behaviors also may include policies affecting other tiers within the pyramid. For example, policies can require the use of evidence-based HIV-prevention interventions (as opposed to interventions that are not scientifically sound) within public schools.

The bottom tier represents *socioeconomic factors*. Reductions in poverty, stable and safe housing, improved education, increased skills, and available jobs can affect HIV exposure. Improvements in socioeconomic factors also can yield reductions in HIV and STIs as well as improvements in other health disparities. Changes at this level also can be influenced and in fact altered by policies designed to intervene on socioeconomic factors [11]. Interventions in this tier have the greatest impact on population and community health.

Because of the role policies have played in highlighted public health successes and the understanding of the potential roles policy can play in the tiers of public health impact, interest in the development of policy initiatives has surfaced in nearly all health content areas and across disciplines. This interest has yielded an emerging literature around the process of policy change. Key stages or components in policy-change frameworks have been described by various researchers and practitioners (Table 8.1).

Kingdon, for example, proposed a 3-process framework used to gain attention from policymakers: (1) convince them that a problem exists, (2) propose a feasible solution, and (3) work to get public support [12]. For the most part, this framework focuses on what needs to happen in order to gain the attention of lawmakers and pressure them to act. Thus, this framework explores the ingredients needed to influence legislative action; it is not a detailed list of steps or processes in policy development.

In turn, Blackwell and colleagues suggested that a more complex series of stages occur in the policy process. These stages are: (1) identifying and refining the policy, (2) setting an agenda and creating awareness, (3) setting policy objectives, (4) designing an alternative course of action, (5) weighing consequences of alternative actions, (6) celebrating victories and preparing for challenges, (7) assigning implementation responsibility, and (8) evaluating policy impact and outcomes. This model is complex and depends heavily on community involvement and engagement [13].

Brownson and colleagues proposed a 4-stage framework for the formulation and evaluation of policy designed to promote health and prevent disease. These stages are: (1) the identification of health risks and preventive options, in which epidemiologic data are gathered to establish and identify health risks and priorities; (2) intervention (program) development, which includes identifying priority populations, examining options and channels, assessing high-risk versus population approach, and determining behavioral science theoretical underpinnings; (3) policy development, in which options are examined, coalitions are established, input from policymakers is obtained, and policy-planning data are collected; and (4) policy enactment and assurance, in which wide-spread support for the policy is the focus through coalition enhancement, media involvement, and the use of data. In this framework, community members and policymakers tend to become involved only at the third stage, after effective interventions have been developed. A key component of this framework is evaluation, which is integrated into each stage [14].

Christoffel proposed a 3-stage framework: information, strategy, and action. In the information stage, similar to the first stage in the framework of Brownson et al.,

Table 8.1 Key policy-change frameworks

Kingdon et al. [12]	Blackwell et al. [13]	Brownson et al. [14]	Christoffel [15]	Minkler et al. [16]
(1) Convince policymakers that a problem exists	(1) Become aware of problem and identify shared cause or vision	(1) Identify health risks and preventive options	(1) Identify, describe, and quantify the public health problem and its patterns, risks, and potential solutions	(1) Identify macro factors contributing to health
(2) Propose a feasible solution	(2) Set the agenda and create awareness	(2) Develop intervention or program by identifying priority populations, examining options, and determining theoretical underpinnings	(2) Disseminate results of previous stage; mobilize community members; develop policy objectives; create policy statement, messages, and campaigns; and build resource and advocacy networks	(2) Build partnership, identify decision-makers; and examine the roles of science, evidence (including data), and community engagement in policy change
(3) Obtain public support so that policymakers will act	(3) Set policy objectives	(3) Develop policies through examining options, establishing coalitions, and obtaining input from policymakers	(3) Move to action, implement strategies, push for policy change	(3) Prioritize problems, raise awareness, construct alternatives, identify policy targets, and advocate for change
	(4) Design alternative courses of action	(4) Enact policy		(4) Examine desired health-related outcomes and unintended consequences
	(5) Weigh consequences of alternative actions			
	(6) Celebrate victories and prepare for challenges			
	(7) Assign implementation responsibility			
	(8) Evaluate			

data about the health risks are gathered. The objective at this stage is to identify, describe, and quantify the public health problem, including its patterns and risks, temporality, and potential solutions. These data may come in many forms and are then disseminated in reports and/or journal articles. Next, during the strategy stage, community needs are identified. This stage includes further disseminating the results of the information stage to both professional and lay audiences; mobilizing the community; developing policy objectives; creating policy statements, public education messages, and campaigns; and building resource and advocacy networks. The action stage includes implementing specific strategies, raising funds, and targeting policymakers and decision-makers to focus on the desired policy goals to yield changes in political and social environments [15].

Although these frameworks recognize the potential roles of community members in the policy-change process at some level, Minkler and colleagues developed a framework that is explicitly based on principles of community engagement [16]. This framework is known as the CBPR contexts, processes, policy strategies, and outcomes model. In this model, community members are engaged throughout all steps of policy development, advocacy, implementation, and evaluation. The process begins with an examination of macro factors that contribute to health (e.g., socioeconomic status, history of collaboration, trust/distrust among partners, and capacity and readiness) in the first stage (context), and then moves into partnership-building activities and identification of stakeholders and decision-makers (CBPR processes). This stage also acknowledges the roles of science, evidence, and community engagement in helping to make the case for policy change. Essential to this stage is the usefulness of understandable and high-quality data and how these data can be adopted and integrated into organizing strategies.

The policy-strategies stage involves working within the partnership to establish priorities, set an agenda, raise awareness, construct policy alternatives, identify policies to target, advocate for change, and work toward implementation. Lastly, the model points to examination of the policy as it is implemented and the impact on the desired health outcomes as well as unintended consequences (evaluation). Thus, this model seems to set a balance between the science of change and the equal inclusion of community.

Overall, these frameworks move from identifying and quantifying a problem in early stages to identifying policy targets and developing strategies to implement them in middle stages, to taking action to put the policies in place and evaluating the impact and revising in the later stages based on outcomes. It is also important to note that despite the seemingly linear description of stages in each of these frameworks, the policy-change process is dynamic and more or less convoluted.

HIV-related Policy Initiatives and CBPR

Communities can and do act to change polices without the involvement of outside experts like academic researchers and practitioners, and this is frequently done, as evidenced by the many successful HIV-related policy initiatives. However, when the passion and strategic thinking of community mobilization are blended with sound research, the result can be powerful. This combination has been proposed to be, and in the few cases in which this combination has been applied has proven to be, highly effective in the overall effort to reduce and eliminate health disparities [16, 17]. However, the application of CBPR approaches to policy-change initiatives is not easy and cannot be conducted without effort, but the payoff can be profound.

Policies developed in partnership with community members, particularly if that partnership is equitable, are more likely to be welcomed, effective, enforced, and sustainable compared with policies made by outside forces making decisions about what they think will work best in a community [16, 18–20]. To effectively promote policy change there must be broad community involvement, ongoing relationships, and communication with people and institutions capable of making the recommended changes [21–25]. CBPR partnerships are well positioned to identify problems and engage with the broader community to identify and develop sustainable policy initiatives to address the particular needs of communities, strategize approaches, and build the necessary networks to promote change.

Policy change initiatives that harness CBPR approaches tend to be most successful when partners, including community members and academic researchers, take the time to foster trust and build relationships with one another. CBPR hinges on building productive relationships and basing engagement and partnership on commonly recognized CBPR principles [16, 26–31] to provide a foundation to begin working toward meaningful policy development, implementation, and evaluation.

Although community engagement within the policy-change literature in general—and within HIV-related policy change in particular—is limited, policy-change initiatives that harness CBPR have addressed a variety of HIV- and non-HIV-related priorities. These priorities include allocation of HIV-prevention funding and programming among sexual minorities [30]; school-based sexual and reproductive education [32]; school funding [33]; reintegration of recently released inmates into society [34]; lead screening and lead exposure [35]; food insecurity [36]; and environmental justice [18, 37]. Although this list is not exhaustive, the studies illustrate broad health priorities that have been addressed blending both policy change and CBPR.

These policy initiatives, whether HIV related or not, provide important insights to guide HIV-related policy initiatives that use community engagement approaches such as CBPR.

Several projects have included the successful use of lay or community health workers [38] or community youth to help engage the community or neighborhood [39] in policy initiatives. Other projects have used publicized reports and town hall meetings to engage community members and policymakers alike [40]. One CBPR project designed to explore sexual risk and identify potentially effective intervention approaches to reduce risk among African-American/black, Latino, and white men who have sex with men (MSM) culminated with an empowerment-based community forum that led to key policy changes in North Carolina. In this project, a well-established CBPR partnership collected, analyzed, and interpreted qualitative data and presented these data during a community forum. Forum attendees included representatives from the lay community, AIDS service organizations, community-based organizations, the North Carolina Department of Health and Human Services, two historically black colleges, and two academic research institutions. The attendees participated in a process that included responding to five sequential empowerment-based triggers: (1) What do you see in these findings? (2) In what ways do these findings make sense to you? (3) In what ways do these findings not make sense to you? (4) What can be done?/What can we all do? (5) What should we be doing "down the road" to reduce risk among MSM? [30].

As a result of the forum, the NC Department of Health and Human Services made three key policy changes. First, they reallocated funds to create safe spaces for gay and bisexual men, MSM, and transgender persons that allowed for tailored programming that went beyond traditional HIV-prevention programming to meet the social support needs of these communities. To date, these safe spaces have been successful in facilitating supportive dialogue around issues of masculinity; family, religious, and societal expectations; and intimacy among men. Second, the NC Department of Health and Human Services changed policies to reduce administrative barriers to increase nontraditional HIV-testing sites across the state. Finally, the NC Department of Health and Human Services applied for and was awarded funding for an annual conference designed to support gay and bisexual men, MSM, and transgender persons; interventionists and preventionists; and health educators in the field through social support and community organizing and advocacy skills development.

Other changes that resulted from the forum included increased use of technology by AIDS service organizations and community-based organizations to promote HIV testing among sexual and gender minorities. It also built partnerships between community members, organization representatives, and academic researchers that have yielded new projects to reduce HIV exposure and transmission among vulnerable populations [30].

Photovoice, a methodology closely aligned with CBPR, also has been used to change policy related to HIV. Photovoice is a qualitative method that can be used to empower community members, gather data related to community health or political priorities, and build relationships between community and academic partners to identify issues particularly important to community members. Photovoice includes providing cameras to community members to document their concerns, promote new knowledge through discussion of the photographs, and translate this new knowledge into action steps through advocacy and public forums [41]; the process has been identified as a key methodology to support policy change [41–43]).

Visions and Voices: HIV in the twenty-first century was a photovoice project conducted to gain insight into the life experiences of persons with HIV. The study uncovered realities of living with HIV though photographic documentation and Freirean-based critical dialogue and facilitated a process for persons with HIV to reach local community members and leaders, policymakers, and advocates to develop plans of action and effect positive change. Based on the prioritized actions agreed on during an empowerment-based community forum (much like the forum described above), four main outcomes occurred. First, a team wrote a funded foundation grant to create a portable gallery exhibition of the photographs, framed with corresponding quotations. Unveiled on World AIDS Day (December 1) at a local art gallery during a community-wide open gallery tour, the exhibition was designed to remind the community that despite the success of health-enhancing treatment options, HIV still exists; to rally support for primary and secondary prevention efforts; to reduce stigma and discrimination against people living with HIV; and to provide education about HIV to those at risk for HIV exposure and transmission. After the opening of the exhibition, four newspapers ran stories on it and interviewed participants and representatives of the CBPR partnership. A local television affiliate conducted two news segments on the project, which included representatives from the partnership and a photographer-participant, that was shown during the early evening news.

Second, a group of persons with HIV partnered with the public health department and took responsibility for expanding and replenishing a portion of the county public health department's offsite free condom distribution sites. Spanish-speaking persons with HIV were recruited to keep local tiendas (grocery stores) stocked with both free condoms and prevention materials.

Furthermore, a speakers bureau made up of persons with HIV was developed in partnership with the county public health department. Finally, an AIDS service organization created a substance use task force to explore ways to better meet the treatment and prevention needs of substance users and those at risk for substance use and relapse. In addition to the changes promoted for the participants and involved community-based organizations, findings from another photovoice project, Windows to Work (described in Chap. 10) were used as formative data in the development of the *National HIV/AIDS Strategy* [44].

Lessons Learned from Existing Community-engaged Policy Initiatives

Two key reports funded by the W.K. Kellogg Foundation provide descriptions of and lessons learned from CBPR policy initiatives [16, 33]. These reports do not focus on HIV-related policy initiatives, but when these reports are combined with the limited HIV-related policy change literature, several factors that facilitate successful policy initiatives emerge. These factors are the importance of (1) the existence of enduring partnerships prior to advocacy efforts or including new partnerships with multiple established community organizations, (2) a salient issue backed by the community, (3) a motivating event, (4) mixed-methods data collection, (5) involvement of media to reach members of the local community, and (6) involvement of policymakers, city councils, local governments, etc., and (7) nonfederal funding.

Effectiveness of Existing Partnerships

Community–academic partnerships require trust building, given the history of mistrust between communities and academic researchers (and the institutions they represent). Even without such history, partnerships require a level of trust to facilitate success and overcome challenges and barriers. For example, community members need to trust that academic researchers are committed to working in partnership with community members for the long-term and not just until the end of research funding, and academic researchers must trust that community members will represent data in a way that aligns with scientific principles. The complexity of identifying policy objectives and crafting policy strategies require partners who work well together and trust one another. Building this trust takes time and must be deliberate.

Identification, development, and implementation of policy initiatives are easier for partners who have a history of working together. Most of the successful partnerships that seek to change policy require that community members trust one another and are willing and able to attend public hearings, knock on doors to raise awareness, and provide input to the collaboration. For these reasons, existing partnerships, with a firm foundation of mutual trust, may be better suited to establishing and pursuing policy initiatives. However, sometimes partnerships must include other community, organizational, or academic partners who have important skills or expertise missing from the partnership.

Furthermore, the length of time and complexity of the early stages of policy initiatives (e.g., raising awareness and developing policy targets) can be challenging, and many partnerships may dissolve before later phases (e.g., setting policy objectives) have been reached. Thus, partners with a history of working together often have established the essential "glue" that can help them move more efficiently through the processes involved in changing policies [45].

Issue Salience and Motivating Events

Issue salience is an important consideration for the policy-initiative process. Often this salience has come from new data indicating inequities. As has been suggested, taking advantage of so-called windows of opportunity can provide a spark to the project and raise issue awareness and salience [13]. For example, HIV infection in actors in the adult film industry, allegedly acquired on set, promoted the establishment and subsequent passage of the County of Los Angeles Safer Sex in the Film Industry Act that mandates the use of condoms as protection from HIV during vaginal and anal sex on adult film sets in Los Angeles County. Like many policies, including ones this Act was modeled after (e.g., safety regulations at tattoo and massage parlors and bathhouses), this policy continues to raise controversy. However, it is important to acknowledge the role of actors becoming infected with HIV on set as a spark and actors coming out publically about their infection that contributed to this policy-related action.

Mixed-methods Data Collection

Many CBPR-policy initiatives have involved the use of a combination of qualitative and quantitative data. In fact, policymakers have reported that the combination of these two types of data often swayed their opinion on policy decisions [16]. Quantitative data can illustrate the impact on a community or population, whereas qualitative data can provide real examples of how lives are affected, putting a face in front of the numbers.

Partnerships have taken advantage of the skills of academic researchers to determine the best evidence and the best methods to collect this evidence to be meaningful for policymakers. These academic partners also brought their strengths and expertise to build community capacity by providing research and advocacy skills development, including guidance and practice on how to collect, analyze, and interpret data and disseminate findings [46, 47] and how to prepare for public speaking and testifying at public hearings.

A public report of study findings has been used effectively in several policy studies [18, 21, 30, 40, 41, 44, 48, 49]. These reports did not use academic language and style in summarizing findings; rather these reports presented key findings within the context of what community members and policymakers care about and how they discuss issues. The partnerships presented the report during town hall meetings and community forums and outlined findings in public hearings. Copies of the report were sent to policymakers and media outlets. Having data from academic sources, whether quantitative or qualitative, also added credibility to reports and weight to subsequent media stories. In addition to these benefits, these data provide a good backstop for counterarguments when corporate or governmental organizations oppose a policy initiative.

Media Involvement

Media can play an important role in policy initiatives by focusing attention on selected issues and perspectives. Media can anticipate problems in advance of public officials, raise awareness about an issue, alert the community to public health problems based on data and/or official warnings, inform the community about the stakes that competing groups have in solving problems, keep various groups and the community abreast of competing initiatives and/or versions of initiatives, contribute to the content of policy, decide the tempo of decision-making, help policymakers decide what priorities to set and how to proceed (e.g., vote), alert the public to how policies are administered, evaluate policy effectiveness, and stimulate policy reviews. However, it is important that media not focus only on describing and raising awareness about a problem like HIV-related disparities, but rather should help move people toward solutions.

Policymaker Involvement

Including experts early on in policy initiatives can be beneficial. For example, members of one partnership included policymakers in photovoice projects, training them and including them throughout the theme-producing process. As a result of working with members of the affected community through photovoice or similar projects, policymakers may be more open to community input and provide more ways for such input into policy initiatives [50]. In these types of cases, the goal is to have a collaborative rather than a combative relationship between community members and policymakers. This approach may build trust and connections and demystify the policymaking process for community members.

Nonfederal Funding

Despite notable exceptions (e.g., W.K. Kellogg Foundation and the California Endowment), there has been little funding for CBPR-policy initiatives in general and HIV-related ones in specific. One reason for the dearth of HIV policy-related initiatives using CBPR approaches may be federal prohibitions against using federal funds, including funds awarded for research, to lobby public officials (http://ethics. od.nih.gov/topics/Lobby-Publicity-Guide.htm). It has been argued that the line between applying knowledge gained through the systematic collection, analysis, and interpretation of empirical data and lobbying for a cause may be somewhat blurry [51–53]. However, given the controversial, emotionally charged, and high-profile nature of most HIV-related policy issues (e.g., needle exchange, condom distribution in prisons, and comprehensive sexual health education in public schools), the likelihood of being perceived as lobbying and then having to defend the research can be too great a barrier.

Furthermore, it must be noted that policy-related research can be time-consuming particularly if health outcomes are expected, and funding may not be adequate for the entire process. It can take a considerable amount of time to move from issue identification to policy change, implementation, and subsequent evaluation. In one study to change policies related to needle sharing, the Urban Research Center at the New York Academy of Medicine was unable to sustain funding for a sufficient length of time to implement and evaluate policy interventions that they developed, although they continue to translate their research findings into advocating for syringe access for those who use injecting drugs [54].

African-American/Black Church Policy and HIV

Faith-based organizations can also play a role in HIV-related policy change. Such organizations are an important and respected resource in the African-American/black community providing well-respected youth development programs and promoting important protective factors key to reduce risk behavior among youth [55–57]. Yet, many researchers and practitioners often perceive that faith-based organizations are reluctant to take an active role in responding to HIV because of factors such as stigma of HIV-related risk behaviors and discomfort discussing sex and sexuality [57].

Given the disproportionate burden of HIV borne by African-American/black communities, a long-established CBPR partnership in North Carolina changed policies at three African-American/black churches. These policy changes led to the implementation and evaluation of a youth-focused, evidence-based HIV-prevention intervention [55]. Lessons learned from this process included the catalyst role of a well-respected "insider" community-based organization, Strengthening the Black Family, Inc. founded in 1980, Strengthening the Black Family is a preeminent coalition of civic and community-based organizations with a single vision: to bring about positive change in the local African-American/black community. Staffed and run by local African-American/black leaders who live and work within the local community, Strengthening the Black Family has played an important role in providing support and programming designed to reduce health disparities and promote health equity in Southeast Raleigh, North Carolina. Their programming also has included a strong HIV-prevention component [58].

Based on ongoing feedback through both systematically collected data and community member recommendations, partners from Strengthening the Black Family and the University of North Carolina at Chapel Hill identified three network churches as potential partners, surmising that pastors from these churches seemed primed for discussing faith-based HIV prevention. Thus, for this partnership, the first step in policy change included assessing "readiness" for change. Although change had to be fostered, members of this partnership wanted to start from a point of some degree of readiness, given that initiating and implementing new HIV-related policies within African-American/black churches can be an ambitious undertaking.

The second step was to establish a diverse and intergenerational community advisory board by bringing together representatives from Strengthening the Black Family, the University of North Carolina, the two churches, and the local community. Strengthening The Black Family's vast network was instrumental to ensure diverse youth, parent, agency, and faith-leader representation. Notably, six youth participated as equal partners on the community advisory board. The ongoing involvement of members of the community advisory board throughout all phases of this project was essential to its success.

Next, the community advisory board participated in focus groups, provided feedback on findings, and examined local data to identify barriers to HIV prevention in African-American/black churches. There was clearly strong support for HIV prevention within churches, but there was disagreement on the type of curriculum that was appropriate: abstinence-only versus a more comprehensive approach. This rich discussion, which included a variety of divergent perspectives, provided crucial input that helped navigate faith-based HIV prevention.

Fourth, community insiders who lived in the local community, attended the churches, and were committed to HIV prevention paved the way for other members of the partnership to attend and participate in church activities (e.g., senior programs, Bible studies, and special events) to gain an understating of the churches' current health-related programming, priorities, customs, values, and cultures. In addition to providing insights into the church contexts, this process facilitated trust and relationships; the process of changing church policies around effective HIV-prevention programming was designed to be collaborative not adversarial.

Because pastors may have "role overload" [59], the partnership also established relationships with other influential church leaders, such as first ladies, associate pastors, deacons, trustees, and health and youth ministry leaders. These leaders had the ear of the pastors and could articulate the benefits that evidence-based HIV-prevention programming could provide to families in their congregations and the wider African-American/black community. Critical to this step was identifying and articulating how an HIV-related policy, such as the implementation of an evidence-based intervention, complemented general church priorities and established policies.

Sixth, key to the process was the openness to alternatives and expanding beyond the initial focus of HIV-related policy change solely within the church. For example, some community advisory board members were not comfortable with condom demonstrations so the partnership developed an alternative activity that could be substituted for condom demonstration. Knowing that there was an alternative eased fears and concerns; in fact, during actual implementation of the intervention, few parents or youth chose the alternative over the condom demonstration, an indication that information sharing, alternative generation, willingness to compromise, and transparency had been effective.

In addition, youth on the community advisory board identified several other needed HIV-related policy changes in the community through a photovoice project and formed an advocacy group Youth Empowered Advocating for Health (YEAH) to raise awareness and galvanize support for policy change. The YEAH youth leaders hosted a community forum to raise awareness of the importance of community and institutional support for African-American/black youth, advocate for youth representation in decision-making activities, and reduce stigma around HIV. This forum was attended by local church, education and political leaders, parents, youth, and adult community members. In addition to local efforts, YEAH leaders garnered support for their policy objectives through networking with national ally organizations (e.g., Advocates for Youth), meeting with political leaders in Washington D.C., and presenting at national science conferences. Further, they are actively mentoring other youth to build their capacity to speak to policymakers, identify and suggest relevant policy changes, and become leaders in their community [60].

Through these steps, the three churches changed their policies around HIV-prevention programming to implement a comprehensive evidence-based HIV-prevention intervention for youth 12–15-years old and a youth advocacy movement was initiated to pursue HIV-related policy change in the local community.

Policy Initiatives and Health Disparities Reduction

Participating in the process of policy change, including the development and advocacy of relevant policies, community members often develop new capacities (e.g., critical and linear thinking) and skills (e.g., self-efficacy and ability to speak at public forums on behalf of their priorities). Partnerships can help community members develop the skills needed to participate in the planning, implementation, and evaluation of policy initiatives in many ways, for example through engaging community members in framing research questions to address community needs and priorities, training them in methods of data collection, using participatory techniques such as photovoice [49], sharing data analysis and interpretation responsibilities [47], and providing opportunities to disseminate research findings through community forums. At the same time, academic researchers who tend to be outside-experts (e.g., scientists from academic, government, and some nongovernment institutions) develop better insights into community priorities and effective processes and solutions that are authentic to the community and its history and context. Thus, while engaged in HIV-related policy initiatives, community members and outside-experts develop skills that are transferrable to understanding and solving other issues facing communities.

A Health-related and Community-engaged Framework for Policy Change

Using developed frameworks as a foundation, lessons learned from the literature [16, 33, 58], and our own experiences with community engagement in policy change [30, 44, 49, 57], we outlined steps that can be used in a carefully orchestrated and community-engaged policy change process (Table 8.2).

Discussion and Conclusion

Some of the early HIV-related policy initiatives were spurred by provocative and high-profile acts of civil disobedience. However, now that communities no longer must "convince" the mainstream to pay attention to a new epidemic, our approach has been able to evolve. We have made great strides in our understanding of the social and biologic causes of HIV; however, we have not made similar strides in addressing HIV-related disparities over the past few decades [27, 31, 61–63]. Within the USA we have become fairly effective in developing, implementing, and evaluating individual- and group-level interventions including those described in the CDC's *Compendium of Evidence-based HIV Behavioral Interventions* (www.cdc.gov/hiv/topics/research/prs/compendium-evidence-based-interventions.htm). However, we now must move the science of health promotion and disease prevention forward by better understanding how policy initiatives can positively affect health and how we can best blend policy initiatives with community engagement including approaches such as CBPR. Representatives from local communities, community-based organizations, and academic and government institutions must work together to consider how we can move our knowledge, perspectives, experiences, and insights into policy initiatives that have the potential to reduce and eliminate the existing (and in some cases growing) profound HIV-related disparities and inequities.

Table 8.2 A health-related and community-engaged framework for policy change

Step	Explanation and/or examples
Existence of an authentic partnership	Comprised of trust and a history of successfully working together, using core values and principles of CBPR
Examining and quantifying community health needs and priorities	Blending the lived experiences of community members with qualitative and quantitative (including epidemiologic) data
Selecting primary health priority to focus efforts	Narrowing focus to one (usually) health priority
Identifying influential actors and institutions	Including those potentially supportive and those not supportive; however, it may not be obvious because it is not always clear whom HIV has touched and how
Analyzing the policy environment	Understanding the history and context of policy change related to the current initiative; conducting a power analysis
Identifying options and targets for policy change	Asking and thoroughly discussing/debating the questions: *what is important and what is changeable*
Setting goals	Determining what policy initiative to engage in, e.g., establishing federal HIV-related priorities; changing needle-exchange policies; revising HIV-prevention funding allocation; and institutionalizing inclusion of HIV prevention within a faith setting
Recognizing, assessing, and preparing for barriers	Preparing for the worst while expecting the best
Developing resources and strategies	Working with stakeholders, gathering and organizing support, and defining activities; using a step-by-step approach that includes short-term objectives to reach long-term policy goal; and harnessing media to focus on promoting health and well-being, correcting an injustice, and saving money
Taking action to promote policy change	Implementing strategies designed to reach objectives
Revisiting and reassessing	Ensuring that data, strategies, and policy objectives and goals remained aligned
Supporting policy implementation and enforcement	Appreciating those who worked behind the scenes and those who were in the spotlight; and rallying behind those who are responsible for enforcement
Evaluating the impact of the policy and disseminating findings	Evaluating the impact and intended and unintended consequences of policy and health outcomes and disseminating process and outcome findings within the community

Evidence suggests that CBPR aligns well with advocacy efforts; we have a foundation. Linking CBPR to policy change has been used to address a broad array of issues. Furthermore, it is clear that community engagement has been integral to the development and implementation of important HIV-related policies; however, these efforts have not been linked with policy intervention research or evaluation. Further research is warranted.

For HIV-related policy initiatives, likely challenges that face partnerships are the attitudes, opinions, and fears still associated with HIV, such as negative attitudes toward homosexuality, needle exchange, drug treatment, comprehensive sexual health education in schools, and condom distribution, as examples. Engaging potential opposition has been found to be an effective strategy for facilitating policy change. For example, identifying potential allies (and gaining understanding of opposition) has been a crucial tactic to gain support for new policies within churches and also beyond the church walls, as church members can generate public opinion against or for advocacy efforts [55].

Furthermore, there are many issues unique to women and men of color; heterosexual women and men; gay and bisexual men, MSM, and transgender persons; and injecting drug users that must be addressed, and policies may be critical in the fight. For example, fear associated with accessing educational and health-related services; the lack of bilingual, bicultural services, particularly in the resource-poor southeastern USA; poverty and harsh working conditions; and institutional racism contribute to increased HIV exposure and transmission among Latinos. Similarly, social networks that have higher rates of HIV, poverty, lack of access to appropriate services, high incarceration rates, and residential segregation that limit opportunities and access to education and prevention efforts contribute to increased HIV exposure and transmission among African-American/blacks. In all of these examples, the use of policy cannot be ignored or understated, and CBPR will be useful in bringing attention to and developing, implementing, and evaluating strategies to address these issues and reduce HIV-related health disparities.

We end by suggesting that academic researchers have focused much of their work on the early stages of policy change, assuming that community and organizational partners will take the torch to the next level. However, congruent to a CBPR approach, like community members, academic researchers should be involved throughout the process—from beginning to end—in order to fully understand the science and reach the public health potential of policy change.

References

1. Callan M, Turner DA. History of the people with AIDS self-empowerment movement. The body [Internet]. 1997. http://www.thebody.com/content/art31074.html. Accessed Feb 28, 2013.
2. Brindis CD. A public health success: understanding policy changes related to teen sexual activity and pregnancy. Annu Rev Public Health. 2006;27:277–95.
3. Mello MM, Wood J, Burris S, Wagenaar AC, Ibrahim JK, Swanson JW. Critical opportunities for public health law: a call for action. Am J Public Health. 2013;103(11):1979–88.
4. McDermott RJ, Glover ED, Glover PN. Merging health behavior and policy to improve population health—a commentary. Health Behav Policy Rev. 2014;1(3–5).

5. Brownson RC, Seiler R, Eyler AA. Measuring the impact of public health policy. Prev Chronic Dis. 2010;7(4):A77.
6. Frieden TR. A framework for public health action: the health impact pyramid. Am J Public Health. 2010;100(4):590–5.
7. Auvert B, Taljaard D, Rech D, Lissouba P, Singh B, Bouscaillou J, et al. Association of the ANRS-12126 male circumcision project with HIV levels among men in a South African township: evaluation of effectiveness using cross-sectional surveys. PLoS Med. 2013;10(9):e1001509.
8. Rhodes SD, Wilkin AM, Abraham C, Backmann LH. Chronic infectious disease management interventions. In: Riekert KA, Ockene JK, Pbert L, editors. The handbook of behavior change. 4th ed. New York: Springer; 2014. p. 331–45.
9. Halkitis PN. Obama, marriage equality, and the health of gay men. Am J Public Health. 2012;102(9):1628–9.
10. Francis AM, Mialon HM. Tolerance and HIV. J Health Econ. 2010;29(2):250–67.
11. Exworthy M. Policy to tackle the social determinants of health: using conceptual models to understand the policy process. Health Policy Plan. 2008;23(5):318–27.
12. Kingdon JW. Agendas, alternatives, and public policies. 2nd ed. New York: Pearson; 2010.
13. Blackwell AG, Thompson M, Freudenberg N, Ayers J, Schrantz D, Minkler M. Using community organizing and community building to influence public policy. In: Minkler M, editor. Community organizing and community building for health and welfare. 3rd ed. New Brunswick: Rutgers; 2012. p. 371–85.
14. Brownson RC, Newschaffer CJ, Ali-Abarghoui F. Policy research for disease prevention: challenges and practical recommendations. Am J Public Health. 1997;87(5):735–9.
15. Christoffel KK. Public health advocacy: process and product. Am J Public Health. 2000;90(5):722–6.
16. Minkler M, Rubin V, Wallerstein N. Community-based participatory research: a strategy for building healthy communities and promoting health through policy change: PolicyLink. 2012. http://www.policylink.org/atf/cf/%7B97C6D565-BB43-406D-A6D5-ECA3BBF35AF0%7D/CBPR.pdf. Accessed Jan 2013.
17. Institute of Medicine. Unequal treatment: confronting racial and ethnic disparities in health care. Washington, DC: National Academy Press; 2003.
18. Vasquez VB, Minkler M, Shepard P. Promoting environmental health policy through community based participatory research: a case study from Harlem, New York. J Urban Health. 2006;83(1):101–10.
19. Sipton P. AIDS and the policy struggle in the United States. Washington, DC: Georgetown University Press; 2002.
20. Beyrer C, Sullivan P, Sanchez J, Baral SD, Collins C, Wirtz AL, et al. The global HIV epidemics in MSM: time to act. AIDS. 2013.
21. Minkler M. Linking science and policy through community-based participatory research to study and address health disparities. Am J Public Health. 2010;100(Suppl 1):81–7.
22. Steckler A, Dawson L. The role of health education in public policy development. Health Educ Q. 1982;9(4):275–92.
23. Roe KM, Berenstein C, Goette C, Roe K. Community building through empowerment: a case study of HIV prevention community planning. In: Minkler M, editor. Community organizing and community building for health. New Brunswick: Rutgers University Press; 2002. p. 308–22.
24. Clark NM, Lachance L, Doctor LJ, Gilmore L, Kelly C, Krieger J, et al. Policy and system change and community coalitions: outcomes from allies against asthma. Am J Public Health. 2010;100(5):904–12.
25. Alinsky S. Rules for radicals. New York: Random House; 1971.
26. Israel BA, Schulz AJ, Parker EA, Becker AB. Review of community-based research: assessing partnership approaches to improve public health. Annu Rev Public Health. 1998;19:173–202.
27. Rhodes SD. Demonstrated effectiveness and potential of CBPR for preventing HIV in Latino populations. In: Organista KC, editor. HIV prevention with Latinos: theory, research, and practice. New York: Oxford; 2012. p. 83–102.

28. Rhodes SD. Community-based participatory research. In Blessing JD, Forister. JG, editors. Introduction to research and medical literature for health professionals. 3rd ed. Burlington: Jones & Bartlett; 2013. p. 167–87.

29. Viswanathan M, Eng E, Ammerman A, Gartlehner G, Lohr KN, Griffith D, et al. Community-based participatory research: assessing the evidence. Evidence report/technology assessment. Rockville, MD: Agency for Healthcare Research and Quality, 2004 July. Report No.: 99.

30. Rhodes SD, Hergenrather KC, Vissman AT, Stowers J, Davis AB, Hannah A, et al. Boys must be men, and men must have sex with women: a qualitative CBPR study to explore sexual risk among African American, Latino, and white gay men and MSM. Am J Mens Health. 2011;5(2):140–51.

31. Rhodes SD, Malow RM, Jolly C. Community-based participatory research: a new and not-so-new approach to HIV/AIDS prevention, care, and treatment. AIDS Educ Prev. 2010;22(3):173–83.

32. Ogusky J, Tenner A. Advocating for schools to provide effective HIV and sexuality education: a case study in how social service organizations working in coalition can (and should) affect sustained policy change. Health Promot Pract. 2010;11(3 Suppl):34–41.

33. Minkler M, Vásquez VB, Chang C, Miller J, Rubin V, Blackwell AG, et al. Promoting healthy public policy through community-based participatory research: ten case studies. Oakland: PolicyLink; 2009.

34. van Olphen J, Freudenberg N, Galea S, Palermo AG, Ritas C. Advocating policies to promote community reintegration of drug users leaving jail: A case study of first steps in a policy change campaign guided by community based participatory research. In: Minkler M, Wallerstein N, editors. Community-based participatory research for health. San Francisco: Jossey-Bass; 2003. p. 371–89.

35. Petersen DM, Minkler M, Vasquez VB, Kegler MC, Malcoe LH, Whitecrow S. Using community-based participatory research to shape policy and prevent lead exposure among Native American children. Progress in community health partnerships: research, education, and action. 2007;1(3):249–56.

36. Vasquez VB, Lanza D, Hennessey-Lavery S, Facente S, Halpin HA, Minkler M. Addressing food security through public policy action in a community-based participatory research partnership. Health Promot Pract. 2007;8(4):342–9.

37. Wing S, Horton RA, Muhammad N, Grant GR, Tajik M, Thu K. Integrating epidemiology, education, and organizing for environmental justice: community health effects of industrial hog operations. Am J Public Health. 2008;98(8):1390–7.

38. Kegler MC, Malcoe LH. Results from a lay health advisor intervention to prevent lead poisoning among rural Native American children. Am J Public Health. 2004;94(10):1730–5.

39. Wilson N, Minkler M, Dasho S, Wallerstein N, Martin AC. Getting to social action: the Youth Empowerment Strategies (YES!) project. Health Promot Pract. 2008;9(4):395–403.

40. Morello-Frosch R, Pastor M, Sadd JL, Porras C, Prichard M. Citizens, science, and data Judo: Leveraging community-based participatory research to build a regional collaborative for environmental justice in Southern California. In: Israel BA, Eng E, Shultz A, Parker E, editors. Methods for conducting community-based participatory research in public health. San Francisco: Jossey-Bass; 2005. p. 371–92.

41. Hergenrather KC, Rhodes SD, Cowan CA, Bardhoshi G, Pula S. Photovoice as community-based participatory research: a qualitative review. Am J Health Behav. 2009;33(6):686–98.

42. Haque N, Eng B. Tackling inequity through a Photovoice project on the social determinants of health: translating photovoice evidence to community action. Glob Health Promot. 2011;18(1):16–9.

43. Wang C, Cash JL, Powers LS. Who knows the streets as well as the homeless? Promoting personal and community action through photovoice. Health Promot Pract. 2000;1(1):81–9.

44. Hergenrather KC, Rhodes SD, Clark G. Windows to work: exploring employment-seeking behaviors of persons with HIV/AIDS through photovoice. AIDS Educ Prev. 2006;18(3):243–58.

45. Tsui E, Cho M, Freudenberg N. Methods for community-based participatory policy work to improve food environments in New York city. In: Israel BA, Eng E, Schulz AJ, Parker

EA, editors. Methods for community-based participatory research for Health. San Francisco: Jossey-Bass; 2013. p. 517–45.

46. Cashman SB, Adeky S, Allen A, Corburn J, Israel BA, Montaño J, et al. Analyzing and interpreting data with communities. In: Minkler M, Wallerstein N, editors. Community-based participatory research for health: from process to outcomes. 2nd ed. San Francisco: Jossey-Bass; 2008. p. 285–302.

47. Cashman SB, Adeky S, Allen AJ, Corburn J, Israel BA, Montaño J, et al. The power and the promise: working with communities to analyze data, interpret findings, and get to outcomes. Am J Public Health. 2008;98(8):1407–17.

48. Streng JM, Rhodes SD, Ayala GX, Eng E, Arceo R, Phipps S. Realidad Latina: Latino adolescents, their school, and a university use photovoice to examine and address the influence of immigration. J Interprof Care. 2004;18(4):403–15.

49. Rhodes SD, Hergenrather KC, Wilkin AM, Jolly C. Visions and voices: indigent persons living with HIV in the southern United States use photovoice to create knowledge, develop partnerships, and take action. Health Promot Pract. 2008;9(2):159–69.

50. Wang CC, Morrel-Samuels S, Hutchison PM, Bell L, Pestronk RM. Flint Photovoice: community building among youths, adults, and policymakers. Am J Public Health. 2004;94(6):911–3.

51. Weitzer R. The mythology of prostitution: Advocacy research and public policy. Sex Res Soc Policy. 2010;7:15–29.

52. Freudenberg N, Tsui E. Evidence, power and policy change in community-based participatory research. Am J Public Health. 2013;104:11–4.

53. Vernick JS. Lobbying and advocacy for the public's health: what are the limits for nonprofit organizations? Am J Public Health. 1999;89(9):1425–9.

54. Israel BA, Krieger J, Vlahov D, Ciske S, Foley M, Fortin P, et al. Challenges and facilitating factors in sustaining community-based participatory research partnerships: lessons learned from the Detroit, New York city and Seattle Urban Research Centers. J Urban Health. 2006;83(6):1022–40.

55. Lightfoot AF, Woods BA, Jackson M, Riggins L, Krieger K, Brodie K, et al. "In my house": laying the foundation for youth HIV prevention in the Black church. Progress in community health partnerships: research, education, and action. 2012;6(4):451–6.

56. Royster MO, Richmond A, Eng E, Margolis L. Hey brother, how's your health?: A focus group analysis of the health and health-related concerns of African American men in a southern city in the United States. Men and Masculinities. 2006;8:389–404.

57. Akers AY, Youmans S, Lloyd SW, Smith DM, Banks B, Blumenthal C, et al. Views of young, rural African Americans of the role of community social institutions in HIV prevention. J Health Care Poor Underserved. 2010;21(2 Suppl):1–12.

58. Yonas M, Aronson R, Coad N, Eng E, RPetteway R, Schaal J, et al. Infrastructure for equitable decision making in research. In: Israel BA, Eng E, Schulz AJ, Parker EA, editors. Methods for community-based participatory research for health. San Francisco: Jossey-Bass; 2013. p. 97–131.

59. Corbie-Smith G, Goldmon M, Isler MR, Washington C, Ammerman A, Green M, et al. Partnerships in health disparities research and the roles of pastors of black churches: potential conflict, synergy, and expectations. J Natl Med Assoc. 2010;102(9):823–31.

60. Woods-Jaeger BA, Sparks A, Turner K, Griffith T, Jackson M, Lightfoot AF. Exploring the social and community context of African American adolescents' HIV vulnerability. Qual Health Res. 2013;23(11):1541–50.

61. Holtgrave D, Hall HI, Rhodes PH, Wolitski R. Updated annual HIV transmission rates in the United States, 1977–2006. J Acquir Immune Defic Syndr. 2009;50(2):236–8.

62. An Q, Prejean J, Hall HI. Racial disparity in U.S. diagnoses of acquired immune deficiency syndrome, 2000–2009. Am J Prev Med. 2012;43(5):461–6.

63. Prejean J, Tang T, Hall HI. HIV diagnoses and prevalence in the southern region of the United States, 2007–2010. J Community Health. 2013;38(3):414–26.

Chapter 9
Communities and Technology: Enhancements in HIV-Prevention Research and Practice Among Adolescents and Young Adults

Sheana Bull, Tarik Walker and Deb Levine

What are Virtual Communities?

Howard Rheingold coined the term "virtual communities" in a 1993 book identifying opportunities for individuals to remain connected in an increasingly digitized world [1]. His suggestion was that geography is not a necessary element for community, but relationships and desire for connection are fundamental for community. A virtual community is a social network of individuals who interact through social media. These individuals are not bound by geography; rather, they usually share an interest or reason to communicate. Virtual communities resemble other types of communities because members provide one another information, friendship, and other types of social support.

Virtual communities take multiple forms that have evolved rapidly over the past two decades. Given ongoing advances in technology, these communities and the methods they use to interact will continue to evolve rapidly. With this ongoing development and evolution, virtual communities have become more common and their reach has expanded; they have become more universally accepted and, in many cases, integrated into nonvirtual communities. Virtual communities include social networks in which individuals can interact with one another online through sites such as Facebook, MySpace, Ning, FourSquare, and Tumblr. Additionally, virtual

S. Bull (✉)
Department of Community and Behavioral Health, Colorado School of Public Health,
University of Colorado Denver, 13001 E. 17th Place, B119, Bldg 500,
Room E3345A, Aurora, CO 80045, USA
e-mail: Sheana.Bull@ucdenver.edu

T. Walker
Department of Family Medicine and Colorado Area Health Education Center,
University of Colorado, Education II South, Room 5108, Aurora, CO 80045, USA
e-mail: tarik.walker@ucdenver.edu

D. Levine
Youth Tech Health (YTH), 409 13th Street, 14th Floor, Oakland,
CA 94612-2607, USA
e-mail: deb@yth.org

S. D. Rhodes (ed.), *Innovations in HIV Prevention Research and Practice through Community Engagement*, DOI 10.1007/978-1-4939-0900-1_9,
© Springer Science+Business Media New York 2014

communities have expanded to the microblogging environment through sites such as Twitter, where users can share brief communications through posts of messages of 140 characters, and Instagram, where users can share photographs and videos.

Many examples exist that underscore the popularity and desire for individuals to connect using social media around a variety of topics, including health. Early examples include online social support groups that helped women address issues related to a breast cancer diagnosis [2] and assisted individuals in managing diabetes [3]. Similarly, existing online chat rooms designed to facilitate social and sexual networking among men who have sex with men (MSM) have been used to facilitate HIV prevention, specifically through moderated question-and-answer sessions designed for educational purposes [4–6]. Another type of online community is a virtual world such as Second Life, where users create avatars and have them interact in multiplayer simulations of various scenarios [7]. An avatar is usually a two- or three-dimensional graphic representation of an Internet user's online character [8–11].

Virtual communities offer the advantage of instant exchange of information, which is not always possible in geographically focused communities. However, debates exist over the potential benefits or harms related to participation in virtual communities. Although virtual communities can share substantive support and work effectively across time, space, and geographic boundaries [4, 12, 13], there are concerns about so-called virtual isolation that can lead to depression or other negative health outcomes [14]; an alteration of personalities online that can lead to misrepresentation [15]; and a potential disintegration of socially appropriate behaviors [16].

Who are Members of Virtual Communities?

Nevertheless, there is overwhelming evidence that virtual communities are popular particularly among adolescents and young adults. In fact, social media use is nearly ubiquitous among adolescents and young adults in the USA. As of May 2012, almost 80 % of adolescents and young adults who are online use a social network website, and 81 % of youth (12–17-years old) use some sort of social media at least once a month. Nearly all (98 %) of 18–24-years-old adolescents and young adults who are online use social media each month, and 81 % of them use social networking sites for e-mail access, online chat, and news [17, 18]. By contrast, older adults have not kept pace with this use; about 40 % of adults 30-years old and over use social media.

Although social media sites regularly compete for users, sites where adolescents and young adults currently spend the greatest time include Facebook, Twitter, LinkedIn, MySpace, and Google+. Experian Hitwise (http://www.experian.com/hitwise/), a resource in digital marketing intelligence, reports that visits to Facebook now account for more than 65 % of all visits to social networking and forums-classified websites in the USA. Over 70 % of teenage youth actively maintain a Facebook profile. Nearly two-thirds (59 %) of youth 13–19-years old have only one social media account, which is Facebook for 89 % of them. Among those who have more than one social media account, 99 % report having a profile on Facebook, compared with 29 % who report using Twitter [7]. Nearly three-quarters (73 %) of adolescents and young adults 18–34-years old who are online visit Facebook monthly, the highest of any adult age group [19].

Most adolescents and young adults use social media to stay connected with their friends, post and share photographs, comment on one another's posts and photographs, and share links within their personal networks [20–22]. Because of the broad and frequent use of social media by certain demographic groups, including adolescents and young adults, many larger organizations use social media as promotion platforms. Social media does much more than connect individuals within virtual communities; social media provides companies, brands, and causes a personalized way to connect with and engage members of virtual communities; at the same time, it provides users with a personalized way to connect with and engage companies, brands, and causes. Thus, social media can be a complex communication channel.

How Can We Capitalize on the Popularity of Virtual Communities and Online Social Media for HIV Prevention?

The latest estimates from the Centers for Disease Control and Prevention (CDC) indicate that approximately 56,300 Americans become infected with HIV annually, and about 16,000 persons with AIDS died in 2008 [23]. A significant proportion of HIV and other sexually transmitted infections (STIs) in the USA occur in adolescents and young adults. Between 2006 and 2009, estimated rates of HIV infection increased 25 % among youth 15–19-years old, and 31 % among youth 20–24-years old; these statistics are disheartening, given that our toolkit for prevention has improved considerably over the course of the HIV epidemic. We know more about health behavior and have made considerable advances in behavioral theory; we have reduced infection rates among some populations, including some subgroups of racial/ethnicity minorities and among injection-drug users, as examples.

However, some subgroups of adolescents and young adults are disproportionately affected by HIV and STIs. For example, African-American/black adolescents represent approximately 17 % of all adolescents, yet they account for about 72 % of HIV infections. Between 2006 and 2009, the rate of new infections among African-American/black young adults increased by 35 %. This rate of new infections was more than five times the rate for Hispanics/Latino young adults and nearly 23 times the rate for white young adults.

As with HIV, there also are profound disparities in the rates of other STIs among racial/ethnic minority adolescents and young adults. In 2007, for example, the rates of gonorrhea among African-American/black females 15–19-years old was 14.7 times greater than those for white females in the same age-group, and the rate for African-American/black males 15–19-years old was 38.7 times higher than that for white males in the same age-group.

Researchers and practitioners have shown that using the Internet to deliver prevention messages can have significant effects on behaviors that reduce HIV risk [6, 13, 21, 24–26] and increase adherence to HIV medication [27–29]. Given the remarkable and unprecedented increase in the number and types of virtual communities and the use of social media in the past decade, it is intriguing, and in fact crucial, to think of ways to capitalize on social media to facilitate HIV prevention. In this section, we discuss our approach to reduce HIV risk among adolescents and young adults through the use of Facebook, clearly one of the most popular and established social networking sites.

Research on Harnessing Social Media to Prevent HIV

The FaceSpace Project was among the first examples of health promotion delivered using social media. This innovative pilot intervention was implemented and evaluated in 2009 and 2010. The project included the delivery of sexual health promotion via social networking sites to key groups at increased risk—adolescents and young adults 16–29-years old and subsequently MSM—through an intervention that was separately branded as Queer As F**K. The interventions used fictional characters to interact and post content (primarily videos known as webisodes) on various social networking sites, with sexual health promotion messages embedded within some of these postings.

Results from both interventions have been published [26, 30–32]; briefly, the pilot of The FaceSpace Project resulted in significant increases in sexual health knowledge among participants between baseline and follow-up using a pretest-posttest design ($p < 0.01$). Thirty-three percent of all participants reported that the project prompted them to discuss or seek more information about HIV and STIs, 22 % reported the project made them more conscious about safer sex practices, and 35 % reported the project led them to seek advice from a health professional or get an HIV and/or STI test [31].

A mixed-methods process evaluation of Queer As F**K indicated that the 32 webisodes that were posted on the project's Facebook and YouTube pages attracted more than 30,000 views; ranging from 124–3,092 views per individual episode. By April 2011, the Queer As F**K Facebook page had 2,929 fans, who were predominantly male. Interview and focus group participants supported the balance of education and entertainment and reported that the narrative soap opera format successfully delivered sexual health messages in an engaging, informative, and accessible manner that encouraged online peer discussion of sexual health and promoted community engagement [32].

Other researchers have similarly shown the potential viability and impact of using social media as an intervention mode. In a pilot study, youth 18–20-years old who disclosed engaging in risky behaviors on their MySpace profile were sent e-mail messages about the potential for harm in doing so; the intervention led to a substantial reduction in mention of sexual behavior and in the removal of public access to profiles [25].

Several other pilot and larger scale studies using the Internet for HIV prevention have produced either evidence of positive effects or promising findings (Table 9.1). These initiatives have reached diverse populations and settings through a variety of technology-based approaches, including the Internet [33], social media [21], chat rooms [4–6], cell phone/text messaging [34–36], and unique websites [37, 38], as well as hybrid interventions [39–42]. Populations reached by these interventions include MSM from diverse racial groups and geographic settings; young adults; and adolescents, including African-American/black male adolescents and homeless adolescents. Although this book focuses on innovations in engagement within the USA, we note an important intervention that was developed, implemented, and evaluated in Mbarara, Uganda [43, 44]. This intervention is particularly relevant, given that the intervention delayed sexual initiation among high-school students. Delaying sexual initiation among adolescents is an important goal, particularly with the broad use of the Internet among preadolescents and adolescents.

Although the potential of social media continues to be advocated within public health and HIV prevention specifically, evaluation of the variety of strategies that can be used is limited; much research is needed. As social media encourages relationships between individuals and content, and the organizations that provide that content, measuring the quality of these relationships is key to quantifying success regarding health behavior change. A deeper understanding and analysis of the demographics of the visitors, length of time spent on the site, referral sources, and measurement of the overall quality of interactions and experiences are necessary. Community engagement provides a vehicle to identify and develop health communication approaches and messages that are meaningful for a target audience.

Furthermore, the success of social media to change knowledge, attitudes, and behaviors depends on our ability to create experiences that raise awareness; educate and inform; earn participant and audience loyalty; and, ideally, connect online experiences with offline behavior change. As a result, in addition to website hits and number of so-called friends (connections within a social network), measures of engagement of virtual community members include the number of times a visitor returns to a website, the number of comments on a blog, and the number of retweets on Twitter (i.e., the number of times a tweet [text message] is forwarded from a recipient to someone else). These examples represent some of many measures of engagement; given the rapidly evolving technology and the ongoing development of social media outlets, there is no exhaustive list of ways to conceptualize engagement.

Just/Us Facebook Page Intervention

Given that Facebook is one of the most popular social networking sites online, we sought to uncover specific strategies to engage adolescents and young adults effectively through this social media site. We focused on adolescents and young adults both because of their prolific use of social media and because of their elevated risk for HIV and other STIs.

Table 9.1 Selected evidence-based and promising technology-based HIV-prevention initiatives. (This list is not exhaustive and studies were selected to represent the variety of technology-based approaches to reach diverse populations)

Authors (reference)	Program name and brief description	Study design	Key findings
Bowen et al. [33]	Wyoming Rural AIDS Prevention Project (WRAPP), an Internet-based HIV prevention initiative for rural white MSM	Randomized controlled trial	The Internet provides a useful and low-cost approach to recruit and assess rural white MSM and to reduce their sexual risks for HIV
Bull et al. [21]	Just/Us, a social media HIV-prevention intervention for adolescents and young adults	Randomized controlled trial	Facebook can be an effective tool to promote and sustain condom use among adolescents and young adults at least in the short-term
Rosser et al. [67, 68]	MiNTs (Men's Internet Study), an Internet-based HIV-prevention program for MSM	Randomized controlled trial	Internet-based HIV-prevention research is possible even with geographically dispersed minority populations. Efficiency appears to be a primary risk associated with meeting partners online
Bull et al. [69, 70]	Youthnet, an Internet-based HIV-prevention initiative for adolescents	Randomized controlled trial with two samples: online and clinic	In the Internet sample, participants exposed to the Internet-based intervention had slight increases in condom norms. There were no intervention effects in the clinic sample
Noar et al. [71]	Systematic review and meta-analysis of existing published and unpublished studies testing computer-based interventions		Statistically significant effect sizes were found for increased condom use, decreased number of partners, and decreased incident STIs. Computer technology-based HIV-prevention interventions have similar efficacy to more traditional human-delivered interventions and are less expensive to deliver, intervention content is easy to customize, and dissemination is flexible

Table 9.1 (continued)

Authors (reference)	Program name and brief description	Study design	Key findings
Fortune et al. [34, 35]	411 for Safe Text, a cell-phone text messaging HIV-prevention intervention for young African-American/black male adolescents	Pilot to test the feasibility of recruiting and enrolling participants 16–20-years old in a text message initiative	Delivering HIV-prevention messages through cell-phone text messages is feasible and acceptable for American/black male adolescents
Rhodes et al. [6]	CyBER/testing, a chat room-based intervention designed to increase HIV testing among online MSM	A quasi-experimental, single-group pilot study design, using cross-sectional pretest and posttest data	Results included increased self-reported HIV testing among "chatters" overall; chatters who reported having both male and female sexual partners concurrently had nearly 6 times the odds of reporting HIV testing at posttest. Internet-based HIV-testing interventions may increase testing among MSM who may be difficult to reach in traditional physical spaces
Levine et al. [36]	SEXINFO, a text messaging intervention in which users text keywords to a central program for STI-prevention information	Pilot; included focus groups to assess feasibility and banner ads for young adults 18–24-years old	Those who saw the campaign were more likely to be concerned about STIs; approximately 10 % sent a text message to the SEXINFO service. Participants reported that the use of cell phones and text messaging caught their attention
Hightow-Weidman et al. [37, 38]	HealthMpowerment.org, a social media site for young African-American/black MSM	Pilot	A targeted social media site is acceptable to African-American/black MSM and feasible to use for delivering HIV-prevention information

Table 9.1 (continued)

Authors (reference)	Program name and brief description	Study design	Key findings
Rice et al. [39–41]	Social network analysis to examine the acceptability of a youth-led, hybrid face-to-face and online social networking HIV-prevention program for homeless adolescents	Pilot intervention used social identity theory to guide the augmentation of prosocial identities among homeless adolescents	Online adolescents were among the most central in their social networks. Younger adolescents were disproportionately connected to those like themselves. The program appears highly acceptable to homeless adolescents
Young et al. [42]	Evaluation of associations between online social networking and sexual health behaviors among homeless adolescents in Los Angeles	Analysis of survey data gathered from 201 homeless adolescents	Results suggest that online social networks usage can be associated with both potential increases and decreases in HIV/STI risk behaviors in homeless adolescents and that using online social networks for partner seeking (compared with not using the networks for seeking partners) can be associated with an increase sexual risk behaviors. Results also suggest that online social network usage is associated with increased knowledge and HIV/STI-prevention behaviors among homeless adolescents
Ybarra et al. [43, 44]	CyberSenga, a 6-session HIV-prevention initiative delivered via the Internet for high school students in Mbarara, Uganda	Randomized controlled trial	Students exposed to CyberSenga were more likely to delay initiation of sex; however, there were no effects on condom use

MSM men who have sex with men, *STI* sexually transmitted infection

Methods

The overarching goal of our research was to determine whether adolescents and young adults exposed to content on the Just/Us Facebook page, which focused on sexual health promotion and the prevention of HIV and STI exposure and transmission, would be more likely to adopt healthy sexual behaviors compared with those who were not exposed to the Just/Us Facebook page and instead only viewed other Facebook pages with other types of content. We used multiple unique approaches to engage racial/ethnic minority adolescents and young adults 16–24-years old. All procedures were approved by institutional review boards at the University of Colorado School of Public Health, Columbia Mailman School of Public Health, and Rutgers University.

Our intended audience was primarily African-American/black and Latino adolescents and young adults because of the disproportionate burden of HIV and STIs within these populations. We engaged these adolescents and young adults to contribute to the development of a Facebook page related to sexual health (Phase 1), to facilitate enrollment of social networks of adolescents as participants in a research study (Phase 2), and to interact with content on the study's Facebook page (Phase 3).

Phase 1 Adolescents and young people were approached online to facilitate development of site content. We conducted synchronous and asynchronous focus groups on MySpace. Participants offered reactions to content ideas, presentation, and wording for the site. Detailed methods for data collection and results from this engagement effort have been published elsewhere [45]. In brief, participants described the social media environment as one in which they engaged in both public and private sharing—similar to hanging out at the mall and keeping a diary. They used the medium to keep in touch with their real-world friends and to share about themselves. On their own pages, they posted links to online content and discussions about content they identified with. They also reported that they enjoyed taking simple online polls and quizzes and seeing the results.

We used feedback from this first phase to develop our Facebook content. A key outcome of this formative work was the naming of our Facebook page. Adolescents wanted a virtual space where they could meet online without "much" adult interference. They also wanted the site to focus on the social justice and human rights aspects of reproductive health (i.e., reproductive justice). To this end, we named our Facebook page Just/Us, a play on words to indicate a space "just for us" (adolescents) and "social justice."

Phase 2 We designed a cluster randomized controlled trial. Inclusion criteria for participation in the trial included an age of 16–24-years old, a Facebook account and informed consent. As in Phase 1, we focused on African-American/black and Latino adolescents and young adults, although no one was excluded from participation because of their race/ethnicity. To recruit participants into the study, we employed a modified respondent driven sampling (RDS) approach. RDS is a systematic approach to identify and recruit members of communities and populations that some community outsiders (e.g., researchers, providers, and practitioners) may label as hard-to-reach. It is not difficult for members of these communities and populations to reach one another; clearly, members of virtual communities are likely to be able to reach one another. Thus, RDS relies on peer-to-peer referrals; an initial "seed" or index participant who is recruited, screened, found eligible, consented, and enrolled identifies and recruits others within his or her social network to participate [46–48]. Community settings were chosen as ideal recruitment sites with anticipation of encountering racial/ethnic minority adolescents and young adults. These settings included community colleges, malls, community-based organizations, and community and street fairs and festivals. We also recruited participants from online sites and through newspaper advertising.

In accordance with RDS methods, we further engaged adolescents and young adults during this phase by asking them to identify and recruit up to three friends in their Facebook network to participate. We conducted three waves of RDS recruitment; this chain-referral process continued until the desired a priori sample size was obtained. Participants received a $ 5 gift card per person recruited for up to three people (possible total of $ 15) for their recruitment effort. All eligible participants, including seeds and all those referred through their social networks, completed informed consent and a baseline behavioral survey of sexual risk via an online tool generated and delivered through Zoomerang, a commercial online survey software program that allows users to easily create and publish surveys online. Zoomerang served as a third-party host for our data, and its hosting agreements comply with our institutional review board requirements related to privacy and data security [49].

All participants were sent a link via e-mail on their Facebook news feed page that would take them to the informed consent and online survey, which they could self-administer on their own computer. The survey took approximately 15 min to complete and included several questions about Facebook use and engagement with our intervention content. Participants were given a $ 15 gift card for completion of the baseline survey. More specific details on how we conducted recruitment and on results from the recruitment have been published elsewhere [21].

After participants enrolled, our intention was to use Facebook in an organic and dynamic manner. This meant we could not simply post static information onto our Just/Us Facebook page that would then be pushed out through a rich site summary feed, commonly known as an RSS feed, to participants' Facebook news feed pages. RSS includes a variety of web-feed formats used to publish in a standardized format online, for example, blogs, news headlines, audio, and video. Instead, we had to post information that addressed topics we believed were important in a way that would encourage response and interaction from participants.

Phase 3 We posted initial content in the form of polls and RSS feeds, on sexual health topics over an 8-week period. Adolescent and young adult moderators were hired and trained to serve as the "face" of Just/Us and facilitate online engagement with the content. Given administrative access to the Just/Us Facebook page, they posted content, engaged participants, encouraged participants to respond with their own postings, and posted their reactions to posted content. These moderators were carefully trained in order to ensure that they posted correct and consistent information. We also established norms for posting and responding to posts on the Just/Us Facebook page.

The content of the Just/Us Facebook page was intended to address specific theoretical constructs and took the form of polls, RSS feed, links, etc. (Table 92). The content identified in Table 9.2 is not exhaustive and is intended to provide insight into the intervention only. Furthermore, participants in our formative research indicated that it was important for the Just/Us Facebook page to be dynamic and regularly updated. We were flexible and agile, posting news items and relevant stories that emerged from the popular media and allowing for participants to engage with the content in a very organic manner and at their own pace. We thought this approach was essential both to adhere to expectations that the Just/Us Facebook page not differ in its operation from other pages on Facebook and also to meet participant expectations that the content be both authentic and up-to-date.

The moderators were encouraged to respond to content daily, and they often posted multiple times each day. This process differs substantially from traditional health promotion programs, which are generally delivered in group or classroom settings at specific times of the day during given days of the week. Each time a moderator posted something on the Just/Us Facebook page, it would automatically be pushed through an RSS feed to participants. All intervention-group participants were required to "like" the Just/Us Facebook page. Thus, they could see all Just/Us Facebook intervention content simply by going to their own Facebook page or their news feed page. If they wanted to, they could click on the RSS feed and go directly to the Just/Us Facebook page, where they could view and engage in greater depth with any of the content over the course of the project (Fig. 9.1).

Results

Of the 36 adolescents who participated in the Phase 1 focus groups, 58 % were female and 60 % were white, although we had participation from Latinos (14 %) and African-Americans/blacks (8 %). Participants were recruited using multiple strategies. Some were recruited from chat room invitations that were sent to 2,354 chatters who subsequently joined a forum created on MySpace. The forum generated about 738 friends, and an initial focus group comprising seven participants was held as a synchronous chat; we held subsequent discussions asynchronously, obtaining input from an additional 29 participants. We learned through this phase that participants take the asynchronous nature of social media seriously and appreciate the ability to exert control over when and where they access information and interact online [12].

For Phase 2, in which we focused on engagement with the content of the intervention, we enrolled 636 participants in the control condition and 942 in the intervention condition. Overall, more than half of those enrolled were female (56 %), 35 % were African-American/black (35 %), and 14 % identified as Latino. This enrollment of Latino participants was lower than expected. The highest proportion of the sample was from the southern part of the USA (39 %), followed by the western part of the country (35 %), with the greatest number of participants coming from Colorado, Georgia, and Louisiana.

Table 9.2 Detailed week-by-week topics covered on the Just/Us Facebook page

Topic and detailed information	Sample content	Theories, theoretical constructs, & relevant outcomes
HIV risk behaviors	*Week 2* *Polls:* "Have you ever been tested for HIV?"; "How many sex partners have you had? Comment + see how you compare"; "How do you know if ur new love is HIV+ or neg? Talk about it." *RSS feed:* "Want to decrease ur risk for HIV: Fewer partners, testing + talking" *Week 3* *Poll:* "Number of sex partners" *RSS feed:* "Pass it back and forth but not around! If u and ur partner both get tested 4 STDs and only have sex w/each other, ur golden." *Week 5* *Video link: Star Squadron: HIV,* available at http://www.youtube.com/watch?v=7Swp5-dVOik *Week 6* *RSS feed:* "Social media linked to rise in syphilis" *Links:* HIV Awareness Day for Women and Girls; Australian STD Campaign for Tourists *Week 7* *Poll:* "What do you think about anal sex?" *Link:* Abstinence education in health care reform *RSS feed:* "1 in 6 have herpes in US" *Blog link:* "'The backdoor': Anal sex" *Week 8* *RSS feeds:* HIV risks; condom use percentages; rates of HIV/AIDS in Washington, DC Detailed information Factors that increase risk for HIV exposure and transmission: Early age at first sex Increased number of sex partners Concurrent partners Unprotected vaginal or anal sex among men and between heterosexual couples Alcohol or drug use and influence on inhibitions and decision making History of STD diagnosis HIV testing as routine every 6 months if you are sexually active but not monogamous Sexual coercion: What constitutes coercion?	Health Belief Model Perceived susceptibility Perceived severity Perceived benefits Perceived barriers (where and how to get tested) Integrated Behavioral Model Attitude Perceived norm (both other's expectations, other's behavior) Personal agency Intention to perform behavior Knowledge & skills to perform the behavior Habit Information, Motivation, Behavior HIV-prevention information/knowledge HIV-prevention motivation Elicitation of existing levels of HIV-prevention information, motivation, behavioral skills, and behavior Elicitation research

Table 9.2 (continued)

Topic and detailed information	Sample content	Theories, theoretical constructs, & relevant outcomes
	How to resist pressure	
	Rape or incest (as risk alone, but also as risk for early sexual debut among those abused as children)	
	Casual sex (with someone now known well)	
	Age difference between partners (where risk is increased for women with partners ages≥5-years older	
	Supplemental material	
	Condom man cartoon to demonstrate proper use of a condom; Youthnet role model stories; animation drama series; and:	
	Abstinence norms: Content promoting abstinence as normative among MySpace and Facebook users	
	Planning for sex as an important step	
	Taking time	
	Becoming well educated about pregnancy, STDs, and HIV before becoming sexually active	
	How to talk to partners about staying abstinent	
	Monogamy norms: Content promoting monogamy as normative among MySpace and Facebook users	
	"Once you decide to have sex, how to talk to your partner about being faithful"	
	Testing for STD and HIV and then staying monogamous	
Forum topics for site: Peer questions and postings on a variety of topics	Week 1	
	Poll: "Why don't you like condoms?"	
	Week 2	
	Poll: "How many partners have you had?"	
	RSS feeds: "Got 1++ sex partners at same time? Ur at risk 4 HIV+STD"; "Have you eva cheated on your bf or gf? Comment+ see what it brings u."	
	Week 4	
	RSS feeds: "Being with only one person at a time keeps you safer from HIV and other STDs"; "Condoms in space"; "Condom design in NYC"; and "Condom machines in Italy"	
	Week 6	
	Links: Australian STD Campaign for Tourists; the Brazilian sustainable rubber condom	
	Blog link: "Getting together, getting it on, getting it online"	

Table 9.2 (continued)

Topic and detailed information	Sample content	Theories, theoretical constructs, & relevant outcomes
	Week 8	
	RSS feed: Condom use percentages	
	Detailed information	
	Age at first sex	
	Benefits of waiting for sex	
	Benefits of being with one person or only dating one person if having sex	
	Disadvantages of one night stands	
	Disadvantages of having multiple sex partners	
	Disadvantages of having concurrent partners	
	Advantages of condom use	
"How to" from experts and/or peers	**Week 1**	
	Poll: "Have you ever talked to your partner about protection b4 u have sex?"	
	Week 2	
	Poll: "How many partners have you had?"	
	RSS feeds: "Got ideas 4 how to talk to ur partners abt safe sex, Tell us"; "Qs about sex? Answers from experts at www.justus411.org" and general information about quality and history of condoms.	
	Video link: *A Condom for Everyone*, available at http://www.youtube.com/watch?v=7d6oqRB79ws	
	Week 3	
	Polls and RSS feeds:	
	"How to use condom"	
	"What's your favorite kind of condom?"	
	"How often do you use condoms during sex?"	
	"Wanna know how often other people use condoms? Find out www.justus411.org"	
	"7 perfect condoms"	
	"Two condoms are not better than one"	
	"Need a bigger condom–size does matter?"	
	"Who puts on the condom in ur relationship?"	
	"Do you never use a condom w/your bf/gf but always with others? OMG-problem"	

Table 9.2 (continued)

Topic and detailed information	Sample content	Theories, theoretical constructs, & relevant outcomes
	"Ever been pressured to have sex without a condom? What do you do"	
	"Anyone tried the female condom? Hear it's good for anal"	
	"Does size matter?"	
	Blog link: Condoms and contraception	
	Video link: *Safe in the City*, available at http://www.stdcentral.org/SitC/about/	
	Video link: *Star Squadron 200X: What is Sex*, available at http://www.youtube.com/watch?v=V_v_Skk6rL8	
	Week 4	
	Article link: Condoms in porn industry	
	Polls and RSS feeds:	
	"Did you know you can put a condom on your partner with your tongue? S-E-X-Y"	
	"Condoms can break when u don't put them on correctly Watch 1–1/2 min video now: [link]"	
	"Two condoms are NOT better than one Two rubbing + friction = tearing. Just one, all the time"	
	"So far xx % of people say they have NOT had a condom break on them. Have you? Take a poll: [link]"	
	"Do u know where to go if ur condom breaks? Text Hookup to 61827"	
	"Do you know what to do if ur condom breaks. U may be at risk for STDs + unplanned pregnancy. Call 8002307526 for srvcs near you."	
	"Can put a condom on using your tongue"	
	"Condoms need to fit right"	
	Video link: *Star Squadron 200X: Condoms*, available at http://www.youtube.com/watch?v=b-5qeYoDhH0	
	Article link: About Roy Ashburn: DUI after leaving gay club	
	Week 5	
	Links: Condoms in a Rome school; Condoms in space; and Female condoms distributed in DC area with high HIV rates	
	RSS feeds: "Anyone have info on the female condom?"; "Britain sending condoms to South Africa for world cup"; "Endangered species condoms"; and "Sex talk during sex play"	
	Week 6	
	RSS feeds: "Arrested for carrying too many condoms" "Condomania store"; and "Pawn shop with condoms in NYC"	

Table 9.2 (continued)

Topic and detailed information	Sample content	Theories, theoretical constructs, & relevant outcomes
	Week 8	
	RSS feeds: Condom use, percentage, Anti-rape condom	
	Detailed information	
	Negotiate safe sex with a partner (from peers—what was your best experience?)	
	Avoid pressure to have sex—conversations about coercion	
	Avoid pressure to have sex without a condom	
	How to use a condom—use of Safe in the City condom man cartoon on how to use a condom	
	Use of Youthnet role model series	
	Coming out	
	Getting help if sexually assaulted	
	Getting help if in an abusive relationship	
	Coping with HIV related stigma	
Support	**Week 1**	
	Status updates: "Is solo sex still sex?"; "Contest: Craziest advice an adult has given you"; "Do you trust advice from adults about sex?"; and "Afraid of unplanned pregnancy"	
	Blog link: You can learn from friends and trusted adults	
	Week 2	
	RSS feeds: "Who gave you the 'talk'?"; "Getting any, Getting lots? Ur at risk 4 HIV + STDs"; "Do u know how often u shud get tested for HIV? Every 6 months if ur sexually active"	
	Week 4	
	RSS feeds: "Masturbation + Safe Sex"; "101 ways to get sexy without having intercourse-add yours"; "Finish the sentence: I felt really close to my sex partner when s/he…"; "Best safer sex experience: When I masturbated w/my partner. Tell us your best safer sex experience…"; "Having sex w/boyz and girlz is fun but isn't safe unless u use a condom (Lesbians can get pregnant from gay friends)"	
	Week 5	
	Links: "Start talking about sex in middle school"; "Sex ed from a teacher's perspective"; "Facebook and Syphilis"	
	Week 6	
	Link: Australian STD Campaign for Tourists	

Table 9.2 (continued)

Topic and detailed information	Sample content	Theories, theoretical constructs, & relevant outcomes
	Week 7	
	Links: "April is STD Awareness Month: Facts you should know"; "Is sex education is a crime?"; "Bristol Palin Delayed Pregnancy Campaign"; "The Onion Pokes fun at Abstinence Pledges"; "Sex education on global scale"	
	Week 8	
	Links: "Men explaining birth control"; "Sex Education is not about pleasure"	
	Blog link: Emergency Contraception vs. Birth Control	
HIV statistics (from CDC fact sheets)	Week 1	
	Blog link: HIV not a blast from the past	
	Week 2	
	RSS feed: Statistics about HIV and STDs among African-Americans and Latinos	
	Week 7	
	RSS feed: April is STD Awareness Month: Facts you should know	
	Week 8	
	RSS feed: Percentages of condom use	
	Detailed Information	
	HIV is the virus that causes AIDS	
	In the US, most men get HIV from other men	
	In 2006, an estimated 1,332 new cases of HIV/AIDS were diagnosed in youth 15–19, and 3,886 cases in young adults 20–24	
	Youth of color are at particular risk for contracting HIV/AIDS and other STDs	
	African-American/black adults and adolescents accounted for 49 % of all HIV/AIDS cases diagnosed in 2005	
	Rates of HIV/AIDS cases were 72.8 per 100,000 among African-Americans/blacks older than 13 years, compared with 28.5 per 100,000 and 9.0 per 100,000 among Latinos and whites of the same age-group	
	The rates of Chlamydia and gonorrhea infections are highest among youth. Chlamydia infections rose in 2007 by 7.7 % for youth 15–19 years old and rose 6.6 % for young adults 20–24 years old	
	Chlamydia disproportionately affects African-Americans/blacks, representing 48 % of Chlamydia cases. The rate of Chlamydia infection is 3 times higher in Latinos than in whites	
	African-Americans/blacks make up only 12 % of the population but represent 70 % of the reported cases of gonorrhea	
	The rate of syphilis is 2 times higher for Latinos than for whites	

Table 9.2 (continued)

Topic and detailed information	Sample content	Theories, theoretical constructs, & relevant outcomes
Information on puberty and reproduction	Week 3	
	RSS feed: Every penis and vagina are different	
	Week 5	
	Links: The Onion article on "Being a woman now"; Canadian sex-ed Super hero	
	Week 6	
	Link: Health Care Reform—Reproductive Health	
	Week 7	
	Link: Talking to kids about sex: When did you first have birds and bees talk	
	Week 8	
	Link: Sex education on a global scale	
	Detailed Information	
	Physical development in males and females	
	Male reproductive system	
	Female reproductive system	
	Pregnancy	

[a] The content noted here is not exhaustive and is intended only to provide insight into the intervention

CDC Centers for Disease Control and Prevention, *STD* sexually transmitted diseases

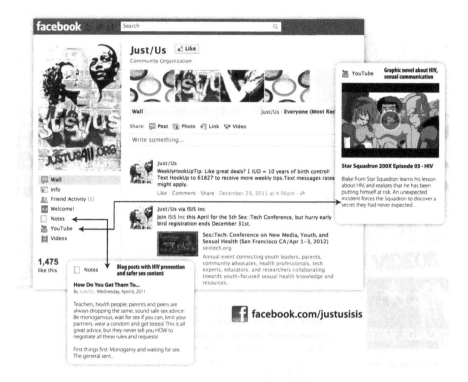

Fig. 9.1 The *Just/Us* Facebook page, with examples of content and elements

We screened 1,017 individuals for the study, and 828 eligible individuals were randomly assigned to the control group ($n = 312$) or the intervention group ($n = 340$), and additional participants were enrolled through referrals (Fig. 9.2). The original sample consisted of 1,578 participants, and 1,092 (69%) completed the 2-month follow-up survey. We had additional attrition at the 6-month follow-up, with 52% of the original sample completing this second follow-up; 59% of participants in the control arm completed the 6-month follow-up compared with 45% in the intervention arm, a statistically significant difference. Additionally, 106 participants completed the 6-month follow-up who had not completed the first follow-up, therefore increasing the proportion of participants with any follow-up data to 75.5%.

Analytic data from Phase 3, during intervention implementation, indicated that the Just/Us Facebook page had an average of 43 unique visitors per week and a high of unique 101 visitors during the week when the content focused on multiple sex partners. The average time spent on the page was 3.16 min, with a high of 7.3 min. There also were 93 loyal visitors (10% of those enrolled in the intervention) who regularly returned to view and post on the Just/Us Facebook page.

During the 8-week intervention, participants were most engaged the week we posted the blog titled, "*Boyfriend? Girlfriend? Or Just Friends with Benefits?*" The

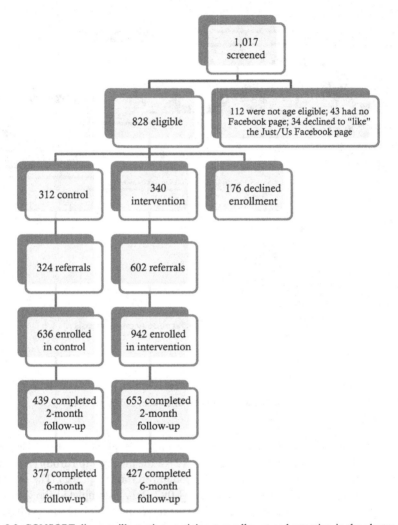

Fig. 9.2 CONSORT diagram illustrating participant enrollment and retention in the cluster randomized controlled trial over time

behavior we were addressing with this blog post was reducing the number of sex partners, making the point that the more partners one has, the more at risk for HIV exposure and transmission. The blog content was provocative and gave tips for navigating the world of "friends with benefits," commonly known as "FWB" on-line, from the vantage point of both reducing HIV and STI risk and maintaining one's emotional health. The poll for the week asked, "Have you ever hooked up with someone at a party and later became friends with benefits?" and the RSS feed covered reminders such as, "When you decide to have sex, you aren't just having sex with that one person…but everyone that person had sex with too!" At the time of the blog posting, a movie was released by the same name, *Friends with Benefits*, with Justin Timberlake and Mila Kunis, and earlier in the same year, *No Strings Attached*, with Ashton Kutcher and Natalie Portman, was in wide release. Clearly, the topic was relevant for many participants, as evidenced by the 400 % spike in number of comments and loyal user engagement when the blog was posted.

Overall, during active enrollment and participation, the moderators made 589 posts and fans made 277 comments, for a ratio of approximately one participant comment for every 2.1 moderator posts. The history of all the posts and content is available online at http://www.facebook.com/justusisis.

At the 2-month follow-up, we asked participants in the intervention arm how often they looked at the content on the Just/Us Facebook page; content here was defined as content that was pushed to them through the RSS feed on their Facebook news feed page as well as content on the Just/Us Facebook page. About 53 % (350 participants) said they looked at the Just/Us content four to six times per week (21 participants) or daily (329 participants). Of these "frequent users," 14 (4 %) were male, indicating that female participants were significantly more likely to be frequently engaged with the content ($p<0.0001$). However, there was no difference in gender for those indicating that they saw content at least once a week (329 participants).

Participants were also asked to write open-ended comments about the Just/Us Facebook page at the 2-month follow-up; we asked them to say what they liked and disliked about the page and to offer any suggestions for how we could improve this intervention (Table 9.3). There were 448 comments from participants in the intervention arm at the 2-month follow-up, indicating that 69 % of all participants had something to say about the Just/Us Facebook page. The overwhelming majority (94 %) of these comments were positive; of the remaining comments, many had to do with wanting to see the results from the study (three comments), complaints about the questions on the survey or not receiving incentives (seven comments), and confusion about the goal of the study (five comments). Only a handful of comments indicated that participants either did not agree with the information or perspectives that were being posted on the Just/Us Facebook page, found it awkward to review this type of material on Facebook, or were annoyed by multiple reminders to participate.

However, given that the overwhelming majority of the comments about the Just/Us Facebook page were positive, and participants said they appreciated having content available on their own Facebook news feed, it seems that participants saw content even if they did not go to the Just/Us Facebook page to post comments or reactions to it.

Moreover, our outcome analyses demonstrated that participants who were exposed to Just/Us Facebook page content were more likely than those who were not exposed to report using condoms consistently at the 2-month follow-up. Unfortunately, at the 6-month follow-up, we saw a decline in study effects, with a decrease to baseline levels of condom use in both the intervention and control groups. These results are reported in detail elsewhere [21].

Table 9.3 Selected comments from user feedback on the Just/Us Facebook page ($N=448$). (Comments are noted verbatim and may include errors in grammar and spelling)

Examples of positive comments ($N=419$)	"I feel that it's a good way to stay informed on sex. It's a little reminder for those who are in sexual relationship(s) to remind them to strap it up"
	"It's really interesting, I've been paying attention to your posts and a video that I saw. If people actually paid more attention to Just/Us, they might actually learn more than what they think they know"
	"Interesting.. ya don't make it awkward"
	"I think its a great project, and I enjoy reading the blogs that get posted on the FB page"
	"Found [this an] interesting way to talk about these topics. Geared towards teens"
	"I like the daily reminders the project posts about cultivating a healthy sexual attitude, and staying safe or abstaining"
Examples of explicitly negative comments	"Although the facts are entertaining and otherwise interesting, I'm not sure how effective the website and Facebook page is as a whole. The people that are looking at the page are the people that already have the facts and are getting tested and taking proper care to avoid STDs and pregnancy"
	"your messages are kinda awkward sometimes when I am sitting in my school's public library and everyone can see..."
Comments on study methods	"Because I know only 2/3 of my CLOSE friends sexual information. And the questions that are asked, for example" how many of your friends on Facebook have had an one night stand" The question should be rephrased " how many of your close friends have had an one night stands" Because when the question is so broad, we are basically being told to stereotype our friends on FB. Because usually only 1/3 of the ppl on FB are ppl we talk to on a regular basis"
	"Some of the questions in the survey are poorly worded and can have double meanings. The survey and Facebook page are heteronormative; e.g. one of the questions asked if I used condoms or a different form of birth control. This question isn't accurate to me because I mostly have sex with men and don't need to use birth control..."
Comments related to confusion about the goal of the study	"Not really sure what it's driving at/what you hope to accomplish"
Neutral comments	"It's OK"
	"Honestly I'm just doing it because of the coupon, and because my friend told me to"

Discussion

Given the disparities in HIV infection and other STIs in the USA among ethnic/racial and sexual minority populations and adolescents and young adults, we are in urgent need of strategies to reach these communities and populations and engage them in effective prevention efforts. However, a history of mistrust of researchers in this country, coupled with potential variation in capacity for researchers to effectively engage with community members [50], suggests that effective engagement of key communities and populations in HIV-prevention interventions remains challenging.

Tindana and colleagues defined community engagement as "the process of working collaboratively with relevant partners who share common goals and interests." This process involves "building authentic partnerships, including mutual respect and active inclusive participation; power sharing and equity; mutual benefit or finding the 'win-win' possibility" in the collaboration [51]. In the USA, community engagement in HIV research has origins in the beginning of the epidemic in the early 1980s. For example, activists, many of whom were gay themselves or closely allied with gay men, lead initial prevention efforts and pushed for the development of a community role in the research in and development of HIV treatments (see Chap. 4). This movement also contributed to the emergence of local community advisory boards, designed to represent diverse voices in the communities where research and prevention practice were taking place. Community engagement has since built on the initial important work of community advisory boards. Increasingly, researchers, funders, health educators, and other types of practitioners have learned the value of engaging members of the community; and along with this engagement comes the transition from community members being viewed as targets to being respected as partners. Community engagement is seen to have broader aims that include improvement of the ethical and scientific integrity of trials; increased transparency and accountability of the research to the community; increased benefits and decreased risks for participants and the surrounding community; and improved local capacity and infrastructure [6, 52–57].

We are only now establishing definitions and expectations for virtual community engagement; although the traditional definition of community engagement may apply to online communities, we lack explicit agreement about what constitutes engagement online. This lack of agreement can be driven in part by what evidence emerges that links community member engagement in the research process to subsequent health outcomes. Ultimately, it will be useful to have a rubric that can assist researchers, funders, health educators, and other types of practitioners to understand what type of engagement, through what strategies and mechanisms, and how much engagement is needed to realize varying level of health outcomes.

Considering the Just/Us Facebook intervention in the context of best processes for community engagement allows us to address a key new factor for community engagement—how to effectively engage in the increasingly important technologic environment of the Internet, mobile technologies, and social media. Here, we consider engagement with the Just/Us Facebook intervention within the three phases previously described: the development of a Facebook page related to sexual health, enrollment of social networks of adolescents as participants in a research study, and interaction with content on the study's Facebook page.

We were able to establish initial engagement of youth through synchronous and asynchronous online focus groups; we and other researchers have demonstrated that engagement not only occurs in the real world through face-to-face interaction but also can be effectively mediated in online settings [21, 25, 58]. Our goal at this phase of the research was to solicit meaningful input on the content and design of our Facebook page. By going beyond the traditional face-to-face approaches, such as focus groups and key informant interviews, and instead, capitalizing on the online environment, we were able to cast our net wider, engaging participants from diverse geographic settings to offer input and ideas that could be incorporated into the intervention. It also ensured that the information gleaned came from those closest to the ultimate user. It was during this process that we generated the concept of Just/Us, with the focus on sexual health as a social right. This is an example of how the virtual environment can generate meaningful engagement.

Our engagement efforts during participant enrollment showed that we could effectively recruit participants using traditional face-to-face methods for research subsequently carried out online. As mentioned above, we relied on face-to-face methods to approach and recruit our initial seeds for a modified RDS approach. After we successfully enrolled seeds and gained their trust, we were able to rely on them to enroll their Facebook friends in the study. Our process suggests that virtual communities may be difficult to work within unless relationships with virtual community members have been established. Our enrollment worked well when we relied on Facebook users to recruit their friends; we suspect that we would never have been able to recruit participants directly online. This finding seems to represent a crucial aspect when considering how to best engage adolescent and young adults within virtual communities.

Furthermore, based on our recruitment experience, social media seems to allow users to stay connected with their real-world friends virtually, but it then means that we compete for their limited attention. For example, a Facebook page promoting sexual health may seem provocative; however, it competes with the other reasons individual are online. It certainly could still be possible to engage participants using banner advertising or targeted advertising within social media sites [13, 59], but it is not clear that this approach would yield access to networks of virtual community members.

Engaging adolescents and young adults after they were enrolled in the study proved enlightening. As this was one of the first intervention research studies of its kind using Facebook for HIV prevention, we had no clear expectations about how participants would engage with the content on the Just/Us Facebook page. We knew that all participants had to "like" our Just/Us Facebook page in order for them to automatically see content, including content that was pushed to them through the RSS feed and automatically posted on their Facebook news feed. The RSS feed served as an opportunity to ensure a minimum exposure to intervention content. We anticipated that some of the content viewed in this manner would be sufficiently compelling for participants to click on it, which would then take them directly to the Just/Us Facebook page for further information and details. However, we also knew that such behavior on Facebook was unusual. Most of the time, adolescents and young people do not leave their own Facebook news feed, so we did not expect participants to click through to the Just/US Facebook page. We strived to make intervention content on the Just/Us Facebook page appealing, following some basic principles related to engagement with adolescents and young people that we believed to be important. These principles included:

- Carefully training moderators to post as representatives from the Just/Us intervention
- Developing content in such a way that was consistent with the expectations voiced by participants during the formative phase, including having content delivered in the form of quizzes, blogs, video links, threaded discussions, and polls
- Ensuring a sufficient number of posts to the page each day to keep participants engaged
- Keeping the Facebook page dynamic
- Evaluating content in real-time to assess what content increased versus decreased monitoring by participants

At the same time, we also wanted to make sure that we did not post so often that participants became annoyed and had a reason to block us or discontinue their fan ("like") status of the Facebook page.

A core group of about 10 % of participants enrolled in the intervention group left their own Facebook news feed page to go to the Just/Us Facebook page to post and interact. An analysis of the top 200 brands on Facebook found that in a given week, less than 0.5 % of fans actively engage with a brand. This was calculated by dividing the "talking about this" feature on a Facebook page (which shows how many fans are actually engaging with content such as sharing or commenting on) by total fans to create a percentage. About 10 % of Facebook pages were reaching an engagement level of 1 % or more; and only one brand page reached a weekly engagement level of 2 % or higher [60]. Thus, we were doing better than most organizations or companies with a Facebook page.

We were surprised and heartened by the idea that we engaged adolescents and young adults, at least for short periods of time, in a Facebook sexual health and HIV-prevention intervention. We hypothesize that this engagement may represent ongoing interest in sexual health, even in the face of competing demands for attention on social media sites. Our outcomes offer promise for other sexual health interventions to replicate and expand on our efforts and work toward sustaining engagement and behavior change over longer periods of time. Indeed, we are confident that sufficient numbers of intervention participants saw content from the Just/Us Facebook page on their own Facebook news feed page and engaged with it in some meaningful way, based on the fact that consistent use of condoms was greater in the intervention group than in the control group.

An important implication from the identification of a group of frequent users is that they could serve as popular opinion leaders (POL) to engage others in their network; as POLs have been established as being effective in the promotion of healthy sexual behaviors [61], it is certainly possible to consider adapting a more traditional POL intervention for the online environment. Future work should focus on understanding whether it is possible, after individuals begin to engage in this more active fashion, to recruit them as POLs to be brought on staff in a part-time fashion. Staff members identified and hired in this sequence may have the potential to have greater influence on those in their own personal networks than the moderators we hired initially. Our moderators had no personal connection to any of the intervention participants.

We do caution, however, that we cannot assume individuals have the same type of connection with their Facebook friends as they have with their real-world friends, as is illustrated in a comment from one participant: ".... Usually only 1/3 of the ppl [people] on FB are ppl [people] we talk to on a regular basis." This comment supports the notion that the hundreds and even thousands of individuals who are friends with any given Facebook user are not all intimate in the way real-world friends are. As recently stated by an author being interviewed on a radio program, "Facebook must up the meaning of the word 'friend'; it really just means someone I am connected to" [62]. Thus, if we want to utilize POLs, for example, we must carefully understand who are true, real-world friends of the POLs as opposed to who they are merely connected to on Facebook; determining whether peers have greater influence on true friends could be an important direction to investigate as we explore and harness virtual communities for health promotion and disease prevention. In analyses to evaluate the relationship between transitioning to obesity and network relationships, researchers found that close intimate relationships were most influential in the transition to obesity [63]. Although our work is an important first step in illustrating that social networking sites, like Facebook, can be used to influence sexual health, we still have much to learn about how to determine influential members within networks and how to activate those members to motivate sexual health behaviors.

Limitations

In this chapter, we provided a brief summary of innovative HIV-prevention interventions for virtual communities. We also offered a case study of one of the first studies of its kind to use Facebook to engage adolescents to reduce HIV exposure and transmission. Although we are pleased with the outcomes of this study and have learned much about what is possible related to engaging adolescents and young adults, we recognize that important limitations of our research remain.

First, given the profound impact of HIV on Latino communities in the USA, we need to do a better job of recruiting Latino adolescents and young adults into HIV-prevention interventions. We can look to our successes in recruiting large numbers of African-American/black adolescents and young adults as a starting place. We believe some of our success recruiting participants from these populations was because one of our recruiters was an African-American/black college-age woman. Our Latina recruiter, however, was older. In addition, studies demonstrate that networks tend to be similar with regard to demographic characteristics, including gender and race/ethnicity; therefore, recruiting more seeds who are Latina or Latino may help in subsequent recruitment of other Latino participants.

Furthermore, it would be valuable to understand more about what motivates individuals to post or respond to Facebook content. Although it may be useful to explore what motivates adolescents and young adults to engage with particular content, it is not completely clear that doing so is necessary to generate behavioral effects. It may also be difficult to encourage individuals to post or interact with this particular kind of content, inasmuch as the public environment of Facebook may thwart or discourage open engagement with content that is sensitive and private, such as sexual behavior. Nonetheless, it would certainly be valuable to have more ethnographic and detailed information about the types of things that generally cause individuals within virtual communities like Facebook to act and move from their own Facebook news feed page to another Facebook page, and whether there are particular triggers; for example, provocative content or particularly timely and current information that gets participants talking about specific content.

Third, given the need to move from research to practice to take interventions developed under research conditions to scale, it may be beneficial to consider whether engagement and sustainability would improve if the Just/Us Facebook page were linked to a real-world organization or entity that had regular and ongoing face-to-face connection with adolescents and young adults. Our project was a stand-alone intervention, where the Facebook page was not linked to any institution or group providing clinical services to adolescents and young adults. It may be worthwhile to explore linking the Just/Us Facebook page intervention to a clinical entity, such as a school-based health clinic or other clinic where adolescents and young adults can seek and receive high-quality, comprehensive reproductive health services. Certainly, there is concern that a page such as this cannot be sustained indefinitely unless it is linked in some way to an organization that is willing to support it.

Research Needs and Priorities in Terms of Prevention and Community Engagement

The Just/Us Facebook page with content to promote sexual health is the first ever to be studied for efficacy using a cluster randomized controlled trial to document improvements in sexual health. An important next step is to replicate findings. By our careful documentation of the specific methods for engaging adolescents and young adults to design, update content, and enroll in this trial, we are confident that replication is possible.

It will be important to attempt replication within the context of the lessons learned related to engagement. If we want to follow recent calls in the literature to pay closer attention to issues of translation and dissemination [64], we should ensure that any replication takes into consideration how to design for dissemination and sustainability. One method to accomplish that would be to do what we have just suggested: Link Just/Us Facebook page content to an organization that already regularly serves adolescents and young adults and is perceived to be a credible trusted source for important information on sexual health. Formalizing a relationship whereby organizations such as Planned Parenthood, school-based health centers, and/or community health centers actively integrate the Just/Us Facebook page content into their patient encounters and educational sessions could be a key next step.

If we do wish to consider approaches to link the Just/Us Facebook page to youth-friendly clinical services, work needs to be done to identify appropriate clinics and train staff and clinic administrators on how to best use social media to establish and maintain relationships with their clients and to share appropriate medical information with them. We can consider strategies to improve both online and offline engagement. For example, after adolescents and young adults have visited information online, they can subsequently go to a clinic where they see content they are familiar with and encounter staff who can reinforce content from the Just/Us Facebook page in a friendly and approachable manner.

Crucial to this work as well as other work that utilizes social media and technology for health promotion is a concern that gold-standard research in these environments happens at such a slow pace that the results may actually be obsolete by the time they are released and disseminated among the scientific and health-practitioner communities [65]. For example, our project was funded in 2006 and our primary outcomes were not under review for publication until 2012 [21]. Six years can be an eternity in the rapidly evolving technologic environment, and we must do better to shorten the timeline in getting prototypes for promising new technology-based initiatives designed quickly and delivered in the market on a much more streamlined timeline.

We also need to ensure that in planning for new prototypes to stay ahead of the technology curve, that we take care to consider dissemination from the very beginning. In the case of the Just/Us Facebook intervention, study partners at ISIS continued to update the Just/Us Facebook page and keep adolescents and young adults engaged in relevant topics after the study was complete. However, questions such as the following remain:

- How do we extend the reach to more people who were not enrolled the study?
- Who will cover maintenance and upgrade costs for both staffing and technology?
- When adaptations are needed, who will do this work?

These questions and related considerations are consistent with the RE-AIM framework established by Glasgow, who, along with Bennett, called explicitly for the need to consider where a technology application for health promotion should be disseminated, by whom, and how many people it could potentially reach, even before any programming of said prototype occurred [66].

We are well into the fourth decade of HIV, and HIV- and STI-related disparities continue to exist for some communities. Thus, we must be creative with both the types of interventions we develop, implement, and test, and the processes we used to develop, implement, and test them. Virtual communities offer seemingly limitless potentials, and we must work within these communities through engagement to ensure that what we do is meaningful and has the greatest potential for successfully reducing HIV and STIs among vulnerable populations.

References

1. Rheingold HT. The virtual community: homesteading on the electronic frontier. Reading: Addison-Wesley Publishing; 1993.
2. Gustafson DH, Hawkins RP, Boberg EW, McTavish F, Owens B, Wise M, et al. Chess: 10 years of research and development in consumer health informatics for broad populations, including the underserved. Int J Med Inform. 2002;65(3):169–77.
3. Glasgow RE, Boles SM, McKay HG, Feil EG, Barrera M, Jr. The D-Net diabetes self-management program: long-term implementation, outcomes, and generalization results. Prev Med. 2003;36(4):410–9.
4. Rhodes SD. Hookups or health promotion? An exploratory study of a chat room-based HIV prevention intervention for men who have sex with men. AIDS Educ Prev. 2004;16(4):315–27.
5. Rhodes SD, Hergenrather KC, Duncan J, Vissman AT, Miller C, Wilkin AM, et al. A pilot intervention utilizing internet chat rooms to prevent HIV risk behaviors among men who have sex with men. Public Health Rep. 2010;125(Suppl 1):29–37.
6. Rhodes SD, Vissman AT, Stowers J, Miller C, McCoy TP, Hergenrather KC, et al. A CBPR partnership increases HIV testing among men who have sex with men (MSM): outcome findings from a pilot test of the CyBER/testing internet intervention. Health Educ Behav. 2011;38(3):311–20.
7. Gorini A, Gaggioli A, Vigna C, Riva G. A second life for eHealth: prospects for the use of 3-D virtual worlds in clinical psychology. J Med Internet Res. 2008;10(3):e21.
8. Gordon R, Bjorklund NK, Smith RJ, Blyden ER. Halting HIV/AIDS with avatars and havatars: a virtual world approach to modelling epidemics. BMC Public Health. 2009;9 (Suppl 1):S13.
9. Gabarron E, Serrano JA, Wynn R, Armayones M. Avatars using computer/smartphone mediated communication and social networking in prevention of sexually transmitted diseases among North-Norwegian youngsters. BMC Med Inform Decis Mak. 2012;12:120.
10. Pereira C, McNamara A, Sorge L, Arya V. Personalizing public health: your health avatar. J Am Pharm Assoc (JAPhA). 2013;53(2):145–51.
11. Roth C, Vermeulen I, Vorderer P, Klimmt C, Pizzi D, Lugrin JL, et al. Playing in or out of character: user role differences in the experience of interactive storytelling. Cyberpsychol Behav Soc Netw. 2012;15(11):630–3.
12. Lipnack J, Stamps J. Virtual teams: reaching across space, time, and organizations with technology. New York: Wiley; 1997.
13. Rhodes SD, Bowie DA, Hergenrather KC. Collecting behavioural data using the world wide web: considerations for researchers. J Epidemiol Community Health. 2003;57(1):68–73.
14. Kraut R, Patterson M, Lundmark V, Kiesler S, Mukopadhyay T, Scherlis W. Internet paradox. A social technology that reduces social involvement and psychological well-being? Am Psychol. 1998;53(9):1017–31.
15. Kaufman M. The internet: a reliable source? Washington Post. 1999; Health Sect. Z17.
16. Shapira NA, Goldsmith TD, Keck PE, Jr., Khosla UM, McElroy SL. Psychiatric features of individuals with problematic internet use. J Affect Disord. 2000;57(1–3):267–72.
17. Lenhart A, Purcell K, Smith A, Zickuhr K. Social media & mobile technology use among teens and young adults. 2010. http://wwwpewinternetorg/~/media//Files/Reports/2010/PIP_Social_Media_and_Young_Adults_Report_Final_with_toplinespdf.
18. Boyar R, Levine D, Zensius N. TECHsex USA: youth sexuality and reproductive health in the digital age. 2011. http://ccasaorg/wp-content/themes/skeleton/documents/Youth-Sexuality-and-Reproductive-Health-in-the-Digital-Agepdf.
19. Tatham M. 15 stats about Facebook. Experian consumer insights. 2012. http://www.experian.com/blogs/marketing-forward/2012/05/16/15-stats-about-facebook/. Accessed: 16 May 2012.

20. Allison S, Bauermeister JA, Bull S, Lightfoot M, Mustanski B, Shegog R, et al. The intersection of youth, technology, and new media with sexual health: moving the research agenda forward. J Adolesc Health. 2012;51(3):207–12.

21. Bull SS, Levine DK, Black SR, Schmiege SJ, Santelli J. Social media-delivered sexual health intervention: a cluster randomized controlled trial. Am J Prev Med. 2012;43(5):467–74.

22. Reich SM, Subrahmanyam K, Espinoza G. Friending, IMing, and hanging out face-to-face: overlap in adolescents' online and offline social networks. Dev Psychol. 2012;48(2):356–68.

23. Centers for Disease Control and Prevention. HIV Surveillance Report, 2011; 2013.

24. Seifer SD, Sisco S. Mining the challenges of CBPR for improvements in urban health. J Urban Health. 2006;83(6):981–4.

25. Moreno MA, Vanderstoep A, Parks MR, Zimmerman FJ, Kurth A, Christakis DA. Reducing at-risk adolescents' display of risk behavior on a social networking web site: a randomized controlled pilot intervention trial. Arch Pediatr Adolesc Med. 2009;163(1):35–41.

26. Gold J, Pedrana AE, Sacks-Davis R, Hellard ME, Chang S, Howard S, et al. A systematic examination of the use of online social networking sites for sexual health promotion. BMC Public Health. 2011;11:583.

27. Ownby RL, Waldrop-Valverde D, Jacobs RJ, Acevedo A, Caballero J. Cost effectiveness of a computer-delivered intervention to improve HIV medication adherence. BMC Med Inform Decis Mak. 2013;13–29.

28. Horvath KJ, Danilenko GP, Williams ML, Simoni J, Amico KR, Oakes JM, et al. Technology use and reasons to participate in social networking health websites among people living with HIV in the US. AIDS Behav. 2012;16(4):900–10.

29. Latkin CA, Davey-Rothwell MA, Knowlton AR, Alexander KA, Williams CT, Boodram B. Social network approaches to recruitment, HIV prevention, medical care, and medication adherence. J Acquir Immune Defic Syndr. 2013;63(Suppl 1):S54–8.

30. Nguyen P, Gold J, Pedrana A, Chang S, Howard S, Ilic O, et al. Sexual health promotion on social networking sites: a process evaluation of the FaceSpace project. J Adolesc Health. 2013;53(1):98–104.

31. Gold J, Pedrana AE, Stoove MA, Chang S, Howard S, Asselin J, et al. Developing health promotion interventions on social networking sites: recommendations from the FaceSpace project. J Med Internet Res. 2012;14(1):e30.

32. Pedrana A, Hellard M, Gold J, Ata N, Chang S, Howard S, et al. Queer as F**k: reaching and engaging gay men in sexual health promotion through social networking sites. J Med Internet Res. 2013;15(2):e25.

33. Bowen AM, Horvath K, Williams ML. A randomized control trial of internet-delivered HIV prevention targeting rural MSM. Health Educ Res. 2007;22(1):120–7.

34. Fortune T, Wright E, Juzang I, Bull S. Recruitment, enrollment and retention of young black men for HIV prevention research: experiences from The 411 for Safe Text project. Contemp Clin Trials. 2010;31(2):151–6.

35. Juzang I, Fortune T, Black S, Wright E, Bull S. A pilot programme using mobile phones for HIV prevention. J Telemed Telecare. 2011;17(3):150–3.

36. Levine D, McCright J, Dobkin L, Woodruff AJ, Klausner JD. SEXINFO: a sexual health text messaging service for San Francisco youth. Am J Public Health. 2008;98(3):393–5.

37. Hightow-Weidman LB, Fowler B, Kibe J, McCoy R, Pike E, Calabria M, et al. HealthMpowerment.org: development of a theory-based HIV/STI website for young black MSM. AIDS Educ Prev. 2011;23(1):1–12.

38. Hightow-Weidman LB, Pike E, Fowler B, Matthews DM, Kibe J, McCoy R, et al. HealthMpowerment.org: feasibility and acceptability of delivering an internet intervention to young Black men who have sex with men. AIDS Care. 2012;24(7):910–20.

39. Rice E, Lee A, Taitt S. Cell phone use among homeless youth: potential for new health interventions and research. J Urban Health. 2011;88(6):1175–82.

40. Rice E, Rhoades H. How should network-based prevention for homeless youth be implemented? Addiction. 2013;108(9):1625–6.

41. Rice E, Tulbert E, Cederbaum J, Barman Adhikari A, Milburn NG. Mobilizing homeless youth for HIV prevention: a social network analysis of the acceptability of a face-to-face and online social networking intervention. Health Educ Res. 2012;27(2):226–36.
42. Young SD, Rice E. Online social networking technologies, HIV knowledge, and sexual risk and testing behaviors among homeless youth. AIDS Behav. 2011;15(2):253–60.
43. Ybarra ML, Bull SS, Prescott TL, Korchmaros JD, Bangsberg DR, Kiwanuka JP. Adolescent abstinence and unprotected sex in CyberSenga, an internet-based HIV prevention program: randomized clinical trial of efficacy. PloS ONE. 2013;8(8):e70083.
44. Ybarra ML, Korchmaros J, Kiwanuka J, Bangsberg DR, Bull S. Examining the applicability of the IMB model in predicting condom use among sexually active secondary school students in Mbarara, Uganda. AIDS Behav. 2013;17(3):1116–28.
45. Levine D, Madsen A, Wright E, Barar RE, Santelli J, Bull S. Formative research on MySpace: online methods to engage hard-to-reach populations. J Health Commun. 2011;16(4):448–54.
46. Heckathorn DD. Respondent-driven sampling: a new approach to the study of hidden populations. Soc Problems. 1997;44(2):174–99.
47. Ramirez-Valles J, Garcia D, Campbell RT, Diaz RM, Heckathorn DD. HIV infection, sexual risk behavior, and substance use among Latino gay and bisexual men and transgender persons. Am J Public Health. 2008;98(6):1036–42.
48. Rhodes SD, McCoy TP, Hergenrather KC, Vissman AT, Wolfson M, Alonzo J, et al. Prevalence estimates of health risk behaviors of immigrant Latino men who have sex with men. J Rural Health. 2012;28(1):73–83.
49. Zoomerang. Zoomerang Privacy Policy. 2012. http://www.zoomerangcom/.
50. Institute of Medicine. Unequal treatment: confronting racial and ethnic disparities in health care. Washington: National Academy Press; 2003.
51. Tindana PO, Singh JA, Tracy CS, Upshur RE, Daar AS, Singer PA, et al. Grand challenges in global health: community engagement in research in developing countries. PLoS Med. 2007;4(9):e273.
52. Rhodes SD, Malow RM, Jolly C. Community-based participatory research: a new and not-so-new approach to HIV/AIDS prevention, care, and treatment. AIDS Educ Prev. 2010;22(3):173–83.
53. Cashman SB, Adeky S, Allen AJ, Corburn J, Israel BA, Montaño J, et al. The power and the promise: working with communities to analyze data, interpret findings, and get to outcomes. Am J Public Health. 2008;98(8):1407–17.
54. Israel BA, Krieger J, Vlahov D, Ciske S, Foley M, Fortin P, et al. Challenges and facilitating factors in sustaining community-based participatory research partnerships: lessons learned from the Detroit, New York City and Seattle Urban Research Centers. J Urban Health. 2006;83(6):1022–40.
55. Rhodes SD, Duck S, Alonzo J, Downs M, Aronson RE. Intervention trials in community-based participatory research. In: Blumenthal D, DiClemente RJ, Braithwaite RL, Smith S, editors. Community-based participatory research: issues, methods, and translation to practice. New York: Springer; 2013. p. 157–80.
56. Rhodes SD, Duck S, Alonzo J, Daniel J, Aronson RE. Using community-based participatory research to prevent HIV disparities: assumptions and opportunities identified by The Latino Partnership. J Acquir Immune Syndr. 2013;63(Suppl 1):S32–5.
57. Viswanathan M, Eng E, Ammerman A, Gartlehner G, Lohr KN, Griffith D, et al. Community-based participatory research: assessing the evidence. Evidence Report/Technology Assessment. Rockville, MD: Agency for Healthcare Research and Quality, 2004 July. Report No.: 99.
58. Moreno MA, Fost NC, Christakis DA. Research ethics in the MySpace era. Pediatrics. 2008;121(1):157–61.
59. Chiasson MA, Shaw FS, Humberstone M, Hirshfield S, Hartel D. Increased HIV disclosure three months after an online video intervention for men who have sex with men (MSM). AIDS Care. 2009;21(9):1081–9.

60. Radwanick S. Facebook blasts into top position in Brazilian social networking market following year of tremendous growth. 2013. http://www.comscore.com/Insights/Press_Releases/2012/1/Facebook_Blasts_into_Top_Position_in_Brazilian_Social_Networking_Market.

61. Kelly JA, St Lawrence JS, Stevenson LY, Hauth AC, Kalichman SC, Diaz YE, et al. Community AIDS/HIV risk reduction: the effects of endorsements by popular people in three cities. Am J Public Health. 1992;82(11):1483–9.

62. NPR Staff. We ask the pros: should you friend your boss on Facebook?. 2012. http://wwwn-prorg/blogs/alltechconsidered/2012/05/21/153213289/we-ask-the-pros-should-you-friend-your-boss-on-facebook. Accessed: 21 May 2012.

63. Christakis NA, Fowler JH. The spread of obesity in a large social network over 32 years. N Engl J Med. 2007;357(4):370–9.

64. Klesges LM, Estabrooks PA, Dzewaltowski DA, Bull SS, Glasgow RE. Beginning with the application in mind: designing and planning health behavior change interventions to enhance dissemination. Ann Behav Med. 2005;29(Suppl):66–75.

65. Riley WT, Glasgow RE, Etheredge L, Abernethy AP. Rapid, responsive, relevant (R3) research: a call for a rapid learning health research enterprise. Clin Transl Med. 2013;2(1):10.

66. Bennett GG, Glasgow RE. The delivery of public health interventions via the Internet: actualizing their potential. Annu Rev Public Health. 2009;30:273–92.

67. Rosser BR, Miner MH, Bockting WO, Ross MW, Konstan J, Gurak L, et al. HIV risk and the Internet: results of the Men's INTernet Sex (MINTS) study. AIDS Behav. 2009;13(4):746–56.

68. Rosser BRS, Gurak L, Horvath KJ, Oakes JM, Konstan J, Danilenko G. The challenges of ensuring participant consent in Internet-based sex studies: a case study of the Men's INTernet Sex (MINTS-I and II) studies. J Comput Mediat Commun. 2009;14:602–26.

69. Bull SS, Vallejos D, Levine D, Ortiz C. Improving recruitment and retention for an online randomized controlled trial: experience from the Youthnet study. AIDS Care. 2008;20(8):887–93.

70. Bull S, Pratte K, Whitesell N, Rietmeijer C, McFarlane M. Effects of an Internet-based intervention for HIV prevention: the Youthnet trials. AIDS Behav. 2009;13(3):474–87.

71. Noar SM, Black HG, Pierce LB. Efficacy of computer technology-based HIV prevention interventions: a meta-analysis. AIDS. 2009;23(1):107–15.

Chapter 10
Employment as a Social Determinant of Health: An Urban Partnership's Experience with HIV Intervention Development and Implementation Using Community-Based Participatory Research (CBPR)

Kenneth C. Hergenrather, Steve Geishecker, Glenn Clark and Scott D. Rhodes

In the USA, more than 1.1 million persons are living with HIV/AIDS. Annually, 74% of new HIV infections occur among men and 63% of new HIV infections occur among MSM. The rate of new HIV infection among MSM is 44 times that of other men and 40 times that of women. Although MSM represent 2–10% of the US male population 13 years of age or older (depending on the study and how MSM behavior is defined and measured), they account for 48% of persons with HIV/AIDS overall, and 64% of men with HIV/AIDS [1–3]. Compared with the rate of HIV infection among white MSM, the rate is approximately three times higher among Latino/Hispanic MSM and is more than seven times higher among African-American/black MSM. Moreover, since 2001, across all racial/ethnic groups, the only transmission group with significant increases in HIV diagnoses is MSM. Of men with new HIV infections, MSM represent more than 80% of white men, more than 70% of Latino/Hispanic men, and more than 60% of African-American/black men [4, 5].

K. C. Hergenrather (✉)
Department of Counseling and Human Development, Graduate School of Education and Human Development, The George Washington University, 2134 G Street, NW, Rm. 312, Washington, DC 20037, USA
e-mail: hergenkc@gwu.edu

S. Geishecker · G. Clark
Behavioral Health Services, Whitman-Walker Health, 1701 14th Street, NW, Washington, DC 20009, USA
e-mail: sgeishecker@whitman-walker.org

G. Clark
e-mail: glennclarkintakomapark@hotmail.com

S. D. Rhodes
Department of Social Sciences and Health Policy, Division of Public Health Sciences, Wake Forest University School of Medicine, Medical Center Blvd., Winston-Salem, NC 27157, USA
e-mail: srhodes@wakehealth.edu

S. D. Rhodes (ed.), *Innovations in HIV Prevention Research and Practice through Community Engagement,* DOI 10.1007/978-1-4939-0900-1_10,
© Springer Science+Business Media New York 2014

The Health and Well-Being of Persons with HIV

The introduction of antiretroviral therapy, which limits the ability of the HIV to replicate itself, has led to profound declines in AIDS-related mortality [6–8]. As persons with HIV live longer, serious non-AIDS-defining illnesses have replaced opportunistic infections as the leading causes of death. These illnesses include cardiovascular disease, diabetes, anxiety, depression, and bipolar disorder [9, 10].

Furthermore, as HIV infection progresses, persons with HIV may experience impairment in three key domains: physical, mental, and neurologic health [11]. Physical health, for example, may be increasingly affected as HIV disease progresses, and persons with HIV can become fatigued, be unable to independently perform activities of daily living (e.g., hygiene, ambulation, meal preparation, and eating), and be less active. The long-term use of antiretroviral therapy also has been linked to body changes that include fat gain concentrated in the abdominal area, peripheral fat loss, and development of metabolic abnormalities (e.g., glucose intolerance, hypercholesterolemia, and hypertriglyceridemia). These bodily changes may induce psychologic distress, increase the risk of cardiovascular disease and diabetes, and impair physical activity [12–15].

Furthermore, CD4+ lymphocyte counts of less than 50 cells/mm^3 of blood are associated with significant functional impairments and increased morbidity and mortality; a normal CD4+ count ranges from 500 to 1,500 cells/mm^3 [16, 17]. Although HIV infection affects the immune system function at any CD4+ count, the risk of opportunistic infections and noninfectious complications of HIV increase as the CD4+ count declines. Current treatment guidelines recommend the initiation of antiretroviral therapy for all persons with HIV, regardless of CD4+, to decrease the risk of disease progression and to reduce the risk of HIV transmission. Disease-specific preventive measures such as prophylaxis of pneumocystis pneumonia when the CD4+ count is less than 200 cells/mm^3 or pneumococcal vaccinations are also indicated to decrease the risk of HIV-associated complications [15, 16].

Among some persons with HIV, mental health can be affected by the strain of living with HIV (e.g., family and/or partner rejection and stigma) and the onset of comorbidities, including mental health disorders and/or substance use or abuse, and may lead to disability and functional impairment. Depression, anxiety, psychologic distress, and posttraumatic stress may also increase as HIV disease progresses. These conditions can reduce the quality of life and increase mortality. Depression has been consistently associated with poor treatment adherence and increased HIV risk behaviors (e.g., substance use and abuse and inconsistent condom use) [18–24]. Posttraumatic stress disorder has been reported in 16–54% of persons with HIV; this comorbidity is associated with both substance abuse disorder and major depressive disorder and has been correlated with a compromised immune system, lower CD4+ count, poor treatment adherence, and increased HIV risk behaviors [25–30].

Neurologic dysfunction may occur among some persons with HIV as a result of HIV infection and/or opportunistic infections. These impairments may range from mild asymptomatic cognitive impairment to severe dementia, presenting as sensory impairments, and neuropathy. As HIV progresses, persons with HIV may experience decreased mental capacity (e.g., forgetting to eat or take medications), visual impairments, and loss of cranial nerve function (e.g., ability to taste, chew, and swallow). The impact of HIV on neurologic health includes impairment of cognitive abilities to plan tasks, learn and process new information, retrieve information, and manage medication. Neurologic impairment also may include deficits in executive functioning and attention [31, 32].

The term "executive functioning" describes a set of cognitive abilities that are necessary for goal-directed behavior. Executive functioning includes the ability to initiate and stop actions, to monitor and change behavior as needed, and to plan future behavior when faced with novel tasks and situations [33]. Executive function deficits are associated with psychiatric disorders that include depression, anxiety, obsessive-compulsive disorder, attention-deficit disorder, and hyperactivity disorder. Higher levels of executive functioning are significantly correlated with effective coping styles when confronting challenges (e.g., adapting to changing demands and/or environments). Persons with HIV who confront distress by using problem-solving and behavior modification techniques (e.g., problem-focused coping) have been found to have significantly better health and a higher quality of life than those who cope by denial. When persons with HIV face stressful life events, their coping responses have been identified as significant moderators to attenuate the disruptive effect of stressors and to improve self-management [34–36]. Self-management has the potential to positively affect the physical, mental, and neurologic health of persons with HIV.

Self-management Interventions

Among persons with chronic health conditions, self-management has been defined as the individual's ability to manage the symptoms, treatment, physical and psychosocial consequences, and lifestyle changes inherent in living with a chronic health condition. Efficacious self-management interventions positively affect the cognitive, behavioral, and emotional responses that a person needs to maintain a satisfactory quality of life and increase his or her ability to effectively monitor the chronic condition to maintain optimal health. In a review of 145 peer-reviewed published interventions designed to improve self-management of chronic health conditions, eight common components were identified that align with the three domains of health (physical, mental, and neurologic) affected by HIV (Table 10.1; [37]).

Self-management has been used to improve health outcomes across a variety of chronic conditions, including depression, asthma, arthritis, and diabetes [37, 38], but few studies have applied self-management concepts to management of HIV, including adherence to antiretroviral therapy. This lack of research is particularly unfortunate because HIV-related mortality is contingent largely on the ability of persons with HIV to adhere to treatment regimens [16, 39, 40]. However, among the limited available HIV-related studies harnessing components of self-management, interventions have improved adherence to treatment regimens and increased CD4+ counts, assisting the human body to fight disease, through lowering anxiety and increasing self-esteem, coping skills, and treatment adherence [6, 16, 36, 41–46].

Table 10.1 Components of self-management

Information (e.g., diagnosis, prognosis, and treatment)

Medication management (e.g., strategies to increase adherence, and identifying and reducing barriers to adherence)

Symptom management (e.g., cognition, fatigue, pain, physiology, and relaxation)

Management of psychologic consequences (e.g., anger, depression management, anxiety management, and stress)

Lifestyle (e.g., exercise, nutrition, leisure, and activities of daily living)

Social support (e.g., family, friends, peers, and significant others/partners)

Communication (e.g., with health- care providers)

Other strategies (e.g., executive functioning, goal setting, planning, decision-making, problem solving, and coping)

HIV and the Effects of Employment on Health

The effect of unemployment on health and psychologic well-being has been well documented in the literature [47–50]. Unemployment has been identified as an independent predictor of depression, mortality, and psychiatric symptomology [51–56]. Several longitudinal studies have presented the correlation between unemployment and poor health [50, 57, 58], mental illness [54, 59], increased maladaptive health behaviors [60], lower executive functioning [61], and increased mortality [62, 63].

Among persons with HIV, employment is associated with better mental health and quality of life, suggesting a therapeutic benefit [64]. In a large-scale study of 2,863 persons with HIV, researchers found that those who were employed reported better mental health (e.g., lower anxiety, lower depression, and increased social functioning) and higher physical functioning and were less likely to have difficulties with activities of daily living than those who were not employed [65]. In a similar study, among 702 men with HIV, those who were employed better handled life difficulties, had lower psychologic stress, and better managed their health than those who were unemployed [66]. Moreover, persons with HIV without stable employment, relative to those with stable employment, are at significantly increased risk for psychologic distress, suicidal ideation, psychiatric symptoms, and anxiety and are more than twice as likely to be hospitalized or die [67–71]. Unfortunately, despite the potential health advantages of employment (or perhaps more precisely, "work,") for persons with HIV, the unemployment rate for this population ranges from 45 to 62 % [59, 72].

HIV and the Effects of Social Support on Health

The psychosocial impact of HIV infection may render persons with HIV susceptible to social isolation and result in a lack of social support. Social support has been defined several ways and measurement remains challenging; however, in general, social support includes emotional, tangible, informational, and companionship support [73–75]. In general, higher mortality has been reported among men who have few close friends or relatives, less frequent contact with people, and reduced participation in social activities [76–79]. Social support may buffer the impact of a variety of stressful life experiences, including those related to illness and unemployment. Among persons with HIV, those with social support have demonstrated less anxiety and depression and had fewer somatic complaints than those without adequate support. Furthermore, social support is important in adjustment to diagnosis and prognosis, and has correlated with slower decline in CD4+ counts, better adherence to treatment, and reduced HIV risk behavior. Moreover, the role of the health-care provider as both informational and emotional support for persons with HIV has been documented in the literature; providers have been identified as being helpful, providing reassurance, validating worth, and preparing for a potential AIDS prognosis [6, 7, 70, 80–86].

The *National HIV/AIDS Strategy*

The effect of employment on the health of persons with HIV has been recognized and addressed by the White House through policy development. In the *National HIV/AIDS Strategy*, for example, the Social Security Administration is designated as the lead agency responsible to assist persons with HIV to access income supports, including job skills and employment. (For a review of domestic US HIV activities for federal departments, see the *Overview of Domestic HIV/AIDS Activities Across Federal Departments* at http://aids.gov/federal-resources/national-hiv-aids-strategy/overview-fed-domestic-hiv-aids-activities.pdf). The *Social Security Administration Operational Plan for Implementing the National HIV/AIDS Strategy* involves three areas: (1) conducting outreach to at-risk communities to educate members of these communities about the assistance of SSA programs; (2) updating policy to ensure more accurate disability determinations and expediting the time for eligible claimants to gain access to health care; and (3) assisting persons currently on disability to return to work through the Ticket-to-Work and Self-Sufficiency Program, Work Incentives Planning and Assistance, and Protection and Advocacy for the Beneficiaries of Social Security initiatives [87]. Ongoing and authentic engagement of and participation by persons with HIV is certainly a strategy that should be utilized, and best processes developed, identified, and implemented within the framework of the *National HIV/AIDS Strategy*.

In 2010, the Institute of Medicine of the National Academies provided recommendations to update the Social Security Administration Listing of Impairment regarding HIV [88]. Recommendations include (1) persons with HIV with CD4+ counts of < 50 cells/mm^3 should be allowed disability and be regularly evaluated, (2) specific types of severe or fatal conditions should be considered as permanent disability among persons with HIV, and (3) persons with HIV with severe HIV-associated conditions that limit functioning also should be allowed disability and be regularly evaluated. The recommendations acknowledge that not all persons with HIV are able to enter employment or re-employment.

Our Community-Based Participatory Research (CBPR) Partnership

Our CBPR partnership was initiated in 2002. The clinical director of Whitman Walker Health (WWH) in Washington, DC, and an academic researcher from The George Washington University (GW) began a dialogue to develop a partnership to explore the needs and priorities of persons with HIV. The idea was that if the needs and priorities were authentically explored and thus better understood, action or intervention would be possible, and these possible actions or interventions would be the most promising to positively affect the health and well-being of persons with HIV. We chose CBPR as an approach to our research to ensure community engagement and full participation in all aspects of the research. Although what is described as CBPR in some of the more recent literature tends to lack key values and principles underlying CBPR, our emerging partnership tried, and continues to strive, to adhere to the ways in which CBPR has been conceptualized and practiced by leading community-academic partnerships in the field; our emerging partnership was founded on and integrated accepted values and principles of CBPR that are widely available and published [89–95].

Members of our ongoing partnership were, and in fact remain, committed to establishing structures for full and equal participation by community members, organization representatives, and academic researchers to improve community health and well-being through individual, group, and community action, and through policy and social change. We also emphasize multidirectional and co-learning, reciprocal transfer of expertise, and sharing of decision-making power. To ensure greater cultural congruence and social relevance of our research, members of our partnership, including African-American/black gay men with HIV, have been directly involved throughout the research processes, including the development of research questions, design and conduct of studies, data analysis and interpretation of results, and dissemination of findings.

A hallmark of CBPR is that a community "outsider" (such as a researcher from a university) can work best in partnership with community members [90–93, 96]. However, such authentic partnership takes time and its development must be systematic. Thus, members of our emerging partnership (i.e., community members, organization representatives, and academic researchers) committed the time and effort to develop the partnership. Partnership members from WWH had a profound understanding of service delivery and the facilitation of interventions and programs designed for persons with HIV. They had valuable experiences trying to meet community needs and a sense of what works and what does not work during service delivery and the implementation of programs.

It is important to note that academic researchers always bring with them the reputation of their academic institutions, favorable or not, as perceived by the community and organizational partners. In our studies, the academic researcher brought the reputation of GW, the reputation of the Graduate School of Education and Human Development (GSEHD), and the reputation of GSHED graduate counseling students completing internship placements at WWH. Furthermore, when community members questioned the academic researcher's interest in working with them, he found it useful to share relevant experiences, which included working as an HIV public health educator, facilitating support groups for persons with HIV, providing HIV testing and counseling services, and managing national AIDS clinical drug trials. These clear links to the concerns relevant to community members increased the academic researcher's credibility. Representatives from WWH also highlighted their overlapping interests and shared their perspectives with persons with HIV to reinforce growing trust and initiate acceptance of the academic researcher as a partner. To further develop trust, the academic researcher volunteered as a facilitator for WWH group counseling sessions; this service allowed community members and organization representatives from WWH to interact with the academic researcher in a setting not influenced by a research agenda.

As trust was established, a network of persons with HIV became more involved in our partnership. Today, our partnership consists of members from local HIV communities in Washington, DC, and members from WWH, a nonprofit community health center serving the metropolitan area with expertise in lesbian, gay, bisexual, and transgender (LGBT) health care and HIV health care; the GW GSEHD, with leadership in educational training and research that is committed to assisting culturally diverse communities, including local HIV communities; and the Wake Forest School of Medicine (WFSM), with leadership in CBPR and commitment to identifying and responding to the needs of the community most affected by HIV through rigorous research methodologies while adhering to CBPR core values and principles.

During the ongoing partnership meetings, persons with HIV, organization representatives, and academic researchers continued to share experiences pertaining to the challenges and priorities of persons with HIV and HIV-service providers and brainstormed ideas and next steps, including the development of meaningful interventions to promote the health and well-being of persons with HIV. As is well described in the CBPR literature, building and nurturing trust and maintaining transparent communication were paramount during this process.

After about a year of partnership development and trust building, members of our established CBPR partnership chose to explore the effect of employment on the health of persons with HIV, based on several factors, including medical advances have increased longevity for persons with HIV, and an increasing number of persons with HIV are seeking employment or re-employment. Members of our partnership wanted to blend our knowledge and perspectives based on the experiences of persons with HIV and the lessons learned in the provision of services to them with what is theoretically understood about self-management and scientifically known about the effects of employment on health and well-being for this population. The process that members of our partnership engaged in included two key questions:

- "What do we want to know about employment among persons with HIV?" and
- "Why do we want to know it?"

These types of questions are frequently used in CBPR studies to ensure that the research focuses on moving to action (i.e., some type of intervention or promotion of positive change to improve health) rather than research for research's sake [96–99]. This movement to action reflects another hallmark of CBPR: research should lead to some tangible form of action to improve the health and well-being of communities. In fact, most often CBPR should improve the health and well-being of the immediate community; participants in research should benefit from research [89–94, 96, 100–102].

During the past decade, members of our partnership conducted four participatory research studies based on the priorities of persons with HIV. The studies were funded and further supported by leveraging intramural and extramural resources. For each study, community members, organization representatives, and academic researchers developed the research protocol using a participatory and iterative approach. To facilitate each study and increase validity, members of our partnership also created, reviewed, revised, and approved study designs and data collection protocols. Furthermore, participants were recruited by community members and organization representatives. Much effort was also placed in analyzing and interpreting data through participatory approaches. For example, together community members, organization representatives, and academic researchers conducted content analysis to finalize preliminary findings. We also identified organizations (e.g., US Social Security Administration, SSA, the American Medical Association, the US Department of Education Rehabilitation Services Administration, and AIDS service organizations) to target for the dissemination of study findings. We used a strategic approach and leveraged networks to reach leaders and members of these organizations. Furthermore, dissemination of study findings included presentations and workshops at conferences and meetings sponsored by local, regional, and national societies and associations, including the National Council on Rehabilitation Education, the National Rehabilitation Association, the National Rehabilitation Counseling Association, and the American Public Health Association, and international societies and associations such as the International AIDS Society and the British Psychological Society. We published papers in peer-reviewed journals such as *AIDS Education and Prevention* and *Journal of Rehabilitation*. The participation of persons with HIV, organization representatives, and academic researchers ensured that the processes and products of our research were authentic, meaningful, and insightful and that the dissemination of findings was broad in order to have an impact on both research and practice.

Our CBPR Partnership's Research History

The four studies our CBPR partnership conducted included an initial study based on our priority to understand the effect of employment on the health and well-being of persons with HIV, two studies that built on the findings of the first study and took us closer to action and intervention, and a fourth study to pilot an intervention.

Employment Beliefs Study

Members of our partnership developed, piloted, and distributed the Employment Interest Survey to persons with HIV receiving services at WWH. The survey was completed by 324 persons with HIV, 204 (63.0%) of whom were unemployed. Regardless of employment status, 287 (88.6%) of the participants reported they wanted help gaining employment or re-employment. Participants identified employment as having positive benefits that they valued, including increased self-esteem, autonomy, social interaction, and quality of life. They also identified groups of persons influencing their decision to become employed (e.g., family, friends, and primary health-care provider) and impediments to employment (e.g., level of job-seeking skills, level of job training, medical instability of HIV prognosis, loss of public assistance, lack of transportation to and from a workplace, and lack of jobs perceived to provide flexible work schedules to accommodate adherence with prescribed medical treatment).

Employment Perspectives Study

In this study, members of our partnership attempted to gain further understanding of the perceived impact of employment among persons with HIV by conducting six focus groups with a total of 54 participants who self-identified as African–American/black and unemployed. Participants reported valuing employment; identified advantages (e.g., increasing one's ability to become self-sufficient, increasing self-esteem, and increasing social interaction) and disadvantages (e.g., exacerbating stress and work environments that stigmatize their HIV status and are not HIV sensitive) associated with employment; identified individuals influencing their decision to become employed (e.g., family and healthcare providers); and delineated facilitators (e.g., job-seeking and job-training skills and job accommodations) and impediments to employment (e.g., HIV discrimination in the workplace, loss of SSA benefits and other public assistance, and side effects of medications) [85].

Windows to Work

Members of our partnership decided that sufficient knowledge had been gained through the first two studies and that it was appropriate to initiate a project that had potential to improve the health and well-being of persons with HIV. The partnership chose to use photovoice, a method of inquiry closely aligned with CBPR, to further the understanding of the impact of employment for persons with HIV.

Photovoice is a qualitative research methodology founded on the principles of critical theory, constructivism, and documentary photography. Basically, critical theory focuses on exploring and intervening upon the social and economic inequalities and promotes system change, and constructivism defines learning through the individual's interactive process of developing and constructing meaning through experiences [41, 86, 103, 104]. The photovoice process involves a series of procedures that include the following [103]:

1. Identification of community topic of interest
2. Participant recruitment

3. Photovoice training
4. Camera distribution and instruction
5. Identification of photo assignments
6. Discussion of photo assignments
7. Data analysis
8. Identification of influential advocates (those who would be allies for change if their consciousness was raised)
9. Presentation of photovoice findings
10. Creation of plans of action for change

Through photovoice, participants photograph issues of concern and participate in group discussions about the photographs taken through empowerment-based facilitated dialogue. The process helps participants from the community to reflect on community needs, priorities, and strengths; engage in critical dialogue; share knowledge; and move toward collective action. The photovoice process typically includes a community forum for participants to share their experiences through their photographs and words. Representatives from community-based organizations and others who are identified by photovoice participants as potential partners (influential advocates) who might support participants after having their consciousness raised are invited to the forum to learn from photovoice participants. By design, influential advocates have some existing power and resources (e.g., job-based or political influence and skills) and may partner with photovoice participants to develop action plans based on needs, priorities, and spheres of influence [41, 86, 103].

Explicit within photovoice is group interaction through which participants are encouraged to discuss their photographs; respond to one another; ask questions; comment on one another's perspectives; and exchange anecdotes, experiences, and ideas. This methodology can identify pertinent variables and nuances that outside researchers may not otherwise be able to foresee and/or identify [86, 103]. Photovoice is well suited as a method within CBPR because it is highly participatory, is a research methodology, and explicitly moves toward action, which, again, is a hallmark of CBPR [86, 103, 105].

A total of 11 men with HIV with a history of full-time work but who were currently unemployed participated in the study. Nine of the participants self-identified as African-American/black and eight self-identified as gay. Participants identified 19 issues important to them when considering employment and grouped these issues into five categories: (1) advantages of employment (e.g., enabling financial responsibility, enabling one to provide for self and others, increasing social skills, and increasing self-esteem); (2) disadvantages of employment (e.g., assimilating into workplaces that are unfriendly to persons with HIV, not being able to adhere to prescribed medical treatment, and losing eligibility for some HIV-related services); (3) referents influencing their employment decisions (e.g., family and health-care providers); (4) facilitators of employment (e.g., motivation, job training, job-seeking skills, work clothing, and transportation to and from the workplace); and (5) impediments to employment (e.g., inability to adhere to prescribed medical treatment, lack of workplace accommodations, loss of Medicare coverage, and lack of HIV education in the workplace). Using their data and interpretations of findings, participants developed an action plan to become employed, which they titled the "Employment Decision-making Model for Persons with HIV/AIDS" (Fig. 10.1). As immediate results of participating in the Windows to Work study, four participants applied for SSA benefits and five explored the viability of the SSA Ticket-to-Work and Self-Sufficiency Program to become employed [106].

The Helping Overcome Problems Effectively (HOPE) Intervention

The process for developing the HOPE intervention was iterative and took several months. For the first few months, members of our partnership held a series of face-to-face meetings to build common understandings. Community representatives presented priorities and perspectives of persons with HIV; organization representatives presented issues affecting persons with HIV receiving services; and academic researchers presented relevant scientific literature and theory. Together, we reviewed the literature; shared the experiences that only community insiders (those living with and most closely affected by HIV) would know; discussed how approaches would be translated into actual intervention components and implementation practice (including activities); and reviewed efficacious interventions for persons with HIV based in health behavior, theory, and self-management. Because theory is intended to explain the processes involved in behavior change, understanding and integrating theory with perspectives on black gay men's experiences were crucial to making informed decisions about the intervention. We established a reciprocal co-learner relationship among community members, organization representatives, and academic researchers to share decision-making responsibilities and support the empowerment of the HIV community's ownership of the entire intervention development and research process.

Members of our partnership also conducted interviews with persons with HIV who were not part of the partnership to further identify strengths, assets, and challenges and to refine and validate partnership ideas for intervention. Partnership members analyzed the interview data. We identified African-American/black gay men with HIV as our priority group, and the results confirmed that employment was a priority among this community. This priority included the impact of employment as a social determinant of health.

We then decided to begin an iterative process to develop a theory-based, group-level intervention to address employment among persons with HIV. Our partnership agreed to base the intervention in social cognitive theory [107], HOPE theory [108], and self-management [37], and locally collected interview data that included the experiences of African-American/black gay men with HIV. To ensure greater cultural, contextual, and educational congruence, partnership members, including African-American/black gay men with HIV, were directly involved throughout development of the intervention and in designing its implementation and evaluation.

Seven unemployed African-American/black gay men with HIV participated in the study. The intervention comprised a 2-hour orientation session, a baseline assessment, seven weekly 3-hour interactive group sessions, and a 3-month postint-

Fig. 10.1 Employment
decision-making model for
persons with HIV/AIDS

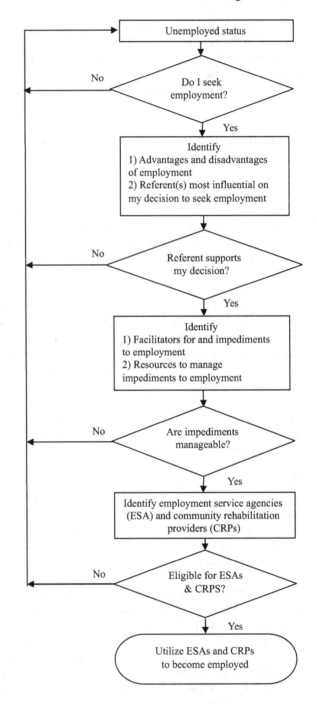

Table 10.2 SPARTAN model

*S*chedule your visit with your health-care provider
*P*lan your questions; log your symptoms on paper and take this with you
*A*sk your questions and present your symptom log to your health-care provider
*R*epeat the health-care provider's responses to each question and use a "check-out" phrase of "Is that right?" or "Did I hear you correctly?"
*T*ake notes and write the health-care provider's response to each question
*A*pply the information to create goals and action plans
*N*avigate through the health-care system with the new information to make informed decisions and better manage your health

ervention assessment with a structured interview. The weekly 3-hour intervention sessions were content specific (e.g., understanding HIV, working with medications, working with health-care providers, HIV tests and treatment, lifestyle management, and employment). Each session included modeling, vicarious learning, and verbal persuasion; exploring physiologic cues; modeling pathway thoughts and agency thoughts (from HOPE theory); and components of self-management. Each session concluded with participant feedback. Participants shared narrative accounts; identified life experiences in which they had successfully created and achieved goals by overcoming barriers; explored potential barriers to goals; and identified supports and resources to overcome barriers and achieve goals.

Members of our partnership also wrote, submitted, and were awarded a pilot grant to implement and evaluate the newly developed intervention. Evaluation of the intervention indicated that among a variety of study findings, participants reported significantly decreased anxiety, depression, and fatigue and increased self-efficacy, treatment adherence, self-esteem, physical activity, and job-seeking skills. Participants also created the SPARTAN model (explained in Table 10.2) to facilitate and enhance communication between persons with HIV and their health-care providers (Table 10.2). Participants reported that the use of the model improved communication with health-care providers and helped them better manage their health care and medical treatment. The results suggest that the HOPE intervention may be promising to enhance health outcomes of persons with HIV.

The successes of our CBPR research studies are attributed to the incorporation of the nine well-recognized principles of CBPR [90, 91, 93, 96, 105, 109]. Within our partnership, for example, we worked with the local HIV community as a unit of identity. Our partnership recognized and built on the strengths, assets, and skills that existed within this community. To address social inequities and share power, we engaged in and facilitated a collaborative and equitable partnership throughout the entire research process. African-American/black gay men with HIV were not merely reduced to intervention targets or recipients of intervention, they were actively involved and engaged in the research process and participated throughout. African-American/black gay men with HIV (as well as other persons with HIV), organization representatives, and academic researchers were involved in study conceptualization, study design and conduct, data analysis and interpretation, and dissemination of findings. All partners shared decision-making power and resources.

We also balanced research and action for the mutual benefit of all partners. As a partnership, we fostered multidirectional and co-learning among members to build capacity. We created transparent processes that embraced clear and open communication. When identifying priorities, we embraced the roles, norms, and processes evolving from the input and agreement of all partners. Building on each partner's strengths and assets, we developed, administered, analyzed, and interpreted study findings, while offering continual feedback among our partnership members. From the CBPR studies conducted, we distributed the findings and knowledge gained to all partners. All partners were involved in the dissemination of findings to community members, research and clinical audiences, and policy makers.

Our four CBPR studies have resulted in a long-term sustainability that has lasted for more than a decade, extending beyond a single research study or funding period, to further explore and intervene on the needs and priorities of persons with HIV in Washington, DC. We also contend that the ongoing work, commitment, and input from all partners have increased the authenticity of the study methods, the trustworthiness of findings, and the development of the most promising interventions possible to meet the needs and priorities while using approaches preferred by communities. Our partnership demonstrates that CBPR is a long-term process, sequentially building on these processes over time.

Community Engagement Lessons Learned

CBPR relies on community engagement and participation to identify community needs and priorities, promote the most accurate understanding of health phenomena, and ensure the development and implementation of meaningful actions or interventions that have the highest potential to improve community health and well-being. Furthermore, CBPR studies are more likely to occur in a culturally, contextually, and educationally congruent manner. Our partnership was able to blend various perspectives and experiences to yield more informed knowledge while building capacity of persons with HIV, organization representatives, and academic researchers. We have learned several lessons to better facilitate our own future CBPR studies and provide insight to other CBPR partnerships.

Time Invested is Substantial

Authentic CBPR partnerships require a substantial investment of time. It takes time to develop trust and build rapport, and over time, the strengths, values, and knowledge of all partners can be better identified, appreciated, and mutually harnessed.

Researchers Must Acknowledge Reflexivity and be Reflective

Often conflated, in this case, reflexivity is a position and reflectivity is a process; reflexivity is the recognition of a researcher being integral and part of what is being observed and integral to what is being studied; the researcher cannot be removed from the research. Reflectivity is the process of reflecting upon one's position as part of the research and one's assumptions and attitudes that influence not only what is known and how it is interpreted but what is occurring. Reflexivity recognizes that researchers affect what is being researched while reflectivity is understanding this impact, interpreting phenomenon in light of this fact. Thus, throughout our CBPR process, the academic researcher, in particular, had to be introspective to be conscious of reflexivity and willing to learn about the nature and essence of local HIV communities. The academic researcher also had to be keenly aware of possible bias toward identifying research questions that aligned with his areas of research that may not align with the priorities of persons with HIV or WWH staff. He had to ensure that his way of conducting research and generating knowledge and understanding did not overshadow other ways that may be more authentic to the community. Academic researchers must acknowledge, and work in a manner that recognizes and appreciates the importance that CBPR assigns to approaches to true community engagement as well as community priorities and community ways of "doing things" and interpreting what is learned.

Power May Not be Balanced

Imbalances of power commonly occur among community members, organization representatives, and academic researchers. When conducting partnership meetings, members did not contribute equally; some members were more vocal than others and tended to lead the decision-making process. We had to establish structures for participation to ensure that those voices that were less "loud" (i.e., less assertive) were heard. We also found it necessary to address groupthink during discussions and decision making [110]. Groupthink occurred when the desire to maintain good relationships became more important that reaching good decisions. During groupthink, input from outside resources may be ignored and decisions may be made without critical analysis. For us, groupthink occurred when there was no real or perceived immutable research timeline and when partners did not apply critical thinking skills.

Furthermore, in some partnerships, when a power differential among members exists because of differences (e.g., language, socioeconomic status, position, title, and level of education), true participation may be reduced to those powerful members who control the communication. Within CBPR, there will always be power differentials; one example is that academic partners often have terminal degrees (e.g., PhDs). Thus, these power differentials are likely to affect group cohesion because those with less power or perceived less power may refrain from authentic engagement and participation and/or those with similar statuses may interact with one another and form alliances, consciously or unconsciously excluding others. Members of our partnership agreed that while the desire to maintain good relationships was important, our "getting along" must not override the importance of reaching good decisions; in fact, we chose to embrace conflict as a form of quality improvement for the good of our research.

Broad Perspectives Should be Included in Review of Study Materials

Members of our partnership agreed that we would work together in teams to develop all study-related materials (e.g., grant applications, protocols, instruments, guides, manuals, and consent forms). Each team required representation from each of the categories of partnership members representing the HIV community, WWH, and GW. After development, all materials would be further validated by members from the broader partnership. At times, members of our partnership also consulted with others in the community (i.e., those who were not members of our partnership) to review materials that we thought needed further insight and/or validation; we recognize that members of our partnership may not always have all the expertise and insights needed as we develop, refine, enhance, and/or adapt materials. We contend that our approach of including diverse voices and perspectives enhanced the quality and content of materials, making them more meaningful and theoretically stronger and improving their scientific soundness. Clearly, materials developed in this manner are more culturally, contextually, and educationally congruent.

Engaging Organization Representatives is Valuable

We found that it was key to engage organization representatives (e.g., case managers and health-care providers) who interact directly with persons with HIV at the site where we recruited study participants. Our partnership met with case managers multiple times prior to each study for their guidance. These case managers did not want to join the partnership but wanted to help, and members of our partnership knew how important they would be to study success. They provided insights on how to more effectively recruit persons with HIV, including which incentives would be effective and where/when (e.g., location, day of week, and time of day) implementation of the intervention should be scheduled to ensure maximum recruitment, participation, and retention of participants.

Next Steps

Based on lessons learned from the pilot test, our partnership is refining the HOPE intervention, and we plan to more rigorously test the intervention among gay men with HIV. We are committed to continuing to involve community members, organization representatives, and academic researchers in all phases of our research to enhance its quality and validity. Currently, members of our partnership are preparing a randomized controlled trial (RCT) to compare mental health and employment outcomes among 50 gay men with HIV, including those in underrepresented ethnic/racial minority populations. Often it is assumed that communities do not want RCTs to be used; however, it has been shown that over time, as communities gain trust and understand how evidence can be used to improve community health and well-being, RCTs are not always out of the question [96].

Community Needs and Priorities Related to Employment

The four research studies conducted by our partnership have identified that persons with HIV have an interest in employment and a strong desire to become employed, and a priority for members of our partnership continues to be the effect of employment on the health and well-being of persons with HIV. More longitudinal studies that explore the effect of employment on the health of this population are clearly warranted.

Across our studies, members of our partnership identified four areas of need for persons with HIV to secure employment. These needs included: (1) education and training about job-seeking skills (e.g., identifying job vacancies, completing applications, creating a resume, and developing interviewing skills) to be competitive in the job market and workplace; (2) treatment adherence interventions; (3) instruction on how to request accommodations while employed, as a person meeting the criteria for disability under the Americans with Disabilities Act (ADA), to ensure that they feel comfortable and are able to adhere to prescribed medical treatment (e.g., requesting leave); and (4) information on the potential loss of public assistance (e.g., Supplemental Security Income, SSI, Social Security Disability Insurance, SSDI, and Temporary Assistance for Needy Families, TANF) while employed.

Concluding Thoughts on CBPR and the Health of Those with HIV

Although our partnership sets a priority on the effect of employment on health and well-being, we recognize that health status may impede employment. Members of our partnership are committed to further research to inform policy at the local and community and national levels to assist those who are able to be employable to have access to available resources and training. As we pursue this, we continue building partnerships to improve health outcomes among persons with HIV and disseminating our research findings to inform policy. We recognize the power of authentic (as opposed to token) engagement and participation of persons with HIV, organization representatives, and academic researchers throughout all phases of the research; working together and blending perspectives, ideas, insights, and experiences will better impact the lives of persons with HIV in our communities and beyond. We contend that our research questions have been more relevant to community needs and priorities and more insightful to action that promotes the health and well-being of persons with HIV. We also contend that CBPR has led to a more developed understanding of health phenomena within this highly vulnerable population and about a social determinant of health (i.e., employment in this population) that has been neglected to date. In fact, just as CBPR has evolved as an approach to reduce health disparities among vulnerable populations, employment is beginning to be recognized as a social determinant of health. Using CBPR as an underlying approach to research has profound potential to improve the lives of persons with HIV. Our partnership is an example of CBPR as a successful approach to community engagement and participation, and we are committed to our continued use of CBPR.

References

1. Lieb S, Prejean J, Thompson DR, Fallon SJ, Cooper H, Gates GJ, et al. Estimating HIV prevalence rates among racial/ethnic populations of men who have sex with men in the southern United States. J Urban Health. 2009;86(6):887–901.
2. Centers for Disease Control and Prevention. HIV Surveillance Report, 2011. Atlanta, GA: US Department of Health and Human Services; 2013.
3. Purcell DW, Johnson CH, Lansky A, Prejean J, Stein R, Denning P, et al. Estimating the population size of men who have sex with men in the United States to obtain HIV and syphilis rates. Open AIDS J. 2012;6:98–107.
4. Prejean J, Song R, Hernandez A, Ziebell R, Green T, Walker F, et al. Estimated HIV incidence in the United States, 2006–2009. PloS ONE. 2011;6(8):e17502.
5. Lansky A, Brooks JT, DiNenno E, Heffelfinger J, Hall HI, Mermin J. Epidemiology of HIV in the United States. J Acquir Immune Defic Syndr. 2010;55 (Suppl 2):S64–8.
6. Rhodes SD, Hergenrather KC, Wilkin AM, Wooldredge R. Adherence and HIV: a lifetime commitment. In: Shumaker SA, Ockene JK, Riekert K, editors. The handbook of health behavior change. 3rd ed. New York: Springer; 2009. p. 659–75.
7. Hergenrather KC, Rhodes SD, Clark G. Employment-seeking behavior of persons with HIV/AIDS: a theory-based approach. J Rehabil. 2004;70(4):21–30.
8. Nakagawa F, May M, Phillips A. Life expectancy living with HIV: recent estimates and future implications. Curr Opin Infect Dis. 2013;26(1):17–25.
9. Buchacz K, Baker RK, Palella FJ, Jr, Chmiel JS, Lichtenstein KA, Novak RM, et al. AIDS-defining opportunistic illnesses in US patients, 1994–2007: a cohort study. AIDS. 2010;24(10):1549–59.
10. Institute of Medicine. The health of lesbian, gay, bisexual, and transgender people: building a foundation for better understanding. Washington: National Academies Press; 2011.
11. Oursler KK, Goulet JL, Crystal S, Justice AC, Crothers K, Butt AA, et al. Association of age and comorbidity with physical function in HIV-infected and uninfected patients: results from the Veterans aging cohort study. AIDS Patient Care STDS. 2011;25(1):13–20.
12. Carr A, Samaras K, Thorisdottir A, Kaufmann GR, Chisholm DJ, Cooper DA. Diagnosis, prediction, and natural course of HIV-1 protease-inhibitor-associated lipodystrophy, hyperlipidaemia, and diabetes mellitus: a cohort study. Lancet. 1999;353(9170):209–39.
13. Lichtenstein KA, Armon C, Buchacz K, Chmiel JS, Buckner K, Tedaldi E, et al. Provider compliance with guidelines for management of cardiovascular risk in HIV-infected patients. Prev Chronic Dis. 2013;10:E10.
14. van Wijk JP, Cabezas MC. Hypertriglyceridemia, metabolic syndrome, and cardiovascular disease in HIV-infected patients: effects of antiretroviral therapy and adipose tissue distribution. Int J Vasc Med. 2012;2012:201027.
15. Panel on Antiretroviral Guidelines for Adults and Adolescents. Guidelines for the use of antiretroviral agents in HIV-1 infected adults and adolescents: Department of health and human services.

16. Thompson MA, Aberg JA, Hoy JF, Telenti A, Benson C, Cahn P, et al. Antiretroviral treatment of adult HIV infection: 2012 recommendations of the International Antiviral Society-USA panel. JAMA. 2012;308(4):387–402.
17. Klimas N, Koneru AO, Fletcher MA. Overview of HIV. Psychosom Med. 2008;70(5):523–30.
18. Boarts JM, Buckley-Fischer BA, Armelie AP, Bogart LM, Delahanty DL. The impact of HIV diagnosis-related vs. non-diagnosis related trauma on PTSD, depression, medication adherence, and HIV disease markers. J Evid-based Soc Work. 2009;6(1):41–6.
19. Boarts JM, Sledjeski EM, Bogart LM, Delahanty DL. The differential impact of PTSD and depression on HIV disease markers and adherence to HAART in people living with HIV. AIDS Behav. 2006;10(3):253–61.
20. Brief DJ, Bollinger AR, Vielhauer MJ, Berger-Greenstein JA, Morgan EE, Brady SM, et al. Understanding the interface of HIV, trauma, post-traumatic stress disorder, and substance use and its implications for health outcomes. AIDS Care. 2004;16 (Suppl 1):S97–120.
21. Keuroghlian AS, Kamen CS, Neri E, Lee S, Liu R, Gore-Felton C. Trauma, dissociation, and antiretroviral adherence among persons living with HIV/AIDS. J Psychiatr Res. 2011;45(7):942–8.
22. Joyce GF, Chan KS, Orlando M, Burnam MA. Mental health status and use of general medical services for persons with human immunodeficiency virus. Med Care. 2005;43(8):834–9.
23. Conyers LM. HIV/AIDS and employment research: a need for an integrative approach. Couns Psychol. 2008;36(1):108–17.
24. Conyers LM. Expanding understanding of HIV/AIDS and employment: perspectives from focus groups. Rehabil Couns Bull. 2004;48(1):51–8.
25. Pence BW, Miller WC, Whetten K, Eron JJ, Gaynes BN. Prevalence of DSM-IV-defined mood, anxiety, and substance use disorders in an HIV clinic in the Southeastern United States. J Acquir Immune Defic Syndr. 2006;42(3):298–306.
26. Fama R, Eisen JC, Rosenbloom MJ, Sassoon SA, Kemper CA, Deresinski S, et al. Upper and lower limb motor impairments in alcoholism, HIV infection, and their comorbidity. Alcohol Clin Exp Res. 2007;31(6):1038–44.
27. Lightfoot M, Rogers T, Goldstein R, Rotheram-Borus MJ, May S, Kirshenbaum S, et al. Predictors of substance use frequency and reductions in seriousness of use among persons living with HIV. Drug Alcohol Depend. 2005;77(2):129–38.
28. Achappa B, Madi D, Bhaskaran U, Ramapuram JT, Rao S, Mahalingam S. Adherence to antiretroviral therapy among people living with HIV. N Am J Med Sci. 2013;5(3):220–3.
29. Sherr L, Nagra N, Kulubya G, Catalan J, Clucas C, Harding R. HIV infection associated post-traumatic stress disorder and post-traumatic growth—a systematic review. Psychol Health Med. 2011;16(5):612–29.
30. Vranceanu AM, Safren SA, Lu M, Coady WM, Skolnik PR, Rogers WH, et al. The relationship of post-traumatic stress disorder and depression to antiretroviral medication adherence in persons with HIV. AIDS Patient Care STDS. 2008;22(4):313–21.
31. Ellis RJ, Calero P, Stockin MD. HIV infection and the central nervous system: a primer. Neuropsychol Rev. 2009;19(2):144–51.
32. Grant I. Neurocognitive disturbances in HIV. Int Rev Psychiatry (Abingdon, England). 2008;20(1):33–47.
33. Rabkin JG, McElhiney M, Ferrando SJ, Van Gorp W, Lin SH. Predictors of employment of men with HIV/AIDS: a longitudinal study. Psychosom Med. 2004;66(1):72–8.
34. Taylor DN. Effects of a behavioral stress-management program on anxiety, mood, self-esteem, and T-cell count in HIV positive men. Psychol Rep. 1995;76(2):451–7.
35. Scott-Sheldon LA, Kalichman SC, Carey MP, Fielder RL. Stress management interventions for HIV+ adults: a meta-analysis of randomized controlled trials, 1989–2006. Health Psychol. 2008;27(2):129–39.
36. Smith SR, Rublein JC, Marcus C, Brock TP, Chesney MA. A medication self-management program to improve adherence to HIV therapy regimens. Patient Educ Couns. 2003;50(2):187–99.

37. Barlow J, Wright C, Sheasby J, Turner A, Hainsworth J. Self-management approaches for people with chronic conditions: a review. Patient Educ Couns. 2002;48(2):177–87.
38. Barlow J, Turner A, Swaby L, Gilchrist M, Wright C, Doherty M. An 8-yr follow-up of arthritis self-management programme participants. Rheumatology (Oxford, England). 2009;48(2):128–33.
39. Granich R, Williams B, Montaner J. Fifteen million people on antiretroviral treatment by 2015: treatment as prevention. Curr Opin HIV AIDS. 2013;8(1):41–9.
40. Emamzadeh-Fard S, Fard SE, SeyedAlinaghi S, Paydary K. Adherence to anti-retroviral therapy and its determinants in HIV/AIDS patients: a review. Infect Disord Drug Targets. 2012;12(5):346–56.
41. Rhodes SD. Visions and voices: HIV in the 21st century. Indigent persons living with HIV/AIDS in the southern USA use photovoice to communicate meaning. J Epidemiol Community Health. 2006;60(10):886.
42. Bontempi JM, Burleson L, Lopez MH. HIV medication adherence programs: the importance of social support. J Community Health Nurs. 2004;21(2):111–22.
43. Golin C, Isasi F, Bontempi JB, Eng E. Secret pills: HIV-positive patients' experiences taking antiretroviral therapy in North Carolina. AIDS Educ Prev. 2002;14(4):318–29.
44. Horvath KJ, Michael Oakes J, Simon Rosser BR, Danilenko G, Vezina H, Rivet Amico K, et al. Feasibility, acceptability and preliminary efficacy of an online peer-to-peer social support ART adherence intervention. AIDS Behav. 2013;17(6):2031–44.
45. Cene CW, Akers AY, Lloyd SW, Albritton T, Powell Hammond W, Corbie-Smith G. Understanding social capital and HIV risk in rural African American communities. J Gen Intern Med. 2011;26(7):737–44.
46. Nel A, Kagee A. Common mental health problems and antiretroviral therapy adherence. AIDS Care. 2011;23(11):1360–5.
47. Cable N, Sacker A, Bartley M. The effect of employment on psychological health in mid-adulthood: findings from the 1970 British cohort study. J Epidemiol Community Health. 2008;62(5):e10.
48. Bartley M. Unemployment and ill health: understanding the relationship. J Epidemiol Community Health. 1994;48(4):33–37.
49. Cho E, Chan K. The financial impact of employment decisions for individuals with HIV. Work. 2013;44(4):383–91.
50. Jin RL, Shah CP, Svoboda TJ. The impact of unemployment on health: a review of the evidence. CMAJ. 1995;153(5):529–40.
51. Cornelius LR, van der Klink JJ, Groothoff JW, Brouwer S. Prognostic factors of long term disability due to mental disorders: a systematic review. J Occup Rehabil. 2011;21(2):259–74.
52. Martikainen PT, Valkonen T. Excess mortality of unemployed men and women during a period of rapidly increasing unemployment. Lancet. 1996;348(9032):909–12.
53. Oliffe JL, Han CS. Beyond workers' compensation: men's mental health in and out of work. Am J Mens Health. 2014;8(1):45–53.
54. Olesen SC, Butterworth P, Leach LS, Kelaher M, Pirkis J. Mental health affects future employment as job loss affects mental health: findings from a longitudinal population study. BMC Psychiatry. 2013;13(1):144.
55. Pelzer B, Schaffrath S, Vernaleken I. Coping with unemployment: the impact of unemployment on mental health, personality, and social interaction skills. Work 2013(Mar 26). doi: Q334417221662457 (To be published).
56. Rueda S, Chambers L, Wilson M, Mustard C, Rourke SB, Bayoumi A, et al. Association of returning to work with better health in working-aged adults: a systematic review. Am J Public Health. 2012;102(3):541–56.
57. Kasl SV, Rodriguez E, Lasch KE. The impact of unemployment on health and well-being. In: Dohrenwend BP, editor. Adversity, stress, and psychopathology. New York: Oxford University Press; 1998. p. 111–31.

58. Price RH, Choi JN, Vinokur AD. Links in the chain of adversity following job loss: how financial strain and loss of personal control lead to depression, impaired functioning, and poor health. J Occup Health Psychol. 2002;7(4):302–12.
59. Burgoyne RW, Saunders DS. Quality of life among urban Canadian HIV/AIDS clinic outpatients. Int J STD AIDS. 2001;12(8):505–12.
60. Hammarstrom A, Janlert U. Early unemployment can contribute to adult health problems: results from a longitudinal study of school leavers. J Epidemiol Community Health. 2002;56(8):624–30.
61. Gifford AL, Laurent DD, Gonzales VM, Chesney MA, Lorig KR. Pilot randomized trial of education to improve self-management skills of men with symptomatic HIV/AIDS. J Acquir Immune Defic Syndr Hum Retrovirol. 1998;18(2):136–44.
62. Sorlie PD, Rogot E. Mortality by employment status in the national longitudinal mortality study. Am J Epidemiol. 1990;132(5):983–92.
63. Morris JK, Cook DG, Shaper AG. Loss of employment and mortality. BMJ. 1994;308(6937):113–59.
64. Rueda S, Raboud J, Plankey M, Ostrow D, Mustard C, Rourke SB, et al. Labor force participation and health-related quality of life in HIV-positive men who have sex with men: the Multicenter AIDS Cohort Study. AIDS Behav. 2012;16(8):2350–60.
65. Bernell SL, Shinogle JA. The relationship between HAART use and employment for HIV-positive individuals: an empirical analysis and policy outlook. Health Policy (Amsterdam, Netherlands). 2005;71(2):255–64.
66. Fogarty AS, Zablotska I, Rawstorne P, Prestage G, Kippax SC. Factors distinguishing employed from unemployed people in the positive health study. AIDS. 2007;21(Suppl 1):S37–42.
67. Albert SM, Marder K, Dooneief G, Bell K, Sano M, Todak G, et al. Neuropsychologic impairment in early HIV infection. A risk factor for work disability. Arch Neurol. 1995;52(5):525–30.
68. Blank MB, Mandell DS, Aiken L, Hadley TR. Co-occurrence of HIV and serious mental illness among medicaid recipients. Psychiatr Serv. 2002;53(7):868–73.
69. Bing EG, Burnam MA, Longshore D, Fleishman JA, Sherbourne CD, London AS, et al. Psychiatric disorders and drug use among human immunodeficiency virus-infected adults in the United States. Arch Gen Psychiatry. 2001;58(8):721–8.
70. Dray-Spira R, Gueguen A, Persoz A, Deveau C, Lert F, Delfraissy JF, et al. Temporary employment, absence of stable partnership, and risk of hospitalization or death during the course of HIV infection. J Acquir Immune Defic Syndr. 2005;40(2):190–7.
71. Heckman TG, Kochman A, Sikkema KJ, Kalichman SC, Masten J, Bergholte J, et al. A pilot coping improvement intervention for late middle-aged and older adults living with HIV/AIDS in the USA. AIDS Care. 2001;13(1):129–39.
72. Kelly B, Raphael B, Judd F, Perdices M, Kernutt G, Burnett P, et al. Suicidal ideation, suicide attempts, and HIV infection. Psychosomatics. 1998;39(5):405–15.
73. Rhodes SD, Daniel J, Song EY, Alonzo J, Downs M, Reboussin BA. Social support among immigrant Latino men: a validation study. Am J Health Behav. 2013;37(5):620–8.
74. Heaney CA, Israel BA. Social networks and social support. In: Glanz K, Rimer BK, Lewis FM, editors. Health behavior and health education: theory, research and practice. 4th ed. San Francisco: Jossey-Bass; 2008. p. 189–210.
75. Israel BA. Social networks and health status: linking theory, research, and practice. Patient Couns Health Educ. 1982;4(2):65–79.
76. Shumaker SA, Hill DR. Gender differences in social support and physical health. Health Psychol. 1991;10(2):102–11.
77. Eng PM, Rimm EB, Fitzmaurice G, Kawachi I. Social ties and change in social ties in relation to subsequent total and cause-specific mortality and coronary heart disease incidence in men. Am J Epidemiol. 2002;155(8):700–9.
78. Barger SD. Social integration, social support and mortality in the US national health interview survey. Psychosom Med. 2013;75(5):510–7.

79. Cohen S, Gottlieb BH, Underwood LG. Social relationships and health. In: Cohen S, Underwood LG, Gottlieb BH, editors. Social support measurement and intervention: a guide for health and social scientists. New York: Oxford University Press; 2000. p. 32–5.
80. Martin DJ, Arns PG, Batterham PJ, Afifi AA, Steckart MJ. Workforce reentry for people with HIV/AIDS: intervention effects and predictors of success. Work (Reading, Mass). 2006;27(3):221–33.
81. Hays RB, Turner H, Coates TJ. Social support, AIDS-related symptoms, and depression among gay men. J Consult Clin Psychol. 1992;60(3):463–9.
82. Seedat S. Interventions to improve psychological functioning and health outcomes of HIV-infected individuals with a history of trauma or PTSD. Curr HIV/AIDS Rep. 2012;9(4):344–50.
83. McIntosh RC, Rosselli M. Stress and coping in women living with HIV: a meta-analytic review. AIDS Behav. 2012;16(8):2144–59.
84. Young J, De Geest S, Spirig R, Flepp M, Rickenbach M, Furrer H, et al. Stable partnership and progression to AIDS or death in HIV infected patients receiving highly active antiretroviral therapy: Swiss HIV cohort study. BMJ. 2004;328(7430):15.
85. Hergenrather KC, Rhodes SD, Clark G. The employment perspectives study: identifying factors influencing the job-seeking behavior of persons living with HIV/AIDS. AIDS Educ Prev. 2005;17(2):131–42.
86. Rhodes SD, Hergenrather KC, Wilkin AM, Jolly C. Visions and voices: indigent persons living With HIV in the southern United States use photovoice to create knowledge, develop partnerships, and take action. Health Promot Pract. 2008;9(2):159–69.
87. US Social Security Administration. Social security administration operational plan for implementing the national HIV/AIDS strategy. http://aidsgov/federal-resources/national-hiv-aids-strategy/nhas-operational-plan-ssapdf (2010).
88. Institute of Medicine. HIV and disability: updating the social security listings. Washington: The National Academies Press; 2010.
89. Israel BA, Lichtenstein R, Lantz P, McGranaghan R, Allen A, Guzman JR, et al. The detroit community-academic urban research center: development, implementation, and evaluation. J Public Health Manag Pract. 2001;7(5):11–9.
90. Israel BA, Schulz AJ, Parker EA, Becker AB. Review of community-based research: assessing partnership approaches to improve public health. Annu Rev Public Health. 1998;19:17320–2.
91. Rhodes SD, Hergenrather KC, Vissman AT, Stowers J, Davis AB, Hannah A, et al. Boys must be men, and men must have sex with women: a qualitative CBPR study to explore sexual risk among African American, Latino, and white gay men and MSM. Am J Mens Health. 2011;5(2):140–51.
92. Hergenrather KC, Rhodes SD. Community-based participatory research: applications for research in health and disability. In: Knoll T, editor. Focus on disability: trends in research and application. New York: Nova Science; 2008. p. 59–87.
93. Rhodes SD. Demonstrated effectiveness and potential of CBPR for preventing HIV in Latino populations. In: Organista KC, editor. HIV prevention with Latinos: theory, research, and practice. New York: Oxford University Press; 2012. p. 8310–2.
94. Minkler M. Community-based research partnerships: challenges and opportunities. J Urban Health. 2005;82(2 Suppl 2):ii31–2.
95. Reece M, Dodge B. A study in sexual health applying the principles of community-based participatory research. Arch Sex Behav. 2004;33(3):235–47.
96. Rhodes SD, Duck S, Alonzo J, Downs M, Aronson RE. Intervention trials in community-based participatory research. In: Blumenthal D, DiClemente RJ, Braithwaite RL, Smith S, editors. Community-based participatory research: issues, methods, and translation to practice. New York: Springer; 2013. p. 157–80.
97. Rhodes SD, Malow RM, Jolly C. Community-based participatory research: a new and not-so-new approach to HIV/AIDS prevention, care, and treatment. AIDS Educ Prev. 2010;22(3):173–83.

98. Rhodes SD, Kelley C, Simán F, Cashman R, Alonzo J, Wellendorf T, et al. Using community-based participatory research (CBPR) to develop a community-level HIV prevention intervention for Latinas: a local response to a global challenge. Womens Health Issues. 2012;22(3):293–301.

99. Rhodes SD, Eng E, Hergenrather KC, Remnitz IM, Arceo R, Montano J, et al. Exploring Latino men's HIV risk using community-based participatory research. Am J Health Behav. 2007;31(2):146–58.

100. Viswanathan M, Eng E, Ammerman A, Gartlehner G, Lohr KN, Griffith D, et al. Community-based participatory research: assessing the evidence. Evidence report/technology assessment. Rockville, MD: Agency for Healthcare Research and Quality, 2004 July. Report No.: 99.

101. Rhodes SD, Vissman AT, Stowers J, Miller C, McCoy TP, Hergenrather KC, et al. A CBPR partnership increases HIV testing among men who have sex with men (MSM): outcome findings from a pilot test of the CyBER/testing internet intervention. Health Educ Behav. 2011;38(3):311–20.

102. Rhodes SD, Daniel J, Alonzo J, Duck S, Garcia M, Downs M, et al. A systematic community-based participatory approach to refining an evidence-based community-level intervention: the HOLA intervention for Latino men who have sex with men. Health Promot Pract. 2013;14(4):6071–6.

103. Hergenrather KC, Rhodes SD, Cowan CA, Bardhoshi G, Pula S. Photovoice as community-based participatory research: a qualitative review. Am J Health Behav. 2009;33(6):686–98.

104. Rhodes SD, Hergenrather KC. Recently arrived immigrant Latino men identify community approaches to promote HIV prevention. Am J Public Health. 2007;97(6):984–5.

105. Israel BA, Eng E, Schulz AJ, Parker EA. Introduction to methods in community-based participatory research for health. In: Israel BA, Eng E, Schulz AJ, Parker EA, editors. Methods in community-based participatory research. San Francisco: Jossey-Bass; 2005.

106. Hergenrather KC, Rhodes SD, Clark G. Windows to Work: Exploring employment-seeking behaviors of persons with HIV/AIDS through photovoice. AIDS Educ Prev. 2006;18(3):243–58.

107. Bandura A. Social foundations of thought and action: a social cognitive theory. Englewood Cliffs: Prentice-Hall; 1986.

108. Snyder C. Hypothesis: There is hope. In: Snyder CR, editor. Handbook of hope: theory, measures and application. San Diego: Academic; 2000. p. 32–4.

109. Rhodes SD. The influence of perceived parental monitoring and perceived peer norms on the risk behaviors of African American seventh-grade intervention participants [Doctoral Dissertation]. Birmingham: University of Alabama at Birmingham; 2001.

110. Janis IL. Groupthink. In: Blumberg HH, Hare AP, Kent V, Davies MF, editors. Small groups and social interaction. New York: Wiley; 1982. p. 39–46.

Chapter 11
Dissemination, Implementation, and Adaptation of Evidence-based Behavioral HIV-Prevention Interventions Through Community Engagement: The US Centers for Disease Control and Prevention (CDC) Experience

Charles B. Collins and Hank L. Tomlinson

HIV continues to pose a serious global threat, and prevention has historically been a primary strategy for reducing the incidence of HIV in the USA. It is estimated that prevention efforts have averted more than 350,000 new HIV infections in the USA over the past 15 years [1]. Since 2002, a major dissemination and implementation project supported by scientists and practitioners at the US Centers for Disease Control and Prevention (CDC) has disseminated evidence-based prevention interventions into community-based prevention practice [2]. Health departments, community-based organizations, and medical settings that provide HIV-prevention services have received evidence-based behavioral intervention curricula and technical support to implement these interventions with fidelity so as to achieve significant reductions in HIV transmission risk behaviors and significant increases in protective behaviors [3]. The CDC's Diffusion of Effective Behavioral Interventions (DEBI) Project has been key to this broad community-based dissemination of evidence-based interventions. Details about the DEBI Project have been published, and the project has received thoughtful critique in the peer-reviewed literature, often with questions about the extent to which principles of community engagement and collaboration have guided key processes associated with the project's dissemination efforts [4–10]. In this chapter, we review the history of this CDC initiative and address specific issues around community engagement and collaboration that underlie this important national dissemination effort.

C. B. Collins (✉)
Division of HIV/AIDS Prevention, National Center for HIV, Hepatitis, STD, and TB Prevention, Centers for Disease Control and Prevention, 1600 Clifton Rd. NE, MS E-40, Atlanta, GA 30333, USA
e-mail: cwc4@cdc.gov

H. L. Tomlinson
Division of HIV/AIDS Prevention, National Center for HIV, Hepatitis, STD, and TB Prevention, Centers for Disease Control and Prevention, 1600 Clifton Rd. NE, MS E-40, Atlanta, GA 30333, USA
e-mail: chjg7@cdc.gov

S. D. Rhodes (ed.), *Innovations in HIV Prevention Research and Practice through Community Engagement*, DOI 10.1007/978-1-4939-0900-1_11, © Springer Science+Business Media New York 2014

The CDC Division of HIV/AIDS Prevention's Research-to-Practice Model

The CDC Division of HIV/AIDS employs a research-to-practice model that involves several key steps:

1. Primary behavioral science research on promising behavioral interventions to reduce risk
2. Meta-analysis and research synthesis to identify interventions with the highest levels of efficacy for changing HIV risk behaviors
3. Translations of that research into user-friendly implementation materials
4. Dissemination of the translated intervention resource materials through educational resource distribution, training, and technical assistance
5. Implementation of the interventions under real-world conditions with at-risk populations
6. Evaluation of the reach and outcomes of such program implementation

The DEBI Project was initiated in response to a report by the Institute of Medicine that urged CDC scientists and practitioners to take the lead to transfer evidence-based HIV-prevention research to community-prevention practice to reduce the public health burden of HIV [11]. This report reflected a growing trend in public health and medicine toward evidence-based prevention practice [12, 13]. An assumption in the Institute of Medicine recommendation is that evidence-based interventions that are found to be efficacious at changing risk behaviors or increasing protective behaviors within research contexts are a better choice for implementation within community-practice settings such as health departments, community-based organizations, and other medical settings than interventions with no evidence of efficacy, including interventions that have not been evaluated and those that have been evaluated but not found to be efficacious [11].

Thus, CDC scientists and practitioners established evidence-based standards for best practice in HIV prevention and began the ongoing work of identifying and disseminating evidence-based HIV-prevention behavioral interventions that meet those standards. CDC scientists select interventions for dissemination through the DEBI Project from those interventions identified through research synthesis and meta-analysis that meet specific efficacy criteria defined by the CDC Prevention Research Synthesis (PRS) Project [14, 15]. Interventions disseminated by the DEBI Project must meet "best or good evidence" criteria, including testing of the interventions through a randomized controlled trial (RCT) and positive, statistically significant effects at reducing an HIV-transmission behavior or increasing an HIV-protective behavior. The interventions also should have no negative effects. This approach supports the assumption that RCT-tested interventions have benefits over interventions that have not been evaluated or found to not be efficacious [16]. Locally developed programs that have been evaluated and meet the CDC's criteria for best or good evidence are eligible for dissemination through the DEBI Project.

As of August 2011, 74 risk-reduction interventions were included in CDC's *Compendium of Evidence-based HIV Behavioral Interventions*. This Compendium includes interventions that emerged from the PRS Project process. Currently, the Compendium includes two chapters. Briefly, the first chapter outlines risk-reduction interventions (e.g., interventions designed to reduce sexual initiation and/or increase condom use) and the second chapter focuses on interventions that address medication adherence. Information about the development of the Compendium and the included interventions is available online   (www.cdc.gov/hiv/topics/research/prs/compendium-evidence-based-interventions.htm).

Determinations about which interventions should be disseminated as part of the DEBI Project are based on both exigent public health needs (e.g., a lack of interventions for members of a particularly vulnerable or high-risk group) and likelihood of uptake by health departments, community-based organizations, and other medical settings. Interventions more likely to be used tend to be those that have fewer sessions, require less training of staff, appeal to organization staff as well as to the target populations, and are affordable. The increased number of evidence-based behavioral interventions in the Compendium reflects the state of the science, whereas selections for dissemination reflect, in part, messages received from staff from community-based organizations about what works in real-world settings, what is compatible with existing practices, and what reflects the needs of the communities they serve.

After an intervention is selected for dissemination through the DEBI Project, toolkits, based on these select evidence-based interventions, are developed and "packaged" by the CDC Replicating Effective Programs (REP) Project [17]. During the REP process, an intervention identified as efficacious is implemented with fidelity in one or more sites different from the original research site so that implementation tools to facilitate replication are field tested and then "translated" into user-friendly products. This development of field-tested implementation tools for those who will replicate the intervention in the future has been referred to as a "packaged intervention." Each new replication site must establish a community advisory group to engage the community and seek guidance on contextual fit of the intervention into the new replication site. Throughout the replication process, each community advisory group offers feedback on the usefulness of the materials developed in real-world implementation. Because most of the interventions identified by the PRS Project and packaged by REP were based on a single efficacy trial, the steps of replicating implementation with the involvement of a community advisory group help ensure that implementation materials are generalizable beyond the original research sites and have utility and feasibility when used for replicating the implementation of an intervention. The selected interventions that are translated and packaged by REP are then disseminated through the DEBI Project [2].

The DEBI Project

In 2002, the CDC Division of HIV/AIDS Prevention (DHAP) embarked on the DEBI Project to enhance the capacity of health departments, community-based organizations, and medical settings to adopt, appropriately adapt, and implement evidence-based behavioral interventions. The DEBI Project is the largest coordinated effort to disseminate evidence-based HIV behavioral interventions in the USA and was designed to ensure that efficacious evidence-based HIV-prevention interventions are widely available to, and implemented by, staff in the aforementioned settings. Within the CDC DHAP, the Capacity Building Branch (CBB) designs and implements the DEBI Project. Currently, 31 behavioral interventions are included in the CBB dissemination portfolio. These interventions were selected from the 74 interventions included in the Compendium, eight of which have been translated into Spanish. Staff at more than 5,000 prevention agencies in the USA have been trained on these interventions, and prevention resource materials have been provided to prevention workers in 127 countries.

The DEBI Project increases use of evidence-based approaches to HIV prevention and increases knowledge utilization by front-line HIV-prevention providers. Thus, those of us working within the DEBI Project at CDC encourage both the utilization of the interventions we disseminate as well as a better understanding of the complexities of changing human behavior.

Information on these interventions is available for community use via a CDC-supported website (http://www.effectiveinterventions.org). The interventions are diverse in terms of target populations (e.g., race, ethnicity, gender, and sexual orientation), intervention settings (e.g., sexually transmitted disease, STD, clinic, drug treatment program, and county jail), and HIV risk behaviors addressed. The target populations in evidence-based interventions include high-risk groups, such as sexually active youth, men who have sex with men (MSM), sexually active heterosexual women, injection-drug users, and HIV-positive persons. The behavioral goals of the evidence-based interventions focus primarily on condom use and other HIV-risk-reduction activities (e.g., injection drug use and inadequate medication adherence). More than 20,000 staff from US health departments, community-based organizations, and other medical settings have been trained in the use of one or more of the interventions disseminated through the DEBI Project [2, 3]. Since its launch in 2002, the DEBI Project has changed the landscape of HIV-prevention services in the USA by providing a systematic approach to reducing the impact of HIV [10].

Community Engagement in the Development, Implementation, and Evaluation of Evidence-based Interventions

There has been some concern regarding the extent to which the DEBI Project, and CDC's research-to-practice model more generally, may have inadvertently eliminated the potential for locally developed interventions to meet the identified local needs and priorities to reduce HIV infections [9]. We offer this case study to illustrate how the dissemination process has embraced locally developed interventions when sufficient strength of efficacy is demonstrated or when there is a gap in the dissemination portfolio.

About 10 years ago, CDC leaders wanted to issue a funding announcement to fund community-based organizations to implement evidence-based behavioral interventions for black MSM, a group significantly affected by the HIV epidemic [18]. In planning that funding and dissemination process, the staff from the PRS Project noted that insufficient evidence-based interventions were available for African-American/black MSM, despite the fact that this population is the most highly affected by HIV in the USA. Thus, a reputationally strong, locally developed intervention for African-American/black MSM, known as Many Men, Many Voices, was selected for dissemination along with other interventions [19]. Many Men, Many Voices was developed by a community-based organization that served African-American/black MSM in Rochester, NY; staff were convinced that the intervention was effective based on their ongoing implementation of the intervention. The intervention also had been identified by administrators within the New York State Health Department as being strong. The community-based organization engaged the consultation services of the Rochester STD/HIV Prevention Training Center to assist with the design, implementation, and evaluation of the intervention. Staff from the Prevention Training Center consulted with teams from around the country that developed efficacious community-based HIV-prevention interventions for other MSM populations. These teams included scientists, practitioners, and community members who had developed, implemented, evaluated, and participated in the Popular Opinion Leader intervention [20] and the Mpowerment intervention [21]. The experiences of these teams further informed the process of intervention design and content. Funds were then allocated to simultaneously test the efficacy of the intervention while dissemination efforts moved forward. The willingness of CDC to include in the DEBI Project, as special exceptions, interventions without typical demonstrations of efficacy—Many Men Many Voices at the time of its inclusion in 2004 (though later demonstrated to be efficacious) and d-up: Defend Yourself!, a cultural adaptation of the Popular Opinion Leader intervention—was a direct response to community priorities and community solutions to an ongoing challenge [19, 20, 22]. Although the methods for diffusion may be perceived to be top–down, these examples provide evidence of the direct connections and feedback loops among community members, practitioners, advocates, and decision-makers at all levels at CDC.

Community Engagement Principles and Processes for Dissemination

The implementation of the DEBI Project requires adherence to key principles and processes associated with the community engagement and collaboration process. In the following sections, we identify five principles and processes and outline how they are implemented in the DEBI Project.

Dissemination Must Work Within a Context of Community Needs and Priorities

Does an entire community define its own problems and priorities or do key community stakeholders with vested interests define the problems and priorities? Do the key stakeholders embrace and utilize empirically derived evidence, epidemiologic data, or sound behavioral theory, or do they have a vested interest in prioritization of issues and possible solutions that fit their ideology or direct resources to them or their constituency? These are not easy questions to answer, as various communities are represented or not represented by a range of formal and informal structures.

There may be communities that follow purely democratic principles in which all voices are heard and have equal weight and influence on the final decisions for the community. Some communities hold regular town meetings of all citizens, and all citizens define problems, debate the definitions and determinants of those problems, gather credible evidence to support setting priorities for the problems, and then move forward with implementation of solutions to the problems according to their priority [23, 24]. In the realm of public health, this scenario, however, is rare. Delivery of public health services requires some specialized knowledge of empirical ways to define the problem using surveillance and epidemiologically derived data and specialized knowledge of innovations or technology-enhanced strategies to address the problem. In general, community members by themselves may lack expertise in the use of public health practitioners' tools for identifying problems as well as knowledge of state-of-the-science programs to address those problems. For the implementation of public health programs to be successful, key elements must be in place:

- Community enthusiasm
- Agreement with the definition of the problem
- Agreement with the identified determinants of risk or factors contributing to the problem
- Motivation to invest resources into a solution
- Agreement on the potential solution

All of these elements are included under the broad category of community engagement and collaboration.

The US government invests in public health infrastructure to protect our citizens. Communities are not asked to hold town meetings around childhood vaccinations, clean water, and food-processing inspections. Thus, there may be a continuum of engagement between the public health infrastructure and the community. Most community-based public health programs, including HIV-prevention interventions and programs, fall somewhere on this continuum between complete control by either the community or the public health infrastructure. In fact, public health programs typically include the use of public health-specific knowledge and technology in combination with community engagement and collaboration.

There are certain underpinning assumptions that the DEBI Project follows in dissemination and implementation of evidence-based interventions. These assumptions include:

1. A belief that interventions demonstrated to be efficacious in controlled trials have the potential to bring about greater HIV-risk reduction than interventions with no evidence of efficacy [25].
2. An understanding that in a time of limited resources devoted to public health, it is more cost effective to reduce HIV incidence by implementation of evidence-based interventions than unproven interventions [26].
3. An appreciation that because evidence-based interventions were developed by highly sophisticated and well-funded academic researchers, most had considerable community engagement, partnership, and collaboration in or with communities in which the interventions were tested, thus increasing the potential for generalization to other settings and populations.
4. A recognition that changing human behavior is not easy and that a body of research around behavior change indicates that core constructs outlined in the behavioral science literature should be harnessed to bring about reductions in risk behaviors and increases in protective behaviors [27, 28].

These assumptions do not imply that the public health field and those working in public health hold all the cards and that a community holds none. In fact, without community engagement and collaboration, there would be no interventions ready for dissemination and dissemination would not be possible. The local public health infrastructure and resources and the goodwill of community-based organizations are key to making dissemination of evidence-based HIV prevention possible.

Although interventions demonstrated to be efficacious are perceived to be the better choice for implementation, some community members have noted that locally developed interventions did not have the opportunity (e.g., resources) to be tested with the rigor of the evidence-based interventions identified by the PRS Project. If tested, however, these locally developed interventions may have proved to be just as efficacious as those in the peer-reviewed research literature. The CDC responded to this concern at the capacity-building, training, and funding policy levels.

In regard to our capacity-building response, we worked with communities to build evaluation capacity to detect intervention effects. Often, community stakeholders indicated that interventions were effective but lacked data to support their assertions. Thus, we worked with staff from health departments, community-based organizations, and other medical settings from across the country to help them move through steps to build their evaluation capacity, including the key steps of outlining and detailing the intervention activities, describing the target audience for the intervention, drawing the causal mechanism(s) for the intervention with a logic model, monitoring the number of persons who enroll and then complete an intervention, and detecting change in risk behaviors for those who completed the intervention with preintervention and postintervention measures. To some, these steps may sound elementary, but we found many locally developed programs that had challenges at various steps. Staff from health departments, community-based organizations, and other medical settings were encouraged to continue to build evaluation capacity and to report behavioral outcomes to funders, including the CDC. Furthermore, having a solid and common foundation was identified by these staff as a requisite to capacity building. Because of the costs associated with RCTs to rigorously establish efficacy, a locally developed intervention would have to demonstrate significant behavior change in basic pretest and posttest monitoring before a control group comparison should be considered.

To support the evaluation of locally developed interventions, we encouraged staff from health departments, community-based organizations, and other medical settings to take trainings offered by the five national CDC-funded STD/HIV Prevention Training Centers on behavior change, behavioral theory, and intervention design. We have learned that the complexity of changing human risk behaviors is not always understood or appreciated by community-based stakeholders [28]. Locally developed interventions often lack important intervention components and activities demonstrated to reduce HIV risk (e.g., role plays of safer-sex negotiation). Moreover, locally developed interventions sometimes lack sufficient dosage to change behavior. Capacity building and technical assistance supports the work of implementation staff so that the locally developed program can be strengthened by inclusion of key activities and supported by behavior change research and theories that increase the probability of reduced risk behaviors or increased protective behaviors. This approach ensures that scientific expertise is blended with local knowledge.

At the policy and funding levels, the CDC has issued program-funding announcements seeking to test locally developed interventions. Through this mechanism, several interventions that were locally developed were identified as meeting the best evidence criteria of the Compendium [19, 22, 29, 30].

Technology Transfer Becomes Technology Exchange Through Co-learning

Co-learning is a concept that covers the exchange of information and experiential knowledge [31]. Training, resources, and technical assistance are offered as part of the DEBI Project's contribution to the co-learning process [32]. Efforts have also been made to learn from community experiences implementing evidence-based interventions so as to provide needed and meaningful capacity building and technical assistance resources, to design new behavioral interventions, and to learn more about the steps that health departments, community-based organizations, and other medical settings take to implement an evidence-based intervention that was not developed locally. During each DEBI Project training of intervention facilitators (the training that supports the implementation of a particular intervention being disseminated by the DEBI Project), the underlying behavior-change theory is discussed so that implementation staff understand the basis of the intervention activities. We have learned that both buy-in and fidelity increases when organizational staff understands why certain activities are included in the intervention and how the interplay of intervention activities is designed to reduce risk and increase protective behaviors [28]. Furthermore, much can be learned about the implementation process by monitoring delivery of an evidence-based intervention under real-world conditions.

Recruitment and Retention Success Depends on Community Insights

Recruitment into and retention in the intervention are essential for successful implementation. Implementation staff must use their knowledge of the target population and community to determine and implement the appropriate incentives and messages to both recruit and retain the target population in the intervention [33]. The incentives for participating in an evidence-based intervention tend to vary from community to community and may change over time within the same community, with some agencies having success with small cash incentives and/or the provision of transportation to attend the intervention and childcare during intervention implementation. Recruitment into the intervention may also be a challenge because more sessions are often needed for evidence-based interventions than for locally developed interventions. Thus, the cultural relevance of the intervention, the incentives for attendance, the atmosphere of the implementing organization as a whole, and the dynamic delivery style of the interventionist all affect retention. The strengths and resources of the organization and community must be focused and brought forward to increase the success of implementation. This process of adoption of an evidence-based intervention involves judgments on the part of local stakeholders as to the value or worth of the intervention for the community. If HIV is viewed as a nonexistent problem or is stigmatized in the community, then recruitment, retention, and implementation in general is undermined.

Community Readiness is Underappreciated and Underexplored

The process of community readiness for an intervention is an underexplored area, but health departments, community-based organizations, and medical settings that can move their respective communities toward readiness receive the most community support and are more successful at implementation [34]. Often, organizations must educate the community at large about the epidemiologic impact of HIV in the community and among the specific intervention target population to establish a foundation on which the intervention is implemented. Referrals to other organizations, donations, formal and informal endorsements, and local news coverage are examples of actions that have added to the dissemination process to ensure movement toward evidence-based prevention practice. Thus, working together in a co-learning process offers CDC scientists and practitioners and local stakeholders an opportunity to share knowledge and experiences to ensure the most successful intervention outcomes.

Adaptation is the Primary Essential Step of Community Ownership

Adaptation is frequently the first concern of staff at a health department, community-based organization, or other medical setting when implementing an evidence-based intervention [35]. Staff frequently report that they have a unique population reached under unique circumstances; thus, they assert that adaptation is necessary to increase the likelihood of success. They often indicate that what worked in one site must be adapted for the unique context of their community or intervention site [36]. This reaction is the beginning of extensive dialogue, co-learning, and equitable partnership between the real-world adopters and those at CDC who are actively disseminating a specific evidence-based intervention. Learning how to implement an intervention in a training session is primarily a passive process but adoption and implementation is a highly active process. Engagement between CDC and the implementing organization can be highly beneficial to both if technology exchange, rather than technology transfer, sets the tone for the dissemination process.

Staff from health departments, community-based organizations, and medical settings who wish to implement one of the interventions disseminated through the DEBI Project are encouraged to attend training on how to implement that specific intervention because implementation that relies just on the content of the packaged intervention is not sufficient for implementation with fidelity. At these trainings, intervention teams from health departments, community-based organizations, and other medical settings are provided with a range of resources on how to implement the intervention with fidelity. Training and technical assistance support implementation and include materials and discussions around the adaptation process, as adaptation of the intervention to fit organization capacities, community context, and population will certainly take place and is encouraged as part of the give-and-take of co-learning and the community-ownership process. To assist staff from health departments, community-based organizations, and other medical settings to implement with fidelity the interventions disseminated through the DEBI Project, core elements of each intervention are identified. These core elements are typically identified by the original efficacy researchers when the intervention is packaged for dissemination by the CDC. Instruction around implementation of core elements takes place in all DEBI Project-sponsored trainings, with explanations and rationales offered as to how intervention activities are causally linked to the behavioral outcomes of the intervention. The core elements of an intervention are usually linked to concepts of fidelity to the intervention and thus serve as intervention standards [27]. Sample core elements include:

- The intervention is run by a core group of 12–20 young gay and bisexual and MSM who, along with other volunteers, design and carry out all project activities (taken from the Mpowerment intervention materials) [21]
- Small-group skill-building sessions are provided to work on overcoming barriers to condom use (taken from the VOICES/VOCES intervention materials) [37]
- Participants' skills are built to enhance problem solving, increase personal assertiveness, and reduce HIV/AIDS harm (taken from the Safety Counts intervention materials) [38].

A natural tension arises between the establishment of core elements for an intervention and the necessary adaptation of an intervention to fit community settings, population and demographic differences, and differing determinants of risk that influence some populations and communities more than others. Adaptation of an intervention is part of the community-ownership process, and throughout the 10 years of implementation of the DEBI Project, we have encouraged staff from health departments, community-based organizations, and other medical settings to adapt interventions to the unique cultural, economic, and demographic features of their communities. Social determinants of risk vary from community to community, with wide variance in poverty rates, rates of addiction to illegal substances, visibility of sex workers, and history of discrimination regarding access to health services for various stigmatized populations. These are all valid reasons to adapt an intervention to increase community relevance and thereby increase intervention efficacy. At national meetings and conferences, we further encourage adaptation by providing a format for information exchange on adaptation processes and results. We even have produced adaptation guides, such as one on how to adapt an evidence-based intervention for black MSM. The guide can be accessed at http://www.effectivein-terventions.org/Libraries/General_Docs/CS218684_CDC_Adapt_Guide_v1.sflb. ashx.

We also have encouraged flexibility and the importance of formative evaluation, as well as process and outcome monitoring to ensure the intervention is meeting its disease-control function (i.e., reducing HIV infection). We strongly encourage adaptation of these interventions for several reasons: (1) to enhance community engagement in the processes prescribed by the intervention; (2) to increase the ownership of the intervention by the community and organizational staff; (3) to increase accessibility, scale, and reach of the intervention through adaptation to local conditions; and (4) to enhance the effects of the intervention by making it more acceptable to and meaningful for community members. This approach to the transfer of research into practice is designed to balance the knowledge gained in the initial efficacy trial with community engagement and collaboration. This approach minimizes a top–down approach and establishes a co-learning environment whereby community stakeholders and behavioral scientists and practitioners engage, work in partnership, and commit to co-learning. We recognize that several extremely relevant factors may undermine the implementation of an evidence-based intervention or enhance the implementation and potential impact of an intervention to reduce HIV exposure and transmission when delivered under real-world conditions. These factors include (1) the quality of intervention delivery, (2) staff training and cultural competence, (3) the acceptability of the intervention to community needs and values, (4) the accessibility of the intervention by the target audience, (5) the capacity of the organization to deliver the intervention, (6) the mix of interventions offered in a local community, and (7) the motivation of an organization to implement an intervention. The degree that the community and organization adjust and adapt for these factors is the degree that the intervention has the highest possibility of achieving its goals for behavior change.

To those who may say that adaptation weakens an intervention, we argue that this issue is an empirical one, and careful, thoughtful adaptation may in fact strengthen rather than weaken intervention effects. Within dissemination and implementation science and practice, there is much to be learned. We now have a broad list of efficacious interventions identified in the Compendium of evidence-based interventions; a key next step is to learn whether these interventions are also efficacious when implemented with or in varying at-risk populations, interventionists, conditions, settings, and contexts, and potential new behavioral outcomes.

We have learned that it is very difficult for a single staff member to implement an evidence-based intervention, even if he or she is a committed advocate and champion for the intervention. Having more than one staff member attend training on an evidence-based intervention increases the chances that the intervention will be implemented. Training on an evidence-based intervention prepares staff members for implementation but does not prepare them to convince others in their organization to attempt the intervention.

Additionally, although we encourage implementation staff to rename the intervention at their local site to increase community and organizational ownership, we have also learned that the methods of adaptation are frequently not known or understood by frontline intervention implementation staff at some health departments, community-based organizations, or other medical settings. Common methods recommended by CDC scientists and practitioners to adapt interventions include standard formative evaluation techniques of community observation, focus groups with potential clients and members of risk populations, surveys, pretesting materials, and piloting of key intervention activities [35, 36, 39–41].

We have introduced our initial concepts around adaptation of the evidence-based interventions disseminated by the DEBI Project [35]. In our approach, adaptation for specific populations is needed and flexibility around intervention content is acceptable, as long as the core elements are not compromised. Most often, the core elements are worded in such a way that local adaptation to meet community-prevention needs is possible.

Adaptation guidance has increased in the published literature around the interventions included in the DEBI Project, and CDC scientists and practitioners have produced adaptation products that ensure community engagement and better guide staff from health departments, community-based organizations, and medical settings in the implementation process [35, 36]. The CDC has also funded a broad range of organizational partners with expertise in helping staff from health department, community-based organizations, and other medical settings adapt the evidence-based interventions for a broad range of community settings (e.g., the STD/HIV Prevention Training Centers, the Capacity Building Assistance Providers). We also know that adaption methods and concepts should be disseminated parallel to the dissemination of the evidence-based interventions.

Dissemination is necessary but not sufficient for successful technology transfer (e.g., implementation of evidence-based interventions by staff from health departments, community-based organizations, and medical settings [9]. Our approach to adaptation of evidence-based-prevention practice to meet contextual considerations and to increase capacity to adopt as well as capacity to adapt allows considerable flexibility. Such flexibility increases ownership and understanding of the causative mechanisms in the intervention design, which in turn increases fidelity to the original intervention model. Local wisdom must be honored in the dissemination process for scientific knowledge to be transferred and/or exchanged [16]. The discipline of implementation science is still very young, and the role that local wisdom plays in the adoption, ownership, recruitment, retention, and evaluation processes has yet to be fully explored.

During initial implementation of the DEBI Project, it became apparent that some community-based organizations would drop a core element or add activities that would constitute a new core element. We used the term "reinvention" for this phenomenon [42]. Staff from community-based organizations have expressed concern over how to make the distinction between an acceptable adapted intervention and a reinvented intervention. This concern is usually related to fear that a funding agency, such as a health department or the federal government, will challenge the organization if it is thought that the intervention has been reinvented. It is extremely difficult to distinguish the fine line where adaptation has gone too far and reinvention has begun [43]. The question can be answered only by empirical evidence that includes the study of the processes and methods by which the intervention was adapted as well as the behavioral outcomes of the intervention. Thus, when staff from an organization asks if they have gone beyond adaptation and moved into reinvention, the dialogue starts with the formative evaluation data they collected to guide adaptation and used to determine what aspects of the intervention required adaptation and the strength of that evidence. Attention to community processes is essential at this stage because the adaptation should be made to bring about change in specific behaviors in a specific target audience, with specific risk determinants, who frequent specific venues in specific communities. If the formative evaluation tasks are done well and lead to logical and appropriate changes in the intervention, then pretesting the various aspects and materials used in the intervention is essential. Pretesting small aspects of an intervention is then followed by piloting the changed intervention to determine if the expected outcomes are obtained. Formative evaluation techniques have informed our recommendations around appropriate empirical approaches to adaptation, and an essential last step is outcome monitoring of the expectations of behavior change as a result of the intervention. If the adapted intervention, in a basic pretest and posttest design, does not demonstrate the expected behavior change, then careful consideration of how the core elements were interpreted and how the adaptation process developed is required in order to make logical corrections.

Based on our broad experiences with monitoring the implementation of evidence-based interventions, there appear to be three considerations to determine whether adaptation or reinvention has occurred. The first consideration is whether a core element has been changed, as such a change implies a reinvention. The second consideration is linked to process; if appropriate and sound formative evaluation methods were employed to enhance the fit and acceptability of the intervention, then changes to the intervention would likely be acceptable and usually labeled as an adaptation. The third consideration is linked to outcomes; if the intervention obtained its intended behavior change outcomes, the deletion or addition of a core element is a secondary concern. In both the second and third approaches, it is the quality of the empirical evidence that facilitates the judgment as to whether the adaptation or reinvention retains its ability to reduce HIV risk. Thus, we recommend active adaptation of evidence-based interventions into community-prevention settings in a thoughtful, systematic manner, with attention to formative evaluation and outcome monitoring to determine if the desired results are obtained by the adapted intervention.

Collaborative and Equitable Partnerships that Build on Stakeholder Strengths and Resources

An essential component of collaboration and equitable partnership is a common vocabulary. One area where this may break down is around concepts of evidence and efficacy. For science-based public health institutions like the CDC, evidence of efficacy is essential to meet the mission of disease prevention. Furthermore, public health agencies funded at the federal, state, county, and city levels are held accountable for tax expenditures and assurances that tax dollars are spent on efficacious methods of disease control. In the area of efficacy research, standards are established with regard to research and evaluation methodology and analyses are used to indicate that outcomes can be attributed to the intervention and not just to chance. This evaluation is in contrast to those of locally developed interventions, where the primary considerations in making judgments are the satisfaction of participants/customers and comfort levels of staff delivering the intervention. Participant/client satisfaction with an intervention and the services provided by an organization are essential to reach and engage large numbers of at-risk persons and cannot be discounted, yet, participant/customer satisfaction does not imply change in risk behavior. Throughout the dissemination process, we have attempted to strike a balance between an implementing organization's concerns about participant/customer satisfaction with an intervention and the CDC's concern that the intervention be adapted for community context while maintaining the core elements of the intervention, and thus increasing the likelihood of the intervention achieving desired results (e.g., consistent condom use and HIV testing). For example, participant satisfaction may increase if mothers are allowed to bring their children with them to an intervention.

A key aspect of collaboration and equitable partnership is respect for the resources brought to bear by each of the stakeholders in the dissemination and implementation process. In the DEBI Project, evidence-based interventions are packaged with well-articulated implementation steps, instructions, and resources. Many intervention products, such as risk assessments, job descriptions, camera-ready promotional materials, evaluation tools, sample budgets, and logic models are included to provide as many concrete tools for successful implementation as possible to those who are implementing an intervention. The process is far more complex than merely developing an "intervention in a box." Because the resources that implementing organizations bring to bear are essential to the dissemination process, dissemination cannot take place without the collaboration of resources from the research synthesis and translation process as well as the community-level implementation process. Dissemination of evidence-based interventions is virtually impossible unless a partnership is established whereby an organization implementing an intervention brings its wisdom of community, including the social determinants of health within a community, to bear in the delivery of the intervention [44].

In the following examples, we demonstrate how community engagement, participation, and collaboration play essential roles in the final step of the dissemination process, which is implementation of the intervention [20–22, 44–46]. In each of these examples, the community-engagement process has moved from an abstract concept to concrete implementation procedures. There are multiple strategies for community engagement, and these examples are not exhaustive of all the methods by which communities were or can be engaged during the intervention-implementation process.

The Mpowerment Intervention

Young gay and bisexual men and MSM constitute a community within a larger community composed primarily of heterosexuals. They may benefit from some of the infrastructure of the larger community (such as schools and employment); they may also face considerable social pressures and prejudices from the larger community. Thus, young gay and bisexual men and MSM must be engaged as a separate community with its own needs, activities, culture, identity, and sense of self-direction. The Mpowerment intervention is an evidence-based approach to HIV prevention for young gay and bisexual men and MSM helps build a healthy community through the community-engagement process [21]. This somewhat "hidden" community is engaged and encouraged to build and strengthen their community so as to support protective behaviors and reduce risk behaviors.

Kegeles and colleagues recognized that few young gay men would voluntarily go to community-based organizations and AIDS-service organizations to participate in an HIV-prevention intervention. In initial focus groups and interviews with key stakeholders, it was evident that an intervention to reduce HIV exposure and transmission among gay and bisexual men and MSM needed to provide social opportunities and community engagement to be successful [21]. Various components or activities of the intervention could be termed community-engagement actions: (1) development of an advisory group of local organization representatives that help advise the project implementation staff, (2) recruiting a core group of young gay men who actively engage in implementation of intervention activities as volunteers, (3) social marketing of the intervention activities, risk-reduction messages, and social opportunities to the risk community, (4) creation of a safe space where young gay men can engage in interactions with each other and project staff, (5) informal outreach to peers by casually endorsing safer sex practices in a nonjudgmental manner, (6) formal outreach by project volunteers to venues where young gay men socialize and can be reached with condoms and social marketing messages about safer sex practices, and (7) supporting social events organized by the core group and other project volunteers to engage community members, create a sense of community, offer condoms and safer sex messages through a social marketing campaign.

Implementation protocols were developed that highlighted the community engagement and collaboration processes. Marketing videos were developed based on real-world implementation. Even though the materials are packaged in a user-friendly and attractive manner, it is made clear that this is not an "intervention in a box" and that community engagement and collaboration are primary drivers of successful implementation. Each of the primary intervention activities involves extensive community involvement for successful implementation.

The Real AIDS Prevention Project (RAPP) and Community PROMISE Interventions

Two interventions disseminated by the DEBI Project are based on community engagement through role-model stories that are distributed by community advocate volunteers. The Real AIDS Prevention Project (RAPP) is an evidence-based intervention that focuses on sexually active heterosexual women in communities with a high prevalence of HIV [44]. The Community PROMISE intervention was originally tested with MSM who do not identify as gay, injecting-drug users, the sex partners of injecting-drug users, and high-risk youth [45]. The intervention is highly adaptable and has now been implemented with additional target audiences [46]. The RAPP and the Community PROMISE interventions were based on the two processes of community engagement and movement of the members of a risk community using the transtheoretical stages of change model [47]. Community engagement is facilitated by passionate and well-trained community volunteers who distribute small media and endorse safer sex practices. The stages of change-based portion of the interventions use small-media stage-based role model stories to show community members moving through the stages of change toward more protective behaviors. The role model stories reflect the real-life experiences of community members as they move away from HIV risk behaviors and move toward protective behaviors.

The RAPP intervention also takes the community engagement and partnership process further; the community facilitators responsible for implementation of the intervention interact with businesses and agencies within the community to identify potential community collaborators in the community-engagement process. The community facilitators visit local businesses where the target communities conduct business and engage these community business leaders in implementation of the intervention through the distribution of condoms and role model stories to the target population. If a business sells condoms, community engagement is fostered by helping community members know where condoms can be purchased and where free condoms may also be found in the community. Social services agencies located within the community are also contacted, and staff members are engaged to distribute condoms and the role model stories. The mixture of business and social service organization partnerships for condom and role model distribution within each community may differ, with some communities having more participation and motivation from the business segment and other communities having more participation and motivation from the social service organizations.

The Popular Opinion Leader and d-up: Defend Yourself! Interventions

The Popular Opinion Leader and d-up: Defend Yourself! interventions use a community-engagement social-networking approach to intervention implementation [20, 22]. In both interventions, engagement in the community is essential to successful implementation and sustainability. These interventions require a period of formative evaluation before implementation, whereby interventionists meet with key stakeholders and informants in venues that are frequented by the intervention target population. This meeting site allows them to observe members of the intervention target population interacting within their own community and increases the likelihood of identifying individuals who are the most persuasive peers within their social network [48]. By watching the community members interact, interviewing the key stakeholders and key informants, and then approaching and interviewing "popular opinion leaders," a cohort of opinion leaders can be recruited from the community. These opinion leaders are generally trusted by other members of the community, and their opinions hold weight in terms of community norms and practices. The opinion leaders are interviewed, and if they are committed to the increase of HIV-protective behaviors, they are asked to become part of the intervention and help endorse risk-reduction practices within their community. They are trained to do this in a casual, relaxed, empathetic manner that does not differentiate them from their peers and is of such subtlety that often community members do not even know that they have been intervened upon by an opinion leader.

The d-up: Defend Yourself! intervention has an element that distinguishes it from the Popular Opinion Leader intervention, although both were intended for MSM audiences [22]. During the formative evaluation phase of the d-up: Defend Yourself! intervention in the original research site in North Carolina, members of the target audience of young African-American/black gay and bisexual men and MSM voiced their concern that they faced considerable homophobia within their communities, and this external homophobia led to their hiding their sexual orientation and identity. This homophobia also made the community harder to reach with intervention activities. In community-based focus groups, these African-American/ black gay and bisexual men and MSM indicated that, whereas family members and friends reinforced resiliency and resiliency strategies for dealing with racism, resiliency strategies for confronting homophobia were often not taught. Thus, as a method of community engagement and community building, the d-up: Defend Yourself! intervention added an intervention element titled "Preparation for Bias," that was designed to help young African-American/black gay and bisexual men and MSM support each other as they struggled with dual identities and faced homophobia in the larger community. Thus, a relatively suppressed hidden at-risk community engaged to support each other in developing resiliency to the prejudices and biases that may arise around the issue of sexual orientation.

These examples of implementation of various evidence-based interventions demonstrate that community engagement, collaboration, and participation play essential roles in the tailoring, adaptation, and implementation of the interventions.

Mode of Dissemination: Addressing Perceptions of Unequal Power

Some have questioned the extent to which staff from health departments, community-based organizations, or other medical settings have a choice concerning the decision to select and adopt an evidence-based intervention. Historically, funds have been provided by the CDC and by health departments to those organizations that wished to adopt and implement one of the interventions disseminated by the DEBI Project. However, no efforts were made to discourage organizations from implementing evidence-based interventions using funds from the CDC while also implementing other locally developed interventions funded through community or foundation funding. The practice of offering more than one intervention within a community was never discouraged. An organization is more likely to meet community needs by offering a full menu of services to persons at risk. The CDC has further encouraged activities, such as HIV testing and linkage to medical care for persons with HIV, to be integrated into the delivery of evidence-based interventions. Persons at risk for HIV often have multiple issues that require support, resources, and intervention. Integrating evidence-based interventions into a full menu of organizational services for at-risk communities has always been and continues to be encouraged. The large number of interventions disseminated through the DEBI Project allowed for considerable intervention choice for organization staff who wished to obtain CDC or health department funding to implement an evidence-based intervention. Increasing choices among evidence-based interventions appeared to decrease perception of coercion. Forty-nine of the 50 state health departments have ever indicated they would fund evidence-based interventions in their geographic jurisdiction [49]. Many also sought to fund locally developed interventions as well, which generally had some evidence of reach and efficacy. Many of these locally developed interventions had been funded for years by health departments, and health department representatives endorsed these interventions as being candidates for more sophisticated evaluation efforts to demonstrate efficacy.

The role of community involvement or community participation in the DEBI Project varies based on which of the Project's phases and activities are being considered. The broad and overarching strategies used for diffusion of HIV-prevention technologies to community-based settings—whether directly from the CDC or through state and local health departments—are distinct from implementation of those technologies by partners on the ground. We contend that, in a modern public health environment, the former necessitates a high degree of centralized planning, decision-making, and coordination—about both resources and science—whereas the latter takes maximum advantage of local knowledge, experience, and wisdom. We acknowledge that HIV-prevention service providers must contend with multiple and sometimes competing directives and messages and that operating within a context where funders make decisions about the acceptable boundaries of an organization's work, but then encourage full expression of local capabilities within those boundaries, leads to a complex set of reactions that must be successfully managed for effective diffusion to occur.

Although the DEBI Project's model for diffusing behavioral interventions draws heavily on diffusion theory, the type of innovation (e.g., multicomponent, multiactivity, and theory-based) and context for adoption do not lend themselves to natural, rapid, and widespread uptake. Before the launch of the DEBI Project, many in the HIV-prevention workforce would not have sought to implement evidence-based practices. It is precisely the ability of funders to influence the policy and resource environments that has been used to advance public health in HIV prevention and in other areas. In all such cases where diffusion requires some degree of manipulation or exertion of external authority, resistance to change is expected. For the DEBI Project, those responses were anticipated and our ability to reduce resistance was improved over time. The perceived barriers to the dissemination process diminished for a number of reasons: (1) improved understanding on the part of HIV-prevention service providers of the behavioral interventions within the DEBI Project, including the similarities to their existing work and opportunities to maximize community engagement, collaboration, and partnership; (2) an expanded number of behavioral interventions in the DEBI Project portfolio—from 4 to 31 in a span of 10 years—which significantly improved the ability of staff at health departments, community-based organizations, and other medical settings to make choices that maximize goodness-of-fit between their organizations and communities and evidence-based interventions; (3) improvements in the quality and quantity of technical assistance resources to help with the selection, adaptation, and implementation of evidence-based interventions in local communities; and (4) enhanced awareness that the DEBI Project could complement, rather than supplant, locally developed interventions and efforts.

Policymakers, scientists, and practitioners at the CDC recognize the value of locally developed interventions and practice and have sought to identify and support them alongside the rollout of the interventions in the DEBI Project. The CDC's Division of HIV/AIDS Prevention Research Branch has funded several projects under its Innovative Interventions initiative, which seeks to identify, test, and standardize promising theory-based interventions developed by community members and organizations. Two of these interventions have now been tested in RCTs, demonstrated efficacy at reducing risk for HIV acquisition, and been packaged for diffusion—Many Men, Many Voices and the Healthy Love Workshop, which was developed and tested by Sister Love in Atlanta, Georgia [19, 30]. In addition, since 2006, CDC's flagship funding opportunities for community-based organizations have included funding categories to support implementation of so-called homegrown interventions (e.g., PA-06–618, PA-10–1003, and PA-11–1113).

In North Carolina, for example, an intervention known as HOLA en Grupos, developed by a community-based participatory research (CBPR) partnership to prevent HIV among Latino gay and bisexual men, MSM, and transgender persons, is currently being implemented and evaluated through a CDC initiative to test homegrown interventions for MSM. The process of developing the intervention was iterative with CBPR partners, specifically staff from a community-based organization and Latino gay men from the community, developing and revising the intervention based on three factors: (1) review of other interventions that target Latinos in general and MSM in particular, (2) learnings from ongoing implementation of the evolving intervention in the real world over time by staff from a community-based organization, and (3) the experiences with other interventions that the CBPR partners and community-based organizational staff had developed for the Latino community including HoMBReS, HoMBReS-2, MuJEReS, and HoMBReS Por un Cambio [50]. These are good-faith efforts on the part of CDC scientists and practitioners to recognize the contributions of local actors and to augment the interventions in the DEBI Project.

Discussion and Conclusion

Our experiences disseminating evidence-based behavioral interventions over the last 11 years has alerted us to the need for a more fully developed science of dissemination and implementation of evidence-based interventions [51]. Admittedly, the community engagement aspects of the various interventions lent themselves more to community participation than did a centralized effort on the part of the CDC to disseminate evidence-based prevention practice. However, the flexibility and partnerships we instituted in the dissemination effort demonstrate the manner in which the community-engagement process may be operationalized in dissemination efforts. Power differences exist in any dissemination process as evidence-based interventions are moved from the realm of scientific and academic inquiry to practice in underserved and vulnerable communities at risk for HIV. However, power differences do not always constitute condescension. The use of local knowledge and community engagement, collaboration, and partnership have been, and continue to be, essential in dissemination and implementation of these evidence-based interventions across literally thousands of prevention organizations.

Disclaimer

The findings and conclusions in this chapter are those of the authors and do not necessarily represent the official position of the Centers for Disease Control and Prevention.

References

1. Centers for Disease Control and Prevention. High impact prevention—CDC's approach to reducing HIV infections in the United States. National Center for HIV/AIDS, Viral Hepatitis, STD and TB Prevention. April 17, 2013. www.cdc.gov/hiv/policies/hip.html. Accessed 19 May 2014.

2. Collins C, Harshbarger C, Sawyer R, Hamdallah M. The diffusion of effective behavioral interventions project: development, implementation, and lessons learned. AIDS Educ Prev. 2006;18(Suppl):5–20.

3. Collins CB, Hearn KD, Whittier DN, Freeman A. Implementing packaged HIV-prevention interventions for HIV-positive individuals: considerations for clinic-based and community-based interventions. Public Health Rep. 2010;125(Suppl 1):55–63.

4. Owczarzak J. Evidence-based HIV prevention in community settings: provider perspectives on evidence and effectiveness. Crit Public Health. 2012;22(1):73–84.

5. Owczarzak J, Dickson-Gomez J. Provider's perceptions of and receptivity toward evidence-based HIV prevention interventions. AIDS Educ Prev. 2011;23(2):105–17.

6. Veniegas RC, Kao UH, Rosales R, Arellanes M. HIV prevention technology transfer: challenges and strategies in the real world. Am J Public Health. 2009;99(51):124–30.

7. Veniegas RC, Kao UH, Rosales R. Adapting HIV prevention evidence-based interventions in practice settings: an interview study. Implement Sci. 2009;4:76.

8. Dolcini MM, Gandelman A, Vogan SA, Kong C, Leak T, King AJ, et al. Translating HIV interventions into practice: community-based organizations' experiences with the Diffusion of Effective Behavioral Interventions (DEBIs). Soc Sci Med. 2010;71(10):1839–46.

9. Dworkin SI, Pinto RM, Hunter J, Rapkin B, Remien RH. Keeping the spirit of community partnership alive in the scale up oh HIV/AIDS prevention: critical reflections on the roll out of DEBI (Diffusion of Effective Behavioral Interventions). Am J Community Psychol. 2008;42(1–2):51–59.

10. Kalichman SC, Hudd K, DiBerto G. Operational fidelity to an evidence-based HIV prevention intervention for people living with HIV/AIDS. J Prim Prev. 2010; 31:235–245.

11. Ruiz, MS, Gable, AR, Kaplan, EH, Stoto, MA, Fineberg, HV, & James Trussell, E. (Eds.). No time to lose: getting more from HIV prevention. Washington, DC: National Academy Press; 2001.

12. Green LW. From research to 'best practices' in other settings and populations. Am J Health Behav. 2001;25:165–78.

13. Kohatsu ND, Robinson, JG, Turner JC. Evidence-based public health: an evolving concept. Am J Prev Med. 2004;27:417–421.

14. Lyles CM, Crepaz N, Herbst JH, Kay LS, HIV/AIDS Prevention Research Synthesis Team. Evidence-based HIV behavioral prevention from the perspective of the CDC's HIV/AIDS Prevention Research Synthesis Team. AIDS Educ Prev. 2006;18(Suppl A):21–31.

15. Lyles, CM, Kay, LS, Crepaz, N, Herbst, JH, Passin, WF, Kim, AS, Rama, SM, Thadiparthi, S, DeLuca, JB, Mullins, MM. Best-evidence interventions: findings from a systematic review of HIV behavioral interventions for US populations at high risk, 2000–2004. Am J Public Health. 2007;97(1):133–43.

16. Miller, RL, Shinn, M. Learning from communities: overcoming difficulties in dissemination of prevention and promotion efforts. Am J Community Psychol. 2005;35(3/4):169–54.

17. Neumann MS, Sogolow ED. Replicating effective programs: HIV/AIDS prevention technology transfer. AIDS Educ Prev. 2000;12(Suppl. A):1–3.

18. Centers for Disease Control and Prevention Subpopulation estimates from the HIV incidence surveillance system—United States, 2006. MMWR. 2008;57:985–89.

19. Wilton L, Herbst JH, Coury-Doniger P, Painter TM, English G, Alvarez ME, et al. Efficacy of an HIV/STI prevention intervention for black men who have sex with men: findings from the Many Men, Many Voices (3MV) project. AIDS Behav. 2009;13:532–44.

20. Kelly JA, St. Lawrence JS, Diaz YE, Stevenson LY, Hauth AC, Brasfield, TL, Kalichman, SC, Smith, JE, Andew, ME. HIV risk behavioral reduction following intervention with key opinion leaders of population: an experimental analysis. Am J Public Health. 1991;81(2):168–71.

21. Kegeles SM, Hays RB, Coates TJ. The Mpowerment project: a community-level HIV prevention intervention for young gay men. Am J Public Health. 1996;86(8):1129–36.

22. Jones KT, Gray P, Whiteside O, Wang T, Bost D, Dunbar E, et al. Evaluation of an HIV prevention intervention adapted for black men who have sex with men. Am J Public Health. 2008;98(6):1043–50.

23. Hinton A, Downey J, Lisoviez N, Mayfield-Johnson S, White-Johnson F. The Community Health Advisor Program and the Deep South Network for Cancer Control: health promotion programs for volunteer community health advisors. Fam Community Health. 2005;28(1):20–7.

24. Green LW, Kreuter MW. CDC's planned approach to community health as an application of PRECEED and an inspiration for PROCEED. J Health Educ. 1992;23(3):140–47.

25. Lyles CM, Crepaz N, Herbst JH, Kay LS. Evidence-based HIV behavioral prevention from the perspective of the CDC's HIV/AIDS Prevention Research Synthesis Team. AIDS Educ Prev. 2006;18(Suppl 21):21–31.

26. Cohen DA, Shin-Yi W, Farley TA. Comparing the cost-effectiveness of HIV prevention interventions. J Acquir Immune Defic Syndr. 2004;37(3):1404–14.

27. Galbraith JS, Herbst JH, Whittier DK, Jones PL, Smith BD, Uhl G, et al. Taxonomy for strengthening the identification of core elements for evidence-based behavioral interventions for HIV/AIDS prevention. Health Educ Res. 2001;26(5):872–85.

28. Dolcini MM, Canin L, Gandelman A, Skolnik H. Theoretical domains: a heuristic for teaching behavioral theory in HIV/STD prevention courses. Health Promot Pract. 2004;5(4):404–17.

29. Wingood GM, DiClemente RJ, Villamizar K, Deja L, DeVarona M, Taveras J, et al. Efficacy of a health educator-delivered HIV prevention randomized controlled trail. Am J Public Health. 2011;101(12):2245–52.

30. Diallo DD, Moore TW, Ngalame PM, White LD, Herbst JH, Painter TM. Efficacy of a single-session HIV prevention intervention for black women: a group randomized controlled trial. AIDS Behav. 2010;14:518–29.

31. Rhodes SD, Malow RM, Jolly C. Community-based participatory research (CBPR): a new and not-so-new approach to HIV/AIDS prevention, care, and treatment. AIDS Educ Prev. 2010;22(3):173–83.

32. Pemberton G, Andia J, Robles R, Collins C, Colon-Cartegena N, Perez Del Pilar O, et al. From research to community-based practice—working with Latino researchers to translate and diffuse a culturally relevant evidence-based intervention: The Modelo de Intervencion Psichomedica (MIP). AIDS Educ Prev. 2009;21(Suppl B):171–85.

33. Noguchi K, Albarracín D, Durantini MR, Glasman LR. Who participates in which health promotion programs? A meta-analysis of motivations underlying enrollment and retention in HIV-prevention interventions. Psychol Bull. 2007;133(6):955–75.

34. Thurman PJ, Vernon IS, Plested B. Advancing HIV/AIDS prevention among American Indians through capacity building and the Community Readiness Model. J Public Health Manag Pract. 2007;13(Suppl):49–54.

35. McKleroy VS, Galbraith JS, Cummings B, Jones P, Harshbarger C, Collins C, et al. Adapting evidence-based behavioral interventions for new settings and target populations. AIDS Educ Prev. 2006;18(4 Suppl A):59–73.

36. Wingood GM, DiClemente RJ. The ADAPT-ITT model: a novel method of adapting evidence-based HIV interventions. J Acquir Immune Defic Syndr. 2008;47(Suppl 1):40–6.

37. O'Donnell CR, O'Donnell L, San Doval A, Duran R, Laves K. Reductions in STD infections subsequent to an STD clinic visit: using video-based patient education to supplement provider interactions. Sex Transm Dis. 1998;25(3):161–68.

38. Rhodes F, Wood MM, Hershberger SL. A cognitive-behavioral intervention to reduce HIV risks among active drug users; efficacy study. Sacramento, California Department of Health Services, Office of AIDS; 2000.

39. Wainberg ML, Gonzalez MA, McKinnon K, Elkington KS, Pinto D, Mann CG, et al. Targeted ethnography as a critical step to inform cultural adaptations of HIV prevention interventions for adults with severe mental illness. Soc Sci Med. 2007;65(2):296–308.
40. Solomon J, Card JJ, Malow RM. Adapting efficacious interventions: advancing translational research in HIV prevention. Eval Health Prof. 2006;29(2):162–94.
41. Tortolero SR, Markham CM, Parcel GS, Peters RJ, Escobar-Chaves SL, Basen-Engquist K, Lewis HL. Using intervention mapping to adapt an effective HIV, sexually transmitted disease, and pregnancy prevention program for high-risk minority youth. Health Promot Pract. 2005;6(3):286–98.
42. Rogers EM. Diffusion of innovations. 5th ed. New York: The Free Press; 2003.
43. Bauman LJ, Stein REK, Ireys HT. Reinventing fidelity: the transfer of social technology among settings. Am J Community Psychol. 1991;19(4):619–39.
44. Lauby JL., Smith PJ, Stark M, Person B, Adams J. A community-level HIV prevention intervention for inner-city women: results of the women and infants demonstration trial. Am J Public Health. 2000;90 (2):216–22.
45. AIDS Community Demonstration Projects. Community-level HIV intervention in 5 cities: final outcome data from the CDC AIDS demonstration projects. Am J Public Health. 1999;89(3);336–45.
46. Collins C, Kohler C, DiClemente R, Wang MQ. Evaluation of the exposure effects of a theory-based street outreach intervention on African-American drug users. Eval Program Plann. 1999;22(3):279–94.
47. Prochaska J, Velicer W. The transtheoretical model of health behavior change. Am J Health Promot. 1997;12:38–48.
48. Valente TW, Pumpuang P. Identifying opinion leaders to promote behavior change. Health Educ Behav. 2007;34(6):881–96.
49. NASTAD and Kaiser Family Foundation. The national HIV prevention inventory: the state of HIV prevention across the U.S.; 2009.
50. Rhodes SD. Demonstrated effectiveness and potential of CBPR for preventing HIV in Latino populations. In: Organista KC, editor. HIV Prevention with Latinos: theory, research, and practice. New York: Oxford University Press; 2012. p. 83–102.
51. Norton WE, Amico KR, Cornman DH, Fisher WA, Fisher JD. An agenda for advancing the science of implementation of evidence-based HIV prevention interventions. AIDS Behav. 2009;13(3):424–29.

Index

S. D. Rhodes (ed.), *Innovations in HIV Prevention Research and Practice
through Community Engagement*, DOI 10.1007/978-1-4939-0900-1,
© Springer Science+Business Media New York 2014

Printed in the United States
By Bookmasters